ACNE AND ACNEIFORM ERUPTIONS

Edited by **Selda Pelin Kartal**
and **Müzeyyen Gönül**

Acne and Acneiform Eruptions
http://dx.doi.org/10.5772/62927
Edited by Selda Pelin Kartal and Müzeyyen Gönül

Contributors

Selda Pelin Kartal, Ozge Keseroglu, Müzeyyen Gönül, Bilgen Gencler, Demet Cicek, Betul Demir, Emin Ozlu, Ayse Serap Karadag, Didem Mullaaziz, Asli Feride Kaptanoglu, Dilek Bayramgurler, Zekayi Kutlubay, Asli Gunaydin Tatliparmak, Erol Koc, Fatma Aksoy Khurami, Murat Alper, M Çiğdem Oba, Server Serdaroglu, Yalçın Tüzün, Burhan Engin, Işıl Kamberoğlu, Sevgi Akarsu, Aysun Sanal Dogan, Funda Kemeriz, Fatma Pelin Cengiz, Nazan Emiroğlu

Published by InTech
Janeza Trdine 9, 51000 Rijeka, Croatia

Publishing Process Manager Romina Skomersic
Technical Editor SPi Global
Cover InTech Design team

First published March, 2017
Printed in Croatia
Legal deposit, Croatia: National and University Library in Zagreb

Additional hard copies can be obtained from orders@intechopen.com

Acne and Acneiform Eruptions, Edited by Selda Pelin Kartal and Müzeyyen Gönül
p. cm.
Print ISBN 978-953-51-2989-9
Online ISBN 978-953-51-2990-5

For EU product safety concerns:
IN TECH d.o.o., Prolaz Marije Krucifikse Kozulić 3, 51000 Rijeka, Croatia,
info@intechopen.com or visit our website at intechopen.com.

Meet the editors

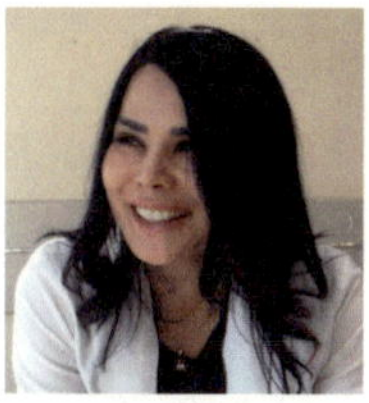

Assoc. Prof. Dr. Selda Pelin Kartal graduated from Hacettepe University School of Medicine. Currently, she is an associate professor in the Department of Dermatology at Dişkapi Yildirim Beyazit Education and Research Hospital in Ankara, Turkey. She has coauthored over 100 published articles and supervised several master and postdoctoral students. Her actual interests are focused on acne, psoriasis, urticaria, autoimmune bullous diseases, Behçet's disease, and cosmetic dermatology.

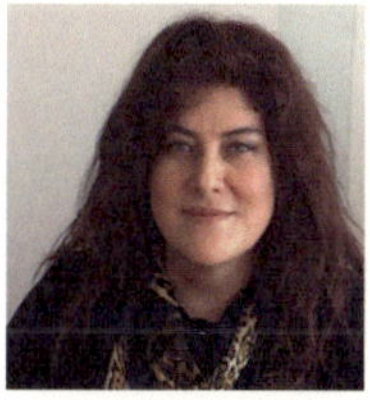

Assoc. Prof. Dr. Muzeyyen Gonul graduated from Ankara University School of Medicine. Currently, she is an associate professor in the Department of Dermatology at Dişkapi Yildirim Beyazit Education and Research Hospital in Ankara, Turkey. She has coauthored over 100 published articles and supervised several master and postdoctoral students. Her research interests are psoriasis, urticaria, autoimmune bullous diseases, and Behçet's disease.

Contents

Preface

The aim of this book is to give readers a broad review of acne vulgaris and acneiform dermatoses, which may affect people from birth to death, and their treatment options.

This book has a total of 14 chapters - Introductory review chapter and 13 chapters created by experts in different fields like dermatology, dermatosurgery, pathology, and ophthalmology. This book is organized to be read in sequence from chapter to chapter, or each can be taken individually, as each chapter centers on different aspects of the content. In the first part, there is a comprehensive introductory review chapter focusing on the terms "acne" and "acneiform," one of which is a multifactorial disease of pilosebaceous unit and the other refers to dermatoses, which resemble acne vulgaris clinically but have different etiopathogenesis. The second part includes the chapters entitled "Acne Vulgaris," "Pediatric Acne," "Occupational Acne," "Drug-Induced Acneiform Eruptions," "Acneiform Eruptions and Pregnancy," "Acneiform Papulopustular Lesions in Patients with Behcet's Disease," "The Use of Topical Retinoids in Acne," "Treatment of Acneiform Eruptions, Acne, and Acne Scars," "Histopathological Evaluation of Acneiform Eruptions," "Acne-Associated Syndromes," "Acne Conglobata," "Acne Rosacea," and "Ocular Rosacea." This book is easy to read, and it includes illustrations, tables, patient photographs, and histopathological slides to support the written text and to enhance the reader's understanding.

We are grateful to all the contributors and leading experts for the submission of their wonderful work, which provides an in-depth view of all aspects of the content, backed with the most current literature in the field. We offer our special thanks and appreciation to Ms. Anita Pribanic and Ms. Romina Skomersic, Publishing Process Manager, for their encouragement and help in bringing out the book in the present form.

We express our heartfeltgratitude to magnificent Ataturk who said "Our true mentor in life is science" .

Assoc. Prof. Dr. Selda Pelin Kartal
Ministry of Health Ankara Diskapi Yildirim Beyazit Education and Research Hospital
Dermatology Clinic,
Ankara, Turkey

Assoc. Prof. Dr. Muzeyyen Gonul
Ministry of Health Ankara Diskapi Yildirim Beyazit Education and Research Hospital
Dermatology Clinic,
Ankara, Turkey

Chapter 1

Introductory Chapter: Acne and Acneiform Dermatoses

Selda Pelin Kartal and Müzeyyen Gönül

Additional information is available at the end of the chapter

http://dx.doi.org/10.5772/66979

1. Introduction

1.1. The definition of 'acne' and 'acneiform'

Acne vulgaris (AV) is a multifactorial disease of pilosebaceous unit and is a prototype of acneiform dermatoses. The term 'acneiform' refers to dermatoses which resemble acne vulgaris clinically but have different etiopathogenesis [1]. Acneiform dermatoses include a wide range of diseases which can occur in all age groups from infancy to elderly. They are so prevalent in all around the world that only AV rate has been reported to be 40–50 million/year in the USA and its prevalence has been estimated as 100% among adolescents in United Kingdom [2, 3]. Acneiform dermatoses have also important economic burden on governments due to high prevalence [2, 4].

2. Acne

AV lesions develop due to increased sebum production, follicular epidermal hyperproliferation, inflammation and *Propionibacterium acnes* (*P. acnes*) colonization [5]. Formation of microcomedones was originally thought to be the first step in AV pathogenesis. However, recent studies supported that inflammation has a role at all stages of acne lesion development, perhaps subclinically even before microcomedone formation. The immunochemical pathways underlying the initiation and extension of the inflammation in AV are not known completely but several inflammatory mediators including cytokines, defensins, peptidases, sebum lipids and neuropeptides may play role in complex pathogenesis of AV [6]. AV is clinically characterized by open and closed comedones, papules, pustules, nodules, cysts and scar formations [4, 7]. It primarily affects adolescents so it has negative psychosocial effects on this age group [8]. Also, there is a risk of postinflammatory hypo/hyperpigmentation and scar formation, so early treatment of AV is important. Topical (retinoids, benzoyl peroxide, antibiotics, salicylic acid, azelaic acid) and systemic (antibiotics, hormonal treatment, isotretinoin) agents and surgical procedures can be used in the treatment of AV [4, 7]. In pregnant women, topical benzoyl peroxide and antibiotics (erythromycin, clindamycin) can be preferred. When necessary, systemic antibiotics such as penicillins, erythromycin and clindamycin can be added. Due to the risk of teratogenicity, retinoids should not be used in pregnant women [9].

Although acne is mostly seen in adolescence period, it may be seen in pediatric age group. Neonatal acne is a temporary and benign acne variant characterized by millimetric inflammatory papules on cheeks and across the nasal bridge which appears usually during the neonatal period [10]. Increased sebum secretion due to stimulation of neonatal sebaceous glands with maternal hormones, and *Malassezia furfur* and *Malassezia smpodialis* colonization have been implicated in the etiopathogenesis of this disease [7, 10, 11]. Lesions usually resolve by 3 months of age without any treatment [10]. Infantile acne usually begins between 3 and 6 months of age. It results from hormonal imbalance in this age period. Clinically, comedones, papules, pustules and nodules may be present similar to adolescent acne. Although it has a tendency to heal spontaneously within 1 or 2 years, it should be treated due to the risk of scar formation [7, 10].

Severity of AV may change from mild to severe. Moreover, in acne fulminans (acute febrile ulcerative acne), which is the most severe acne form, systemic symptoms such as fever, arthralgia, myalgia, fatigue, hepatosplenomegaly and osteolytic bone lesions may accompany to skin lesions that are characterized by suddenly appeared multiple, tender, inflammatory nodular, suppurative lesions and ulcers with hemorrhagic crusts on the back and chest. Increased sedimentation rate, proteinuria, leukocytosis and anemia may also be seen. Acne conglobata is another severe nodulocystic acne form; however, in contrast to acne fulminans, it is not accompanied by any systemic symptoms. It is characterized by comedones, papules, pustules, nodules, abscesses and scars on the chest, back, buttocks, face, shoulders and thighs. Solid facial edema (Morbihan disease) is an important complication of acne characterized by woody enduration and erythema on midface and cheeks [7, 10].

Acne lesions sometimes may occur due to chronic friction, and this form is named as acne mechanica. It is characterized by comedones, which occur secondary to mechanic obstruction of pilosebaceous unit [7, 12]. Cosmetic acne is most commonly seen among young females and is associated with the application of cosmetics containing comedogenic substances. It is characterized by multiple comedones at the sites of cosmetic used [11, 12]. Excessive heat exposure may cause inflammatory nodulocystic acneiform lesions on body and arms and this entity is named as tropical acne [4, 7]. Acne aestivalis (Mallorca acne) is characterized by multiple papular lesions on cheeks, sides of the neck, chest, shoulders and upper arms that develop after sun exposure. UV radiation, especially UVA, is the responsible factor in the development of these lesions. Recurrences are common in successive years [1]. Radiation acne refers to eruption, consisting of multiple comedone-like papules on the sites that are previously exposed to ionized radiation for treatment. Acne *excoriee des jeunes filles* is an acne form that is mainly seen among young women and characterized by crusted, excoriated papules. It is generally accompanied by psychiatric disorders [4, 7].

Another form of acne, occupational acne, occurs as a result of occupational exposure to follicular occlusive compounds such as chlorinated hydrocarbons, coal tar derivatives. It is characterized by especially comedones on exposure sites, but inflammatory papules, pustules and cysts may be seen. Chloracne is the main example of occupational acne. It is characterized by multiple cysts, papules and nodules on malar, retroauricular, mandibular, aksillar regions and scrotum [7, 12].

With an increasing frequency in recent years, drug-induced acne characterized by a monomorphic eruption composed of inflammatory papule and pustules which occurs after usage of certain drugs. The distribution of lesions may be similar to AV; on the contrary, the onset is mostly acute, lesions are predominantly inflammatory and monomorphic and comedones are usually absent [1]. Involvement of unusual localizations for AV (e.g. distal extremities), occurrence at an unusual age for AV, the history of exposure to one of the known causative drugs and regression of lesions after the cessation the offending agent are other clues for diagnoses [1, 13]. Steroid acne is the best known example of drug-induced acne. It may occur on chest and back as a result of systemic steroid usage or on face due to inappropriate or prolonged usage of topical steroids [7]. Anabolic steroids, fenitoin, lithium, vitamins, cyclosporine, isoniazid, azathioprine, iodides, bromides and epidermal growth factor receptor inhibitors are the other major drugs which are responsible from acneiform eruptions [1, 13]. Lesions regress after the cessation of responsible agent [1].

Acne lesions are mostly seen in isolated manner however may develop as a component of some syndromes. SAPHO syndrome is characterized by any combination of *s*ynovitis, *a*cne, *p*ustulosis, *h*yperostosis and *o*steitis. Characteristic skin lesions in SAPHO syndrome include acne fulminans, hidradenitis suppurativa and palmoplantar pustulosis [7, 14]. PAPA syndrome is an autosomal dominantly inherited, autoinflammatory disorder characterized by *p*yogenic *a*rthritis, *p*yoderma gangrenosum and *a*cne, which is usually in severe nodulocystic type. Apert syndrome (acrocephalosyndactyly type I) is an autosomal dominant congenital disorder characterized by craniofacial deformities, dental abnormalities, syndactyly and hypertelorism. Early onset, widespread, severe, comedonal and inflammatory acne involving the face, chest, back and unusual sites like forearms is a common clinical feature of this syndrome [14]. AV is also seen more frequently in patients with *p*oly*c*ystic *o*vary *s*yndrome (PCOS) due to hormonal disturbances. HAIR-AN syndrome, a subset of PCOS, is characterized by *h*yperandrogenism, *a*cne, *i*nsulin *r*esistance and *a*canthosis *n*igricans [7, 14].

3. Acneifom dermatoses

The characteristic papulopustular lesions of Behcet disease are indistinguishable from AV clinically, but arms and legs involved preferentially in contrast to AV [14]. Histologically vasculitis might be seen [15]. It was reported that these lesions are usually observed in combination with arthritis [14].

Rosacea is a multifactorial disorder presented with acneiform lesions. It generally affects individuals with fair skin and older age compared to AV. There is a female predilection, but phymatous type occurs mostly in men. Vascular hyperreactivity and *P. acnes* and *Demodex folliculorum* colonization have been proposed in the etiopathogenesis. Food and drugs that can cause vasodilatation and thermal stimulation may precipitate rosacea development. It is clinically characterized by erythema, papule, pustule and telangiectasias with subjective symptoms such as burning and stinging. Four main clinical subtypes have been described, namely erythematotelangiectatic, papulopustular, phymatous and ocular. In addition to them, there are other rosacea types such as, granulomatous rosacea, periorificial dermatitis and pyoderma faciale. Typically, it starts as a transient erythema attacks (flushing) on cheeks and nose. Erythema becomes permanent with time and telangiectasias occur. After that, millimetric papules, pustules, plaques and nodules with varying severities may occur. Granulomatous rosacea is a variant of rosacea characterized by red-brown papules which show granulomatous inflammation histopathologically. In phymatous type rosacea, follicular orifices become prominent, nodularities and irregularities occur on the thickened skin due to sebaceous hyperplasia. These phymatous changes most often develop on the nose (rhinophyma), but may also occur on chin (gnatophyma), ear (otophyma), forehead (metophyma) and eyelids (blepharophyma). Ocular symptoms such as burning, stinging, dryness, tearing, blepharitis and corneal damage may be present in the nearly half of the patients independently severity of cutaneous signs (Ocular rosacea) [12, 16–18].

Perioral and periorbital dermatitis is characterized by discrete, erythematous papules, plaques and pustules on erythematous base around mouth and eye, which characteristically spare the vermillion border. Although the relationship with rosacea is not clear, it has similar histopathological findings. Also, it responses to similar treatments. Pyoderma faciale is another entity that resembles rosacea histopathologically and responds similar treatment modalities. This disease is characterized by inflammatory papules, pustules and plaques on the midface. Systemic symptoms, such as fever, myalgia and laboratory findings (increased sedimentation rate and white blood cell count) may accompany with cutaneous symptoms in these patients. Inappropriate or long-term steroid usage may also cause rosacea formation or exacerbation (Steroid rosacea) [17, 18].

Usage of sun protection and avoidance from the factors that cause vasodilatation and irritation should be recommended to rosacea patients. Topical (metronidazole, sodium sulfacetamide, azelaic acid, tretioin) and systemic (antibiotics and retinoic acid) agents can be used in the treatment. Vascular lasers and intense pulsed light therapy can be used in the treatment of telangiectasias. Electrosurgery and carbon dioxide laser are the treatment options for the rhinophyma [19].

Demodicosis is a disease of the pilosebaceous unit associated with human *Demodex* mites (*D. folliculorum and Demodex brevis*). *Demodex* mites can be found in normal adult skin with a density of less than 5 mites per cm^2. Demodicosis may occur if the density of these mite increases due to the defect in host immune mechanism, in association with systemic disease or immunosuppressive drug usage (topical corticosteroids, topical calcineurin inhibitors). There are different clinical manifestations of demodicosis that can mimic many other skin disorders, such as rosacea, perioral dermatitis and folliculitis. Spinulate demodicosis (pityriasis folliculorum) characterized by facial erythema with follicular plugs, scaling and sandpaper-like appearance. There is a pronounced inflammation in papulopustular/nodulocystic demodicosis (rosacea-like demodicosis), and it is most commonly affects perioral and periorbital areas. Ocular and auricular types of demodicosis were also described [12, 20].

4. Conclusion

Acne and acneiform eruptions are frequent disorders in dermatology practice and the severity of diseases may change from self-limiting, benign condition to fulminant systemic disease. Etiopathogenesis of them are different. They may be seen as isolated or as a component of any syndrome. So, differential diagnoses of these diseases are important. Patient's age, occupation, cosmetic usage, drug history, concomitant diseases, menstrual cycle irregularities and morphology and localization of lesions are important clues for diagnoses. To make an accurate diagnoses, detailed history, physical examination and, if necessary, histopathological examinations are essential. In this book, acne vulgaris and acneiform eruptions will be discussed in detail.

Author details

Selda Pelin Kartal* and Müzeyyen Gönül

*Address all correspondence to: pelin@dr.com

Department of Dermatology, Ministry of Health Ankara Diskapi Yıldırım Beyazıt Education and Research Hospital, Ankara, Turkey

References

[1] Plewig G, Jansen T. Acneiform dermatoses. Dermatology. 1998;**196**:102–7.

[2] Bhate K, Williams HC. Epidemiology of acne vulgaris. Br J Dermatol. 2013;**168**:474–85. DOI: 10.1111/bjd.12149

[3] Gollnick HP, Zouboulis CC. Not all acne is acne vulgaris. Dtsch Arztebl Int. 2014;**111**:301–12. DOI: 10.3238/arztebl.2014.0301

[4] Zaenglein AL, Thiboutot DM. Acne vulgaris. In: Bolognia JL, Jorizzo JL, Rapini RP, editors. Dermatology. 2nd ed. Spain: Mosby; 2008. p. 495–508.

[5] Suh DH, Kwon HH. What's new in the physiopathology of acne? Br J Dermatol. 2015;**172**:13–9. DOI: 10.1111/bjd.13634

[6] Tanghetti EA. The role of inflammation in the pathology of acne. J Clin Aesthet Dermatol. 2013;**6**:27–35.

[7] Zaenglein AL, Graber EM, Thiboutot DM, Strauss JS. Acne vulgaris and acneiform eruptions. In: Wolff K, Goldsmith LA, Katz SI, Gilchrest BA, Paller AS, Leffell DJ, editors. Fitzpatrick's Dermatology in General Medicine. 7th ed. New York: McGraw-Hill; 2008. p. 690–702.

[8] Revol O, Milliez N, Gerard D. Psychological impact of acne on 21st-century adolescents: decoding for better care. Br J Dermatol. 2015;**172**:52–8. DOI: 10.1111/bjd.13749.

[9] Kartal Durmazlar SP, Eskioglu F. Cosmetic procedures in pregnancy: Review. Turkiye Klinikleri J Med Sci. 2008;**28**:942–6.

[10] Mengesha YM, Bennett ML. Pustular skin disorders: diagnosis and treatment. Am J Clin Dermatol. 2002;**3**:389–400.

[11] White GM. Recent findings in the epidemiologic evidence, classification, and subtypes of acne vulgaris. J Am Acad Dermatol. 1998;**39**:34–7.

[12] Dessinioti C, Antoniou C, Katsambas A. Acneiform eruptions. Clin Dermatol. 2014;**32**:24–34. DOI: 10.1016/j.clindermatol.2013.05.023.

[13] Du-Thanh A, Kluger N, Bensalleh H, Guillot B. Drug-induced acneiform eruption. Am J Clin Dermatol. 2011;**12**:233–45. DOI: 10.2165/11588900-000000000-00000.

[14] Lolis MS, Bowe WP, Shalita AR. Acne and systemic disease. Med Clin North Am. 2009;**93**:1161–81. DOI: 10.1016/j.mcna.2009.08.008.

[15] Kartal Durmazlar SP. Venous Thrombosis in Behcet's Disease, Venous Thrombosis - Principles and Practice, Dr. Ertugrul Okuyan (Ed.), InTech, DOI: 10.5772/28082. Available from: http://www.intechopen.com/books/venous-thrombosis-principles-and-practice/venous-thrombosis-in-behcet-s-disease.

[16] Two AM, Wu W, Gallo RL, Hata TR. Rosacea: part I. Introduction, categorization, histology, pathogenesis, and risk factors. J Am Acad Dermatol. 2015;**72**:749–58. DOI: 10.1016/j.jaad.2014.08.028.

[17] Pelle MT. Rosacea. In: Wolff K, Goldsmith LA, Katz SI, Gilchrest BA, Paller AS, Leffell DJ, editors. Fitzpatrick's Dermatology in General Medicine. 7th ed. New York: McGraw-Hill; 2008. p. 703–8.

[18] Webster GF. Rosacea and related disorders. In: Bolognia JL, Jorizzo JL, Rapini RP, editors, Dermatology, Elsevier. 2nd ed. Spain: Mosby; 2008. p. 509–16.

[19] Two AM, Wu W, Gallo RL, Hata TR. Rosacea: part II. Topical and systemic therapies in the treatment of rosacea. J Am Acad Dermatol. 2015;**72**:761–70. DOI: 10.1016/j.jaad.2014.08.027.

[20] Chen W, Plewig G. Human demodicosis: revisit and a proposed classification. Br J Dermatol. 2014;**170**:1219–25. DOI: 10.1111/bjd.12850.

Chapter 2

Acne Vulgaris

Zekayi Kutlubay, Aysegul Sevim Kecici,
Burhan Engin, Server Serdaroglu and Yalcin Tuzun

Additional information is available at the end of the chapter

http://dx.doi.org/10.5772/65639

Abstract

Acne vulgaris is a multifactorial disorder of the pilosebaceous unit. The clinical picture can range from mild comedones to fulminant, scarring cases. Approximately 83–100% of all adolescents experience acne vulgaris at some point of their lives. Although acne often tends to resolve following the adolescent period, many men and women continue to suffer from either active acne or postinflammatory scars into their twenties and thirties. Most patients with acne vulgaris are in the complicated adolescence period and thus carry a distinctive psychosocial burden. They possess a disease stigma on their skin for the external world to criticize every day. For all these reasons, acne is a disease which should be treated promptly and efficiently in all age groups. This chapter will provide a comprehensive and up-to-date review of pathophysiology of acne vulgaris, new molecular mechanisms on the evolving acne lesions, epidemiology of the disease, and latest treatment options. The molecular biology of acne lesions, novel treatment options including cosmetic approaches, their role in acne pathogenesis, pathophysiology, and mechanism of actions of the drugs, safety, and efficacy issues, and various treatment regimens will be discussed along with novel discoveries and areas in which further research is needed.

Keywords: acne vulgaris, acne vulgaris pathophysiology, treatment of acne vulgaris, systemic treatment of acne vulgaris

1. Introduction

Acne vulgaris is a disease of the pilosebaceous unit. The disorder has a very broad spectrum of clinical picture, from mild comedones to deep inflamed nodules with systemic findings. Acne vulgaris is mainly observed during the adolescent period. Although all age groups may be affected, being primarily a disorder of adolescence, it has a big psychosocial effect leading to low self-esteem, social isolation, and major depression [1].

2. History

The source of the word acne is controversial. It may be derived from the Greek *achne*, a word meaning efflorescence, or the Greek *acme* (Latin acme), which implies a summit or peak. Others have pointed to a hieroglyphic for the word AKU-T as the first written record referring to acne, a symbol interpreted to mean "boils," "pustules," or "a painful swelling" [2]. In the sixth century AD, the term "acne" was first used by the Emperor Justinian's physician, Aetius Amidenus [3]. Its use became obsolete by the 1800s, when "acne" regained a place in medical dictionaries. In 1842, Erasmus Wilson separated acne simplex (acne vulgaris) from acne rosacea [4].

3. Epidemiology

Between 30 and 50% of adolescents experience psychological difficulties associated with acne, including body image concerns, embarrassment, social impairment, anxiety, frustration, anger, depression, and poor self-esteem [5]. The prevalence of body dysmorphic disorder among acne patients has been measured to be as high as 21% in some office settings [6], and these patients are more likely to report dissatisfaction with dermatologic treatment, attempt suicide, and threaten health-care providers both legally and physically [7, 8].

Acne vulgaris affects approximately 40–50 million individuals each year in the USA, with an estimated cost of $2.5 billion annually. The disease affects approximately 85% of young people between 12 and 24 years of age and often tends to continue into the adulthood. In a survey-based study, 35% of women and 20% of men reported having acne in their thirties, while 26% of women and 12% of men were still affected in their forties [9]. Males of Caucasian origin have a tendency to have more severe nodulocystic disease than other groups. Individuals with XYY karyotype or endocrine disorders such as polycystic ovarian syndrome, hyperandrogenism, hypercortisolism, and precocious puberty are at increased risk for acne development, with a more resistant clinical course.

4. Pathogenesis

The development of acne involves a complex interaction of multiple factors within the pilosebaceous gland. Understanding the anatomy and physiology of this unique structure is vital to understanding the pathogenesis of acne and important for formulating effective treatment regimens.

Acne vulgaris is a disease of pilosebaceous units. Major hypotheses on its pathophysiology include the following [10, 11]:

1. Altered follicular keratinization (hyperkeratinization) of the pilosebaceous unit [12]
2. *Propionibacterium acnes* (*P. acnes*) follicular colonization and activity [13]
3. Hormonal influence [14, 15]

4. Sebum production [16]
5. Release of inflammatory mediators [13, 17]

4.1. Genetic factors

The pathogenesis of acne is multifactorial, and the precise role of genetic predisposition is uncertain. The number, size, and activity of sebaceous glands are inherited. In addition, the concordance rate for the prevalence and severity of acne among identical twins is very high. Variable studies have shown strong association between moderate to severe acne and family history [18]. However, because of the high prevalence of acne, it is difficult to attribute its presence only to genetic factors.

4.2. Sebum production

The sebaceous gland is controlled primarily by hormonal stimulation. After the first 6 months of life (when sebum production is relatively high), the rate decreases and remains stable throughout childhood. At adrenarche, sebum production dramatically increases. Although the overall composition of sebum is the same in persons with or without acne, those with acne have variable seborrhea [19].

The sebaceous glands exude lipids by disintegration of entire cells, a process known as *holocrine secretion*. The life span of a sebocyte from cell division to holocrine secretion is approximately 21–25 days [20]. Human sebum, as it leaves the sebaceous gland, contains squalene, cholesterol, cholesterol esters, wax esters, and triglycerides. During passage of sebum through the hair canal, bacterial lipases from *P. acnes* hydrolyze some of the triglycerides, so that the lipid mixture reaching the skin surface contains free fatty acids (FFA) and small proportions of mono- and diglycerides in addition to the original components. The precise function of sebum in humans is unknown. Cunliffe and Shuster proposed that sebum's solitary role is to cause acne [21]. Another theory suggests that sebum reduces water loss from the skin's surface and functions to keep skin soft and smooth. The sebaceous gland-deficient mouse (Asebia) model provides evidence that glycerol derived from triglyceride hydrolysis in sebum is critical for maintaining stratum corneum hydration [22], but there is no evidence for this in humans as stratum corneum hydration is normal during periods, such as, childhood when the gland is quiescent. Similarly, vitamin E delivery to the upper layers of the skin protects the skin and its surface lipids from oxidation; thus, sebum flow to the surface of the skin may provide the transit mechanism necessary for vitamin E to function [23]. Recent evidence suggests that sebaceous glands and sebum play a role in the skin's innate immunity. Sebum is known to have mild antibacterial action, presumably due to the presence of immunoglobulin A [24]. Recent studies show that FFA in human sebum is bactericidal against Gram-positive organisms as a result of its ability to increase antimicrobial peptide, b-defensin 2 (HBD2) expression [25]. Additional antimicrobial peptides including cathelicidin, psoriasin, b-defensin 1, and b-defensin 2 are expressed within the sebaceous gland. Functional cathelicidin peptides have direct antimicrobial activity against *P. acnes* but also initiate cytokine production and inflammation in the host organism [26, 27]. Innate immune Toll-like receptors 2 and 4 (TLR2, TLR4) and CD1d and CD14 molecules are also expressed in sebaceous glands [28]. All these findings provide evidence that the sebaceous gland may play an important role in pathogen recognition and protection of the skin surface.

The exact mechanisms underlying the regulation of human sebum production are not fully defined. Results from a variety of experimental models clearly indicate that sebaceous glands are regulated by androgens and retinoids. Recent evidence suggests that peroxisome proliferator activated receptors, melanocortins, corticotropin-releasing hormone, and fibroblast growth factor receptors play a role as well.

The role of sebum in the pathogenesis of acne is closely associated with the activity of *P. acnes*. The microenvironment within the sebaceous gland is anaerobic and favors the survival of *P. acnes* bacteria over others (i.e., *Staphylococcus epidermidis*). The *P. acnes* bacterium relies on sebaceous lipids as a nutrient source and breaks down triglycerides into FFA, which can be irritating and contribute to the inflammatory response [29, 30]. Furthermore, it is demonstrated that *P. acnes* is capable of stimulating the production of both proinflammatory cytokines/chemokines and antimicrobial peptides from keratinocytes and cultured sebocytes, indicating that keratinocytes and sebocytes themselves may play a role in the inflammatory aspects of acne [31, 32].

4.3. Comedo formation

First step of acne production is the formation of microcomedo, which begins in the infundibulum, the keratinized lining of the upper portion of the follicle. The corneocytes are normally shed into the lumen of the follicle and extruded through the follicular ostium. When they are retained and accumulated, this leads to hyperkeratosis. Lamellar granules, cell membranes, epidermal lipids, and intercellular cementing substances all play a role in the increased adhesiveness of these cells. In addition to increased intercellular cohesiveness of the corneocytes, their production is also accelerated. In the proximal portion of the infundibulum, the infrainfundibulum, combination of increased cellular cohesion, and proliferation creates a bottleneck phenomenon and subsequent microcomedo formation. In the underlying follicular epithelium, keratohyaline granules are increased in size and number, whereas lamellar granules and tonofilaments are decreased. As the comedo expands, the sebaceous lobule undergoes regression. Because of the very narrow opening to the skin surface, there is initially an accumulation of loosely packed shed keratinocytes and sebum. With expansion of the comedo, the contents become closely packed, creating whorled lamellar concretions. With increased pressure, rupture of the comedo wall leads to extrusion of the immunogenic keratin and sebum, with resultant inflammation.

4.4. Inflammatory responses

Inflammation is not always a result of comedo rupture and can also be observed in early acne lesions. Prior to hyperkeratinization, the number of CD4+ T cells and levels of interleukin-1 (IL-1) have been shown to be increased perifollicularly, especially in acne-prone sites [33]. If neutrophils predominate (typical of early lesions) in the lesion, a suppurative pustule is formed. Neutrophils also promote the inflammatory response by releasing lysosomal enzymes and generating reactive oxygen species, which directly correspond with acne

http://dx.doi.org/10.5772/65639

severity [34]. Influx of lymphocytes (predominately T-helper cells) and foreign body-type giant cells, together with neutrophils result in inflamed papules, nodules, and cysts. Genetics are likely to play a role as not all patients with inflammatory acne will scar and patients often report that their parents also have severe scarring from acne in their youths. Data suggest that the likelihood of scarring is associated with the type of inflammatory response. Early, nonspecific inflammation results in less scarring whereas delayed and specific inflammatory response lead to permanent scar tissue [35]. Holland et al. observed that in inflammatory lesions from patients who have less scarring, there is a brisk inflammatory cellular infiltrate composed of T-helper lymphocytes, macrophages, and Langerhans cells, with accompanying angiogenesis that quickly resolves compared with patients who are prone to scarring, where the inflammation and angiogenesis start slowly but is maintained over a longer period. It is speculated that the prolonged inflammatory response in patients prone to scarring is a delayed-type hypersensitivity reaction to persistent antigenic stimulus that they were initially unable to eliminate [36]. As there is no tool to predict who will develop this delayed-type reaction, treating early inflammation is the best approach to prevent acne scarring.

4.5. *Propionibacterium acnes* and the innate immune system

These Gram-positive, non-motile rods which contributes significantly to the pathogenesis of acne are found deep within the sebaceous follicle, along with *Propionibacterium granulosum* and, rarely, *Propionibacterium parvum*. They are anaerobic/microaerophilic and naturally produce porphyrins (primarily coproporphyrin III) that fluoresce with Wood's lamp illumination. These microorganisms release enzymes contributing to comedo rupture, lipases and chemotactic factors, and stimulate host response by inflammatory cells and keratinocytes leading to production of proinflammatory mediators and reactive oxygen species. In acne patients, the number of P. acnes cases is increased, but their numbers do not correlate with clinical severity [37]. Different strains of *P. acnes* have been shown to induce varying degrees of sebocyte differentiation and proinflammatory cytokine/chemokine responses [32].

Interactions between the skin's innate immune system and *P. acnes* play an important role in acne pathogenesis. One mechanism is via Toll-like receptors (TLRs), a class of transmembrane receptors that mediates the recognition of microbial pathogens by immune cells such as monocytes, macrophages, and neutrophils as well as by keratinocytes. TLR2 is found on the surface of macrophages surrounding acne follicles, and *P. acnes* has been found to increase expression of TLR2 and TLR4 on keratinocytes. *P. acnes* has been shown to stimulate the release of proinflammatory mediators (e.g. IL-1α, IL-8, IL-12, tumor necrosis factor-α [TNF-α], matrix metalloproteinases) through the TLR2 pathway [38–40]. IL-8 results in neutrophil recruitment, the release of lysosomal enzymes and subsequent disruption of the follicular epithelium, whereas IL-12 promotes Th1 responses. The degree to which IL-8, IL-12, and interferon-γ production is augmented does not appear to depend upon the strain of *P. acnes* that is present [40, 41]. In contrast, certain strains of *P. acnes* may have an increased propensity, to upregulate expression of human β-defensin-2 by the pilosebaceous unit via a TLR-dependent mechanism [42]. Beta-defensin-2 cathelicidins and other antimicrobial peptides such as psoriasin work synergistically to protect the pilosebaceous unit from *P. acnes* [26, 43]. Histone H4, which is secreted in a holocrine manner by sebocytes, also directly kills *P. acnes* and may function together with free fatty acids to augment innate immune defenses [44]. Lastly, *P. acnes* can induce monocytes to differentiate into two distinct innate immune cell subsets: (1) CD209+ macrophages (development of which is promoted by tretinoin) that more effectively phagocytose and kill *P. acnes* and (2) CD1b+ dendritic cells that activate T cells and release proinflammatory cytokines [45].

All these new findings about the role of innate immunity on acne formation build upon traditionally known pathogenetic factors can be summed up as follows;

1. Inflammatory events mediated by interleukin-1 precede hyperkeratinization
2. *P. acnes* activates the innate immune system via Toll-like receptors
3. *P. acnes* induces matrix metalloproteinase and antimicrobial peptide production
4. Sebaceous gland lipids influence the innate immune system.

4.6. Hormonal influences

Sebum secretion is under direct influence of hormonal factors. Androgens are produced primarily from the gonads and adrenal glands but also locally via the enzymes of 3β-hydroxysteroid dehydrogenase (HSD), 17β-HSD and 5α-reductase. Androgen receptors, found in the cells of the basal layer of the sebaceous gland and the outer root sheath of the hair follicle, are responsive to testosterone and 5α-dihydrotestosterone (DHT). DHT is the principal androgen mediating sebum production and has a 5–10-fold greater affinity than testosterone for the androgen receptor. The role of androgens in sebaceous gland activity begins during the neonatal period. With the onset of adrenarche (typically at 7–8 years of age, usually heralding menarche by several years), circulating levels of DHEAS begin to rise due to adrenal production. This hormone can serve as a precursor for the synthesis of more potent androgens within the sebaceous gland. The rise in serum levels of DHEAS in prepubescent children is associated with an increase in sebum production and the initial development of comedonal acne [46]. The exact mechanism of how estrogens modulate sebum production is not known. Any estrogen given systemically in sufficient amounts will decrease sebum production. However, the dose of estrogen required to suppress sebum production is greater than the dose required to suppress ovulation. Although acne may respond to treatment with lower-dose oral contraceptives containing 0.035–0.050 mg of ethinyl estradiol or its esters, higher doses of estrogen are often required to demonstrate a reduction in sebum secretion [47]. Estrogens may inhibit the effects of androgens locally within the sebaceous gland or via a negative feedback loop whereby pituitary gonadotropin release is inhibited.

4.7. Dietary factors

It has long been posited that diet has no impact on acne, but recent clinical trials have suggested that a relationship does indeed exist. The relationship between diet and acne has always been controversial. The association between glycemic load and acne is especially convincing. Prospective studies have documented a link between a high glycemic-load diet and acne risk [48]. Further clinical trials among a wider patient base could better define recommendations

http://dx.doi.org/10.5772/65639

for modifying carbohydrate intake, but until then, it is appropriate for dermatologists to recommend a lower glycemic load diet among patients with acne.

Although the link between dairy and acne is less convincing than high glycemic load diet, a recent case control study showed a positive association between low-fat/skim milk consumption and acne [49]. The exact mechanism by which dairy may impact acne, whether it is via a hormonal pathway or upregulated IGF-1, remains to be further clarified. If physicians choose to counsel their patients that dairy consumption may indeed exacerbate their acne, it is reasonable to simultaneously advise patients to supplement their diets with vitamin D and calcium. The role of o-3 fatty acids, antioxidants, zinc, vitamin A, and iodine in acne vulgaris remains to be elucidated. Given the level of evidence available if a particular patient notes an association between a certain dietary factor and acne severity, it is best to support that patient's dietary supplementation or restriction and to encourage the patient to keep a food diary to test his or her hypothesis.

5. Clinical features

Acne is mostly observed on the facial area and upper trunk, areas with increased number of sebaceous glands (**Figure 1**). Comedones constitute non-inflammatory lesions of acne.

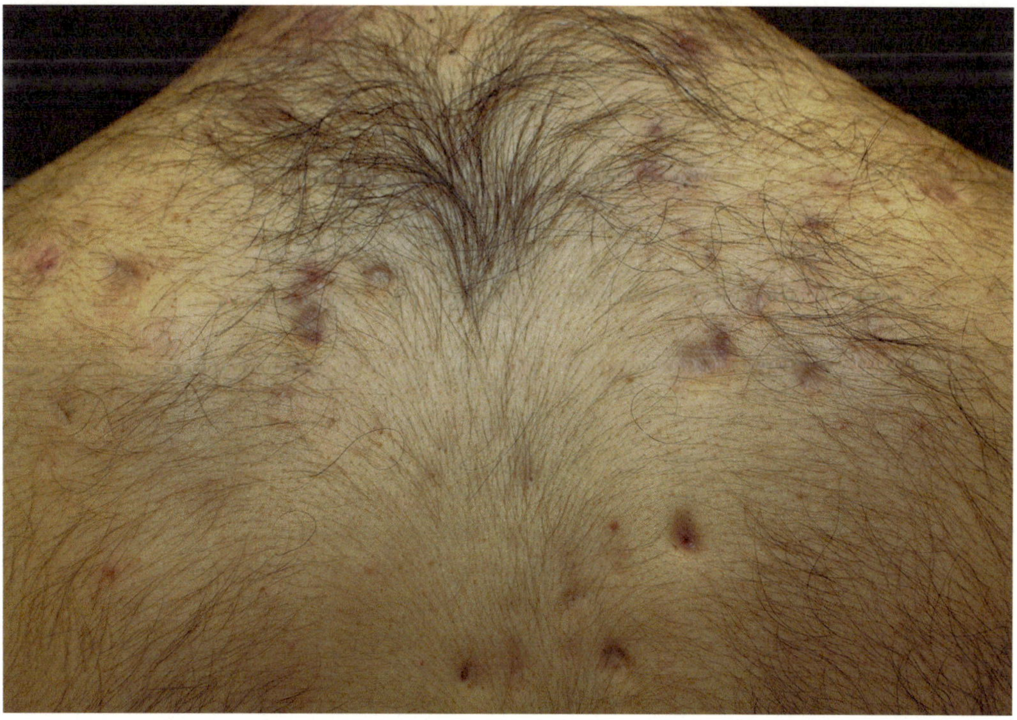

Figure 1. Acne lesions and scars are seen on the back of the patients.

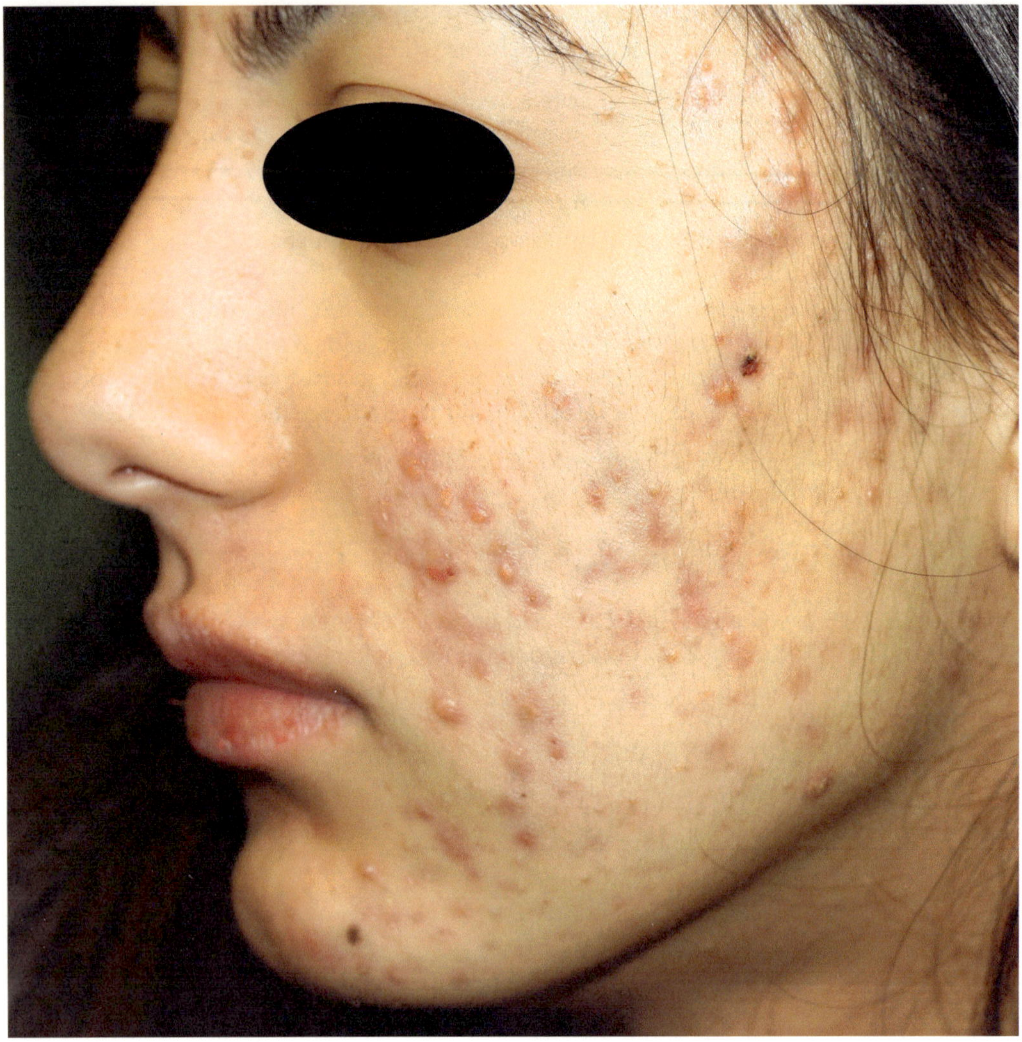

Figure 2. Marked papules, pustules, and comedones are noticed.

Closed comedones are small skin-colored papules with no apparent follicular opening. These lesions may be subtle and best diagnosed via palpation, stretching or side-lighting of the skin. Open comedones, on the other hand, mostly referred as blackheads, are dome-shaped papules with dilated follicular openings filled shed keratin. Black coloration is due to melanin deposition and lipid oxidation within the debris. Inflammatory acne also originates with comedo formation, followed by the development of papules, pustules, nodules, and cysts (**Figure 2**).

Erythematous papules typically range from 1 to 5 mm in diameter. Pustules tend to be approximately equal in size and are filled with white pus and normal flora. As the severity of lesions progresses, nodules form and become markedly inflamed, indurated, and tender.

http://dx.doi.org/10.5772/65639

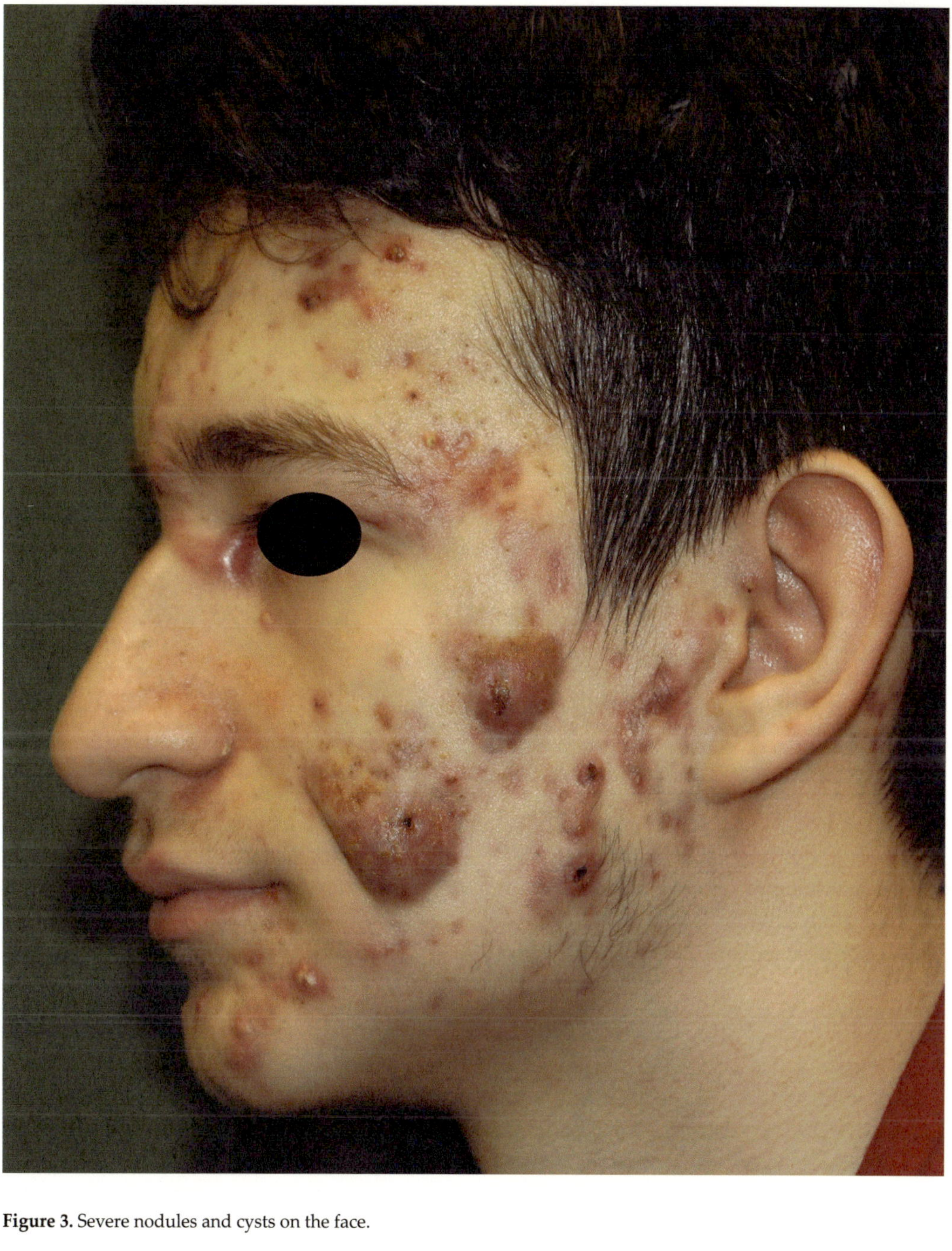

Figure 3. Severe nodules and cysts on the face.

The cysts of acne are deeper and filled with a combination of pus and serosanguineous fluid. In patients with severe nodulocystic acne (**Figure 3**), these lesions frequently coalesce to form large, complex inflamed plaques that can include sinus tracts.

Early treatment of acne is essential for the prevention of lasting cosmetic disfigurement due to scarring. Erythema and postinflammatory hyperpigmentation often persist after resolution of inflammatory acne lesions. Pigmentary changes usually fade away in months whereas pitted or hypertrophic scars are often permanent.

5.1. Acne variants

5.1.1. Postadolescent acne

This form of acne mostly affects women older than 25 years of age with signs of hyperandrogenism and increases in severity prior to menstruation. The lesions consist of tender, deep-seated papulonodules on the lower third of the face, jawline, and neck [50]. Hormonal therapy is often effective regardless of androgen levels.

5.1.2. Acne fulminans

It is the most severe form of acne and is characterized by nodular and suppurative acne lesions with systemic manifestations. It primarily affects adolescent boys who typically have mild to moderate acne prior to the onset of acne fulminans. Numerous microcomedones suddenly erupt and become markedly inflamed. Most commonly affected areas are the face, neck, chest, back, and arms. Lesions tend to ulcerate and can lead to significant scarring. Osteolytic bone lesions may accompany the cutaneous findings; the clavicle and sternum are most commonly affected, followed by the ankles, humerus, and iliosacral joints. Systemic manifestations include fever, arthralgias, myalgias, hepatosplenomegaly, and severe malaise. The related *s*ynovitis, *a*cne, *p*ustulosis, *h*yperostosis and *o*steitis can be seen and is defined as SAPHO syndrome. Erythema nodosum may also arise in association with acne fulminans. An elevated ESR, proteinuria, leukocytosis, and anemia mostly accompanies and may be related with the clinical course and response to therapy.

Treatment of acne fulminans usually includes initial oral corticosteroid treatment, followed by systemic isotretinoin, after the acute inflammation subsides. During the first few weeks of isotretinoin therapy, acne fulminans-like flares can be observed [51]. Oral antibiotics, TNF-α inhibitors, and immunosuppressive agents (e.g. azathioprine) can also be used. Acne fulminans associated with erythema nodosum responds well to dapsone therapy [52].

5.1.3. Acne conglobata and associated conditions

Acne conglobata is also a severe form of nodulocystic acne that may have a sudden onset but without systemic manifestations. The nodules are usually found on the chest, shoulders, back, buttocks, upper arms, thighs, and face (**Figure 4**). It is a part of the follicular occlusion tetrad, along with dissecting cellulitis of the scalp, hidradenitis suppurativa, and pilonidal cysts. The association of sterile *p*yogenic *a*rthritis, *p*yoderma gangrenosum, and *a*cne conglobata can occur in the context of an autosomal dominant autoinflammatory disorder referred to as PAPA syndrome [53]. This syndrome is caused by mutations in the gene that encodes *p*roline–*s*erine–*t*hreonine *p*hosphatase *i*nteracting *p*rotein 1 (PSTPIP1) which leads to the disruption of the physiologic signaling required for maintenance of a proper inflammatory response [53].

http://dx.doi.org/10.5772/65639

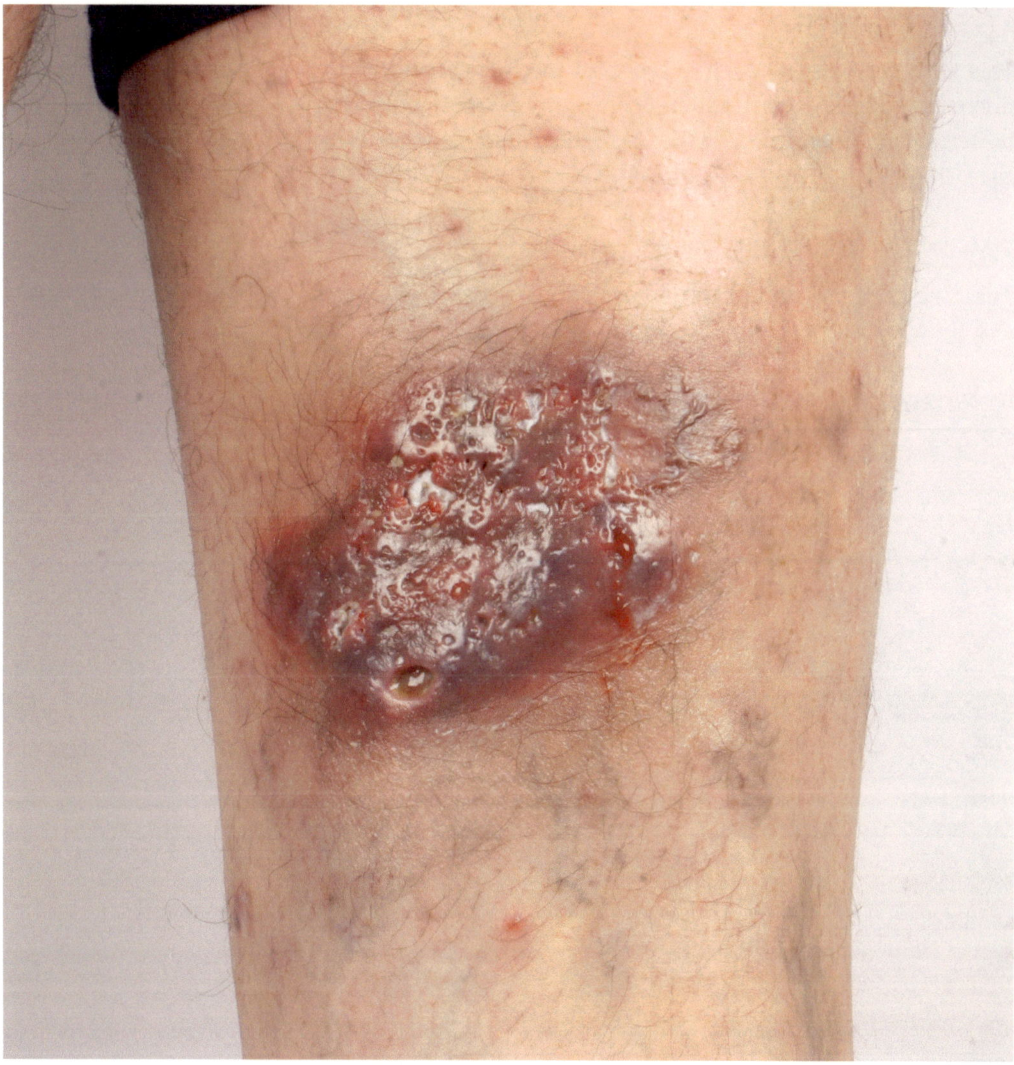

Figure 4. A closer view of draining sinuses and nodules on the lower extremity.

5.1.4. Solid facial edema

An unusual and disfiguring complication of acne vulgaris is solid facial edema (Morbihan's disease). Clinically, there is a distortion of the midline face and cheeks due to soft tissue swelling and accompanying erythema. Due to chronic inflammation and mast cell activation, lymphatic drainage is impaired resulting in fibrosis. Similar changes have been described in patients with rosacea and Melkersson-Rosenthal syndrome. The degree of the edema may change but solid facial edema does not usually resolve spontaneously. Treatment options include systemic isotretinoin alone or together with ketotifen or systemic corticosteroids [54, 55].

5.1.5. Acne mechanica

This form occurs secondary to repeated mechanical and frictional trauma causing obstruction of the pilosebaceous outlet. Rubbing by helmets, chin straps, suspenders or collars can be responsible for acne mechanica. Linear and geometrically distributed comedones are characteristic.

5.1.6. Acne excoriée des jeunes filles

Typical comedones and inflammatory papules are systematically excoriated, leaving crusted and linear erosions (**Figure 5**). An underlying psychiatric component should be considered.

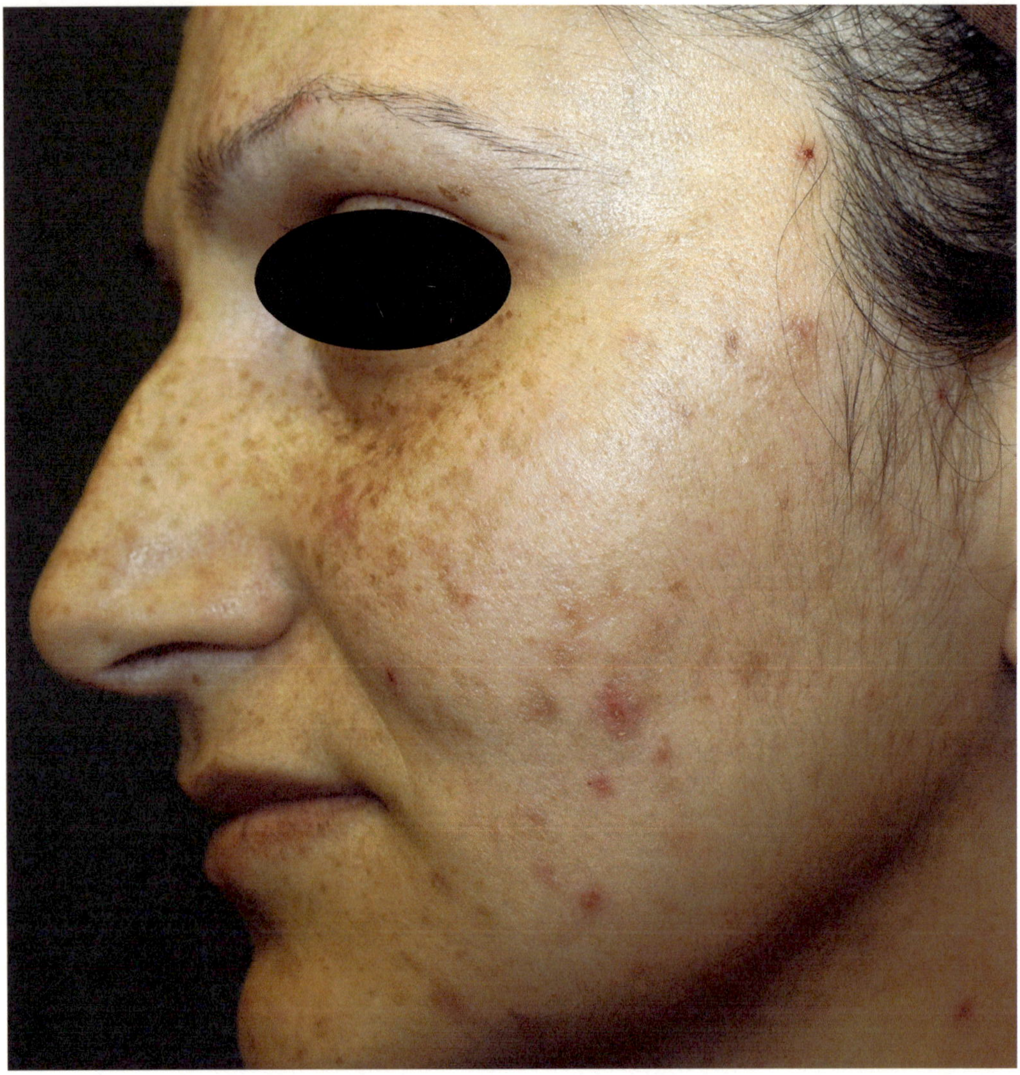

Figure 5. Excoriated inflammatory lesions are seen.

Individuals with an anxiety disorder, obsessive–compulsive disorder or personality disorder are particularly at risk.

5.1.7. Drug-induced acne

Acne or eruptive acneiform lesions can be seen as a side effect of certain drugs. Characteristically abrupt, mono morphous eruption of inflammatory papules and pustules are observed. High-dose intravenous or oral corticosteroids commonly induce characteristic acneiform eruptions with a concentration of lesions on the chest and back. Steroid-induced acne (and rosacea) can also result from the inappropriate use of topical corticosteroids on the face. Inflamed papules and pustules develop on a background of erythema that favors the distribution of corticosteroid application. Lesions eventually resolve following discontinuation of the corticosteroid, although "steroid dependency" can lead to prolonged and severe flares postwithdrawal.

5.1.8. Occupational acne, acne cosmetica

Occupational acne results from exposure to insoluble, follicle-occluding substances. Cutting oils, petroleum-based products, chlorinated aromatic hydrocarbons, and coal tar derivatives can be responsible. Comedones together with papules, pustules, and cystic lesions distributed in exposed as well as typically covered areas. *Acne cosmetica* is mostly seen as closed comedones, due to chronic occlusion of follicles with the use of cosmetics.

5.1.9. Chloracne

It is caused several weeks after the exposure to chlorinated aromatic hydrocarbons. Most commonly affected areas are the malar, retroauricular, and mandibular regions of the head and neck, axillae, and scrotum. Small cystic papules and nodules are seen and healing with scar tissue formation is not uncommon. The following agents, found in electrical conductors and insulators, insecticides, fungicides, herbicides, and wood preservatives, have all been implicated: polychlorinated naphthalenes, biphenyls, dibenzofurans, and dibenzodioxins; polybrominated naphthalenes and biphenyls; tetrachloroazobenzene; and tetrachloroazoxybenzene.

5.1.10. Neonatal acne (neonatal cephalic pustulosis)

Neonatal acne can be observed in more than 20% of healthy newborns. Lesions usually start appearing 2 weeks after birth and generally resolve within the first 3 months of life. Small, inflamed papulopustules without comedones on the cheeks and nasal bridge are typical for neonatal acne. The disease responds well to topical imidazoles, and this also supports the inflammatory response to *Malassezia* spp. as a pathogenetic mechanism. The active sebaceous glands and high sebum excretion rate in neonates are also thought to play a role. The substantial decline in sebum production after the first few months of life helps to explain the limited period of susceptibility to neonatal acne.

5.1.11. Infantile acne

Infantile acne occurs after 3 months of age and usually persists until the end of first year. In contrast to neonatal acne, comedo formation is prominent and pitted scarring can develop.

Deep cystic lesions and suppurative nodules are occasionally seen. Androgen production due to elevated levels of LH stimulating testicular production of testosterone in boys and elevated levels of DHEA produced by the infantile adrenal gland in both boys and girls is responsible from acne formation. These androgen levels normally decrease substantially by 12 months of age and remain at low levels until adrenarche. Thus infantile acne typically resolves within 1–2 years and remains quiescent until around puberty. Topical retinoids (e.g., tretinoin, adapalene) and benzoyl peroxide are first-line treatments for infantile acne. Oral antibiotics (e.g. erythromycin, azithromycin) can be helpful for patients with a more severe inflammatory component, and isotretinoin is occasionally required for recalcitrant cases [56].

5.1.12. Endocrinologic abnormalities

Hyperandrogenism should be suspected in female patients with hirsutism or irregular menstrual periods, as well as in children who develop acne between 2 and 7 years of age. Hyperandrogenism-originated acne is often severe and resistant to therapy. Other signs and symptoms of hyperandrogenism in women and children include coarsening of the voice, a muscular habitus, androgenetic alopecia, clitoromegaly with variable posterior labial fusion, and increased libido. Insulin resistance and acanthosis nigricans can occur in association with hyperandrogenism in the HAIR-AN syndrome. These patients are at increased risk for accelerated cardiovascular disease and diabetes mellitus. Initial laboratory tests of serum levels of total and free testosterone, DHEAS, and 17-hydroxyprogesterone can give an idea about the source of excess androgens. An elevated serum DHEAS or 17-hydroxyprogesterone level indicates an adrenal problem such as congenital adrenal hyperplasia or an adrenal tumor. If the testosterone levels (total and free) are elevated and the DHEAS level is relatively normal, an ovarian source is likely. Polycystic ovary syndrome (PCOS) is the most common condition associated with an elevated serum testosterone level.

6. Pathology

Histopathologic stages of acne lesions show a parallel course with the clinical findings. In early lesions, microcomedones are seen. A mildly distended follicle with a narrowed follicular opening is impacted by shed keratinocytes. In closed comedones, the degree of follicular distension is increased and a compact cystic structure with eosinophilic keratinaceous debris, hair, and numerous bacteria is formed. Open comedones have broad, expanded follicular ostia and overall an increased follicular distension. Perivascular mononuclear cell infiltrate circles the expanding follicle. As the follicular epithelium distends, highly immunogenic cystic contents rupture into the dermis, inducing a marked inflammatory response. Neutrophils first appear, creating a pustule. As the lesion matures, scarring due to foreign body granulomatous inflammation can be seen.

7. Differential diagnosis

Differential diagnosis of acneiform eruptions is broad and depends upon the age of onset, lesional morphology, and location. During the neonatal period, acne must be differentiated

http://dx.doi.org/10.5772/65639

from other similar dermatoses including sebaceous hyperplasia and miliaria rubra. Predominantly comedonal acne vulgaris needs to be differentiated from comedonal eruptions caused by follicular occlusion or friction, including pomade and occupational acne, acne cosmetica and acne mechanica. Multiple open comedones are clustered in the lateral malar region in Favre-Racouchot disease or appear in a linear array in nevus comedonicus. Angiofibromas and appendageal tumors of follicular origin like trichoepitheliomas, trichodiscomas, and fibrofolliculomas, often present as multiple noninflammatory facial papules. Steatocystoma multiplex is also characterized by noninflammatory, closed cystic papules and nodules on the central chest and back. The follicle-based inflammatory papules and pustules of acne vulgaris must be distinguished from the many forms of folliculitis, including staphylococcal, Gram-negative, and eosinophilic variants. Folliculitis lesions are typically monomorphous and comedones are not present. Acne vulgaris treated with oral antibiotics for a prolonged period can complicate with Gram-negative folliculitis. The papular component of rosacea favors the malar region, chin, and forehead; the presence of telangiectasias, absence of comedones and a history of easy flushing can lead to diagnosis. Prolonged use of topical corticosteroids on the face may lead to rosacea-like lesions or perioral/periorificial dermatitis, and patients treated with oral corticosteroids can develop an eruption of monomorphous papulopustules that favors the trunk.

8. Treatment

Acne can have devastating physical as well as emotional effects and the treatment course of acne vulgaris requires a high degree of compliance. Thus it is critical that the patient be made aware of the nature of the disease process and what is to be expected from the treatment regimen prescribed. A complete history and physical examination are key to developing an appropriate and effective treatment plan. A review of all prescription and over-the counter medications used for acne or other conditions, and clinical responsiveness to them, together with cosmetics, sunscreens, cleansers, and moisturizers is also helpful. In female patients, a menstrual and oral contraceptive history is important in determining hormonal influences on acne. On physical examination, careful note should be taken of lesion morphology, including the presence of comedones, inflammatory lesions, nodules, and cysts. Secondary changes such as scarring and postinflammatory pigmentary changes are also important clinical findings. The patient's skin color and type can also influence the chosen formulation of a topical medication.

8.1. Topical treatments

8.1.1. Topical retinoids

Topical retinoids used for the treatment of acne vulgaris will be discussed in elsewhere.

8.1.2. Benzoyl peroxide and other topical antibacterial agents

Benzoyl peroxide (BPO) is still the gold standard for mild-to-moderate acne. It is the leading over the counter anti-acne agent in the United States. Different preparations including bar soaps, washes, gels, lotions, creams, foams, and pads with concentrations ranging from 2.5

to 10% are available as well as products which combine benzoyl peroxide with clindamycin, erythromycin, or adapalene. BPO is a bleaching agent, thus whitening of clothing and bedding can occur. İrritant or allergic contact dermatitis can develop to benzoyl peroxide, presenting with marked erythema. BPO is a potent bactericidal agent that reduces *P. acnes* within the follicle. It also has mild comedolytic properties and is particularly effective when used in combination with other therapies.

The mechanism of action is presumably due to its strong oxidizing property. The release of free oxygen radical causes oxidation of bacterial proteins and the development of oxygen creates a milieu in the follicle, where anaerobic bacteria like *P. acnes* cannot survive [57–60]. BPO has a broad-spectrum and rapid activity against Gram-positive and Gram-negative bacteria, yeasts, and various fungi [58]. Significant and fast reduction in the number of propionibacteria from the skin surface and follicular casts can be achieved with topical use of BPO, starting within days after the initiation of the therapy. However, long-term use of the agent does not provide further decrease in the bacterial population [61–63].

Unlike common antibiotics, BPO is effective and can be readily used against antibiotic-resistant propionibacteria strains [60]. This agent shows its antibacterial action via powerful oxidation. This nonspecific mode of antibacterial action does not lead to the development of resistant strains and thus makes long-term use of the drug possible [62]. Therefore, in order to sustain long-lasting efficacy in acne therapy, broad-spectrum antibacterial agents such as BPO can be used concomitantly or sequentially with antibiotics. Unlike bacterial burden, BPO has a lack of direct effect on sebum production and does not reduce skin surface lipids, but it is effective in reducing the free fatty acids, known as comedogenic agents, and triggers of inflammation in sebum [64, 65]. BPO is thought to have weak comedolytic activity [66].

Another supplementary benefit of BPO in acne therapy is its anti-inflammatory action. BPO, however, does not have significant direct *in vivo* anti-inflammatory potency. A potential explanation for the anti-inflammatory effects of BPO could be the mediation by the antibacterial or oxidizing action of BPO. Following the decrease in the population of *P. acnes* in the follicles and the reduction of free oxygen radicals, one source of inflammation is cut and therefore inflammatory reactions are suppressed. The anti-inflammatory benefit of BPO, regardless of being direct or indirect, is reflected in several studies [67].

BPO products are indicated for mild-to-moderate acne with occurrence of predominantly inflamed lesions. One study tested different BPO formulations with different concentrations and at the end of 4 weeks treatment, they were all shown to decrease the number of papules and pustules and, to a smaller degree, the number of comedones [68]. Not only efficacy in mild-to-moderate acne but also a rapid onset of action can be observed after BPO application, which accompanies the quick antibacterial action within the first week of therapy [69].

8.1.3. Topical antibiotics

Topical antibiotics have been an integral component of the topical acne treatment. Over time, the most common topical antibiotics used for acne treatment have been erythromycin and clindamycin, with the latter being favored over the past several years, primarily

http://dx.doi.org/10.5772/65639

due to widespread emergence globally of *P. acnes* strains resistant to erythromycin [70]. Sulfacetamide with or without sulfur has also been used topically for treatment of acne vulgaris but data regarding the efficacy of these agents are limited. It is thought to restrict the growth of *P. acnes* through competitive inhibition of the condensation of para-aminobenzoic acid with pteridine precursors.

The principal mechanism of action of topical antibiotics appears to be through reduction in *P. acnes* organisms, which reduces the subsequent triggering of inflammatory activities [71, 72]. The use of benzoyl peroxide in combination with erythromycin or clindamycin augments reduction in *P. acnes*, reduces the emergence of resistant *P. acnes* strains, and may improve efficacy over use of either agent alone [71].

Concerns regarding emergence of clinically significant antibiotic-resistant bacteria primarily focus on systemic antibiotic use but topical antibiotic use can also change the cutaneous flora as application of topical antibiotics for treatment of acne is usually continued over several months to years [73, 74]. Thus, progressive emergence of normal bacterial flora that are less antibiotic sensitive such as macrolide-resistant *Staphylococcus epidermidis* and erythromycin- and tetracycline-resistant *P. acnes* strains has an estimated prevalence of 40% globally over approximately three decades [74]. Additionally, antibiotic-resistant *P. acnes* strains have been demonstrated on skin of untreated contacts of acne patients treated with topical antibiotic therapy, supporting interpersonal spread [75]. The clinically relevant effects of these changes in normal bacterial flora secondary to antibiotic use are not entirely clear. However, there is evidence for a correlation between antibiotic-resistant *P. acnes* and a reduction in efficacy with antibiotic therapy [73, 74]. Potential issues of concern that have been raised in this manner include increased prevalence of *P. acnes* strains less responsive to antibiotics, alterations in cutaneous flora, decreased therapeutic responsiveness to antibiotic therapy, and promotion of other clinical infections among treated patients and/or their close contacts. Apart from these, pharyngeal colonization with *Streptococcus pyogenes* and a possible increased risk of an upper respiratory tract infection have been associated with chronic use of antibiotics for acne, including topical agents [76, 77].

A report analyzing several monotherapy studies using either topical erythromycin or topical clindamycin for acne vulgaris demonstrated that the efficacy of topical erythromycin in reducing acne lesions has markedly decreased over time; however, the efficacy of topical clindamycin has not diminished on the basis of the same parameters of acne lesion reduction [78].

Topical antibiotics remain an important part of acne treatment and are recommended as a component of combination topical therapy; monotherapy with a topical antibiotic for acne is not recommended. At present, topical clindamycin remains the predominant topical antibiotic used for acne treatment; however, other agents such as erythromycin, sulfacetamide with or without sulfur, and azelaic acid are also options. Overall, the tolerability and safety profiles of topical antibiotics used for the treatment of acne vulgaris, are very favorable.

8.1.4. Azelaic acid

Azelaic acid is a naturally occurring dicarboxylic acid found in cereal grains. It is available as a topical 20% cream formulation, which has been shown to be effective in inflammatory and comedonal acne [10]. By inhibiting the growth of *P. acnes*, azelaic acid reduces inflammatory acne. It also reverses the altered keratinization of follicles affected by acne and thus demonstrates comedolytic properties. The activity of azelaic acid against inflammatory lesions may be greater than its activity against comedones. Overall, the position of azelaic acid in the treatment algorithm of acne vulgaris has been as an alternative to other topical agents. Initial improvement in acne with topical azelaic acid has been reported to be observed in 4–8 weeks, with maximum benefit generally noted after approximately 16 weeks of use [79]. Azelaic acid is applied twice daily, and its use is reported to have fewer local side effects than topical retinoids. In addition, it may help to lighten postinflammatory hyperpigmentation.

8.1.5. Salicylic acid

Salicylic acid (SA) is a comedolytic and mild anti-inflammatory agent, widely used as a topical therapeutic agent for a variety of skin diseases, including acne, psoriasis, dandruff, and ichthyosis. Concentrations ranging from 0.5 to 10% have been recommended for acne, in numerous delivery formulations, including gels, creams, lotions, foams, solutions, and washes. The action of SA may occur due to the reduced cohesion between corneocytes, resulting in the shedding of epidermal cells, rather than "lysing" of keratin [80]. The antibacterial action of SA against *P. acnes* has also been demonstrated in both *in vitro* and *in vivo* studies. Side effects of topical salicylic acid include erythema and scaling.

Many clinical studies have proven the anti-acne efficacy of SA-containing products. SA can induce a more rapid effect on noninflamed lesions, when compared to inflamed lesions, which strengthens the suggestion that it has a primary effect on comedogenesis [81]. According to cross-over studies, SA is slightly more effective than BPO for the treatment of comedonal acne, as well as inflammatory lesions [82, 83]. The observed superiority of SA might be due to its mode of action. Since the primary lesion of acne is the microcomedo, a treatment that is effective in preventing its formation will be effective in preventing inflammatory lesions into which the microcomedo can progress. As the action of SA is mainly keratolytic, it interferes in an earlier stage than BPO, and in consequence it seems to be superior in acting against later steps, the inflamed lesions.

8.1.6. Topical dapsone

Topical *dapsone* 5% gel is approved for the treatment of acne vulgaris. Of note, a temporary yellow-orange staining of the skin and hair occasionally occurs with concomitant use of topical dapsone and benzoyl peroxide.

8.2. Oral treatments

8.2.1. Antibiotics

Current basic clinical research including identification of the *P. acnes* genome, analysis of innate-immune response in acne inflammation, evaluation of the role of inflammation in comedogenesis, and microbiologic studies correlating *P. acnes* with specific treatments and therapeutic benefit, all support the goal of *P. acnes* suppression with antimicrobial therapy as

http://dx.doi.org/10.5772/65639

a component of acne management [72]. In addition to *P. acnes* suppression, some antibiotics such as the tetracycline derivatives also exhibit anti-inflammatory properties that appear to contribute to their therapeutic benefit in acne vulgaris [84].

Conventionally, the predominant oral antibiotics used for treatment of acne vulgaris in most countries have been tetracycline, doxycycline, minocycline, erythromycin, azithromycin, and rarely trimethoprim. Doxycycline and minocycline are used more frequently than tetracycline and erythromycin due to resistance issues but over time there has been a trend toward an increase in *P. acnes* strains becoming less sensitive to doxycycline and minocycline as well [74, 85, 86] (**Table 1**).The greatest decrease in *P. acnes* colony counts has been demonstrated with minocycline, followed in order of magnitude by doxycycline, tetracycline, trimethoprim-sulfamethoxazole, and erythromycin [87]. The clinical efficacy of oral antibiotic therapy for acne vulgaris is well established and recognized as a conventional component of rational acne treatment.

The main indication for oral antibiotic therapy in acne vulgaris is moderate-to-severe inflammatory involvement on the face and/or trunk [72]. Antibiotic monotherapy should be avoided due to promotion of antibiotic-resistant bacterial strains, with oral antibiotic therapy best utilized in combination with a topical regimen, namely benzoyl peroxide or a topical retinoid [88]. It has also been suggested that a short course of benzoyl peroxide therapy prior to initiating antibiotic therapy assists in the eradication of antibiotic-resistant *P. acnes* strains, thus enhancing the overall efficacy of antibiotic treatment. The combination therapy may also allow for better ability to discontinue the oral antibiotic at some point based on response to treatment, and hopefully allow the topical regimen alone to maintain control of acne.

If not enterically coated, doxycline, especially the hyclate salt, is best administered with food and a large glass of water when the patient is upright and not prior to anticipated reclining for at least a few hours, to reduce the risk of gastrointestinal side effects such as esophagitis. Concomitant administration of doxycycline and minocycline with iron supplements and metal ions may decrease absorption of both agents. Azithromycin, on the other hand, does not as commonly cause gastrointestinal side effects, and is best taken on an empty stomach to maximize absorption.

In case of resistance challenges, it is important to recognize that a direct correlation between prevalence of *P. acnes* resistance and poor therapeutic response to antibiotic therapy has not always been consistent [74]. Factors potentially associated with a reduced response to antibiotic therapy may include pre-existing antibiotic resistance, the quantity of antibiotic-resistant

Drug	Usual dosage range
Minocycline (immediate release)	50–100 mg once or twice daily
Minocycline (extended release)	1 mg/kg/day (45–135 mg once daily)
Doxycycline	75–100 mg once or twice daily 150 mg once daily

Table 1. The recommended dosing schedule is seen.

P. acnes strains in the individual patient, resistance to multiple antibiotics, use of antibiotics without concomitant use of benzoyl peroxide, repeated courses of antibiotic therapy especially without concomitant use of benzoyl peroxide, unnecessary switching of oral antibiotic agents despite previous efficacy, individual drug characteristics such as GI absorption and lipophilicity, relative effects on serum and tissue levels due to interference of GI absorption by co-administered chelating metal ions, and existence of *P. acnes* in a protective extracellular biofilm *in vivo*.

When oral antibiotic therapy is incorporated with a topical regimen for acne, it has been suggested that it be administered over a minimum period of 6–8 weeks and a maximum of 12 weeks–6 months. In the initial follow-up 6–8 weeks after the start of therapy, if a substantial lack of efficacy is observed despite adequate compliance, a change in oral antibiotic therapy is reasonable [72, 74, 89]. If partial improvement is observed, it may be reasonable to continue with the current therapy for an additional 6–8 weeks to evaluate if further progress is achieved. Changing a regimen too frequently often results in suboptimal outcomes as a given regimen is never afforded a true opportunity to initiate its therapeutic effect. Once control of acne is felt to be stable, which is usually achieved over a duration of 3–6 months assuming compliance is adequate, discontinuation of the oral antibiotic therapy may be suggested, with continuation of the topical regimen for long-term maintenance. Stabilized control of acne does not necessarily imply complete clearance but may be defined as the observation that new inflammatory lesions have stopped or markedly decreased. Despite the alleged use of a topical maintenance regimen, some patients return with an acne flare within a few weeks to months after discontinuation of the oral antibiotic. In such cases, it is suggested to reinitiate therapy with the same oral antibiotic that was previously effective.

Use of systemic antibiotics may cause some adverse reactions. Doxycycline is associated with dose-related phototoxicity, whereas minocycline causes acute vestibular adverse events, lupus-like syndrome, together with cutaneous and/or mucosal hyperpigmentation, including brown, gray, or blue pigmentation of skin and/or mucosa and blue discoloration of acne scars. There are no specific recommendations to routinely perform baseline or periodic laboratory testing with oral antibiotics used to treat acne vulgaris; however, medical history of the individual patient may prompt the clinician to avoid use of a specific oral antibiotic or to incorporate baseline and/or periodic laboratory monitoring.

Overall, the efficacy and safety of conventional oral antibiotic therapy used for acne have been very favorable based on available studies and extensive clinical experience over many years.

8.2.2. Hormonal therapy

Hormonal therapy is an established second-line treatment for female patients with acne and can be very effective, irrespective of whether or not the serum androgen levels are abnormal. Hormonal therapies are most effective in adult women with inflammatory papules and nodules of the lower face and neck that tend to flare prior to menstruation. These lesions are usually resistant to oral antibiotherapies, thus hormonal therapy with oral contraceptives to block both ovarian and adrenal production of androgens can be initiated. Due to potential long-term risks associated with oral contraceptive use consultation with a gynecologist is recommended. Most oral contraceptive formulations combine an estrogen with a progestin in

http://dx.doi.org/10.5772/65639

order to minimize the risk of endometrial cancer, which is known to occur with unopposed estrogen administration. Second-generation progestins with low intrinsic androgenic activity such as ethynodiol diacetate, norethindrone, and levonorgestrel are preferred in the combinations. Newer, third-generation progestins like desogestrel, norgestimate, and gestodene have even less androgenic activity and other progestins like drospirenone, cyproterone acetate, and dienogest have *anti*androgenic properties.

Three oral contraceptives are currently FDA-approved for the treatment of acne, although others also have evidence of efficacy. The first is a triphasic oral contraceptive composed of a norgestimate-ethinyl estradiol (35 mcg) combination. The second contains a graduated dose of ethinyl estradiol (20–35 mcg) in combination with norethindrone acetate, while the third contains a stable dose of ethinyl estradiol (20 mcg) plus drospirenone (3 mg) with a 24-day dosing regimen [90]. Side effects of oral contraceptives include nausea, vomiting, abnormal menses, weight gain, and breast tenderness; agents containing drospirenone can lead to elevations in serum potassium levels, but this is generally not clinically significant in otherwise healthy individuals. Rare but more serious complications include hypertension and thromboembolism [91–93]. The progestational antiandrogen cyproterone acetate primarily makes androgen receptor blockade. The standard formulation combines cyproterone acetate (2 mg) with ethinyl estradiol (35 or 50 mcg) in an oral contraceptive formulation, which is the treatment of choice for sexually active women with hormonally responsive acne [94].

Spironolactone functions as both an androgen receptor blocker and an inhibitor of 5α-reductase. In doses of 50–100 mg twice daily, it has been shown to reduce sebum production and improve acne [95]. Side effects are dose-related and include potential hyperkalemia, irregular menstrual periods, breast tenderness, headache, and fatigue. However, hyperkalemia is rare in young healthy patients. Because it is an antiandrogen, there is a risk of feminization of a male fetus if a pregnant woman takes this medication. The potential risk to a fetus and the symptoms of irregular menstrual bleeding can be alleviated by combining spironolactone with an oral contraceptive. Side effects can also be minimized if therapy is initiated with a low dose (25–50 mg/day). Effective maintenance doses range from 25 to 200 mg/day. As with other hormonal therapies, a clinical response may take up to 3 months.

Flutamide, a nonsteroidal androgen receptor blocker that is approved by the FDA for the treatment of prostate cancer, can also be an effective treatment for acne in women at doses of 62.5–500 mg/day. In addition to side effects similar to those of other antiandrogens severe dose-related hepatotoxicity occasionally occurs.

8.2.3. Isotretinoin

Currently, isotretinoin (13-*cis*-retinoic acid) is the drug of choice for the management of severe, treatment-resistant acne vulgaris. Treatment with isotretinoin can lead to both marked improvement and long-lasting remission. It was not until 1979 when Peck et al. conducted an open-label trial for treatment-resistant cystic and conglobate acne with isotretinoin [96] and shortly thereafter the Food and Drug Administration (FDA) approved isotretinoin for the treatment of severe nodulocystic acne. Isotretinoin, though a vitamin A derivative, is a relatively water-soluble molecule. Peak plasma levels are achieved between 1 and 4 hours [97].

Importantly, the magnitude of this peak level is increased by co-administration with lipids. Thus, patients are instructed to take their doses with a small, fatty meal. Given the half-life of 10–20 hours, it is best to take isotretinoin twice a day [97, 98]. Isotretinoin is metabolized in the liver, where it is oxidized to 4-oxo-isotretinoin via CYP450 3A4 substrate and then excreted in urine and feces.

The primary mechanism of isotretinoin is its effect on sebaceous glands, inhibiting sebaceous gland activity, proliferation, differentiation, function, and production of sebum. *In vitro* studies conclude that isotretinoin induces apoptosis and cell cycle arrest of human sebocytes [99]. This effect seems to persist indefinitely upon completion of a full course (120–150 mg/kg) of isotretinoin, and this is thought to be the mode by which treatment with isotretinoin can cure acne. Unlike other retinoids used in dermatology, isotretinoin does not bind retinoic acid receptors (RARs), but functions via an RAR/RXR-independent mechanism. Secondary mechanisms that contribute to the efficacy of isotretinoin include anti-inflammatory, antibacterial (secondary to sebum reduction/alteration), and antikeratinizing effects.

Isotretinoin is indicated for the treatment of severe recalcitrant nodular acne, and its use for less severe acne is often indicated provided such cases are treatment-resistant and especially if the disease is leading to scarring, whether physical or emotional. In only the severest cases should it be considered as initial therapy.

Isotretinoin should be dosed at 0.5–1 mg/kg/day divided BID. Commonly, an initial dose of 0.5 mg/kg/day for the first month is preferred to acclimate the patient to mucocutaneous xerosis, minimize initial inflammatory response, and monitor for any adverse effects. The dose should then be increased to approximately 1 mg/kg/day. In patients with severe acne in which explosive flares may occur, pre-treatment for one or two weeks with daily prednisone is advised. After this pretreatment, 0.5 mg/kg/day of isotretinoin is initiated-vwhile gradually decreasing the steroid dose. What is more important than the daily dose, is achieving a total cumulative dose of 120–150 mg/kg, ensuring the prolonged remission of acne [100].

Relapses can be observed after the completion of the therapy, especially in cases of younger patients, males, and truncal acne. However, acne that recurs after isotretinoin therapy is more responsive to less aggressive acne treatments such as topical agents or oral antibiotics. If still severe, a repeat course of isotretinoin can be tried with success rates similar to that of initial treatments. Purported relapse rates following treatment of acne with isotretinoin varies between 5.6 and 65.5% [101]. The most likely reasons for this large discrepancy are small sample size, short follow-up, retrospective design, and/or subtherapeutic cumulative dosage.

Absolute contraindications for isotretinoin use include pregnancy, breast-feeding, and hypersensitivity to parabens, soybean oil, or other retinoids. Relative contraindications include psychiatric disorders, skeletal disorders, seizure disorder, hyperlipidemia, pancreatitis history, diabetes mellitus, hyperuricemia, gout, and anorexia nervosa.

http://dx.doi.org/10.5772/65639

Concomitant use of isotretinoin and tetracycline can induce intracranial hypertension, leading to pseudotumor cerebri, via idiosyncratic reaction. Severe and persistent headaches with nausea, vomiting, and blurred vision can be signs of pseudotumor cerebri.

Treatment with isotretinoin can have various adverse effects since RARs are ubiquitous throughout the body. These side effects mimic the effects of hypervitaminosis A and almost all are reversible upon discontinuation of isotretinoin. The first, and essentially universal, side effect of isotretinoin is cheilitis and its absence is often considered a marker of non-compliance or insufficient dosage. Any mucocutaneous site can be affected including the skin, conjunctiva, oropharynx, nasopharynx, and genitalia. Treatment for mucocutaneous dryness consists of artificial tears for the eyes, emollients for the lips and body. Other rarely reported dermatological side effects of isotretinoin include photosensitivity, exuberant granulation tissue, abnormal wound healing, telogen effluvium, nail plate fragility, paronychia, and onycholysis.

Transient dyslipidemia is the second most common side effect after mucocutaneous xerosis. About 20% of acne patients treated with isotretinoin experience hypertriglyceridemia [102]. LDL may also be increased, while HDL may be decreased. These alterations typically occur early in treatment during the first month or two, stabilize, and then revert to pretreatment levels upon discontinuation of isotretinoin. Substantially increased triglyceride levels can have risks including pancreatitis and eruptive xanthomas. Since triglyceride elevations are dose related, one can decrease the dose of isotretinoin. If dose reduction is not sufficient, apart from lifestyle changes pharmacologic therapy is indicated. The drug of choice for isotretinoin-induced hypertryglyceridemia is gemfibrozil, 600 mg twice daily. For triglyceride levels greater than 800 mg/dL, discontinuation of isotretinoin is appropriate.

Increased transaminase levels are seen in some 11–15% of acne patients treated with isotretinoin, whereas development of severe hepatotoxicity is extremely rare [103].

Other occasionally reported adverse effects of isotretinoin include nausea, diarrhea, abdominal pain, gastritis, proctocolitis, flares of inflammatory bowel disease, decreased white blood cell count, hemoglobin, and platelets, arthralgias, or myalgias.

The most serious side effect of isotretinoin is teratogenicity. It affects organogenesis; therefore, its greatest risk to a fetus is early in pregnancy, during the first trimester. Even one dose is thought to be able to induce congenital defects or spontaneous abortion [104]. The rate of birth defects ranges from 18 to 28%, including craniofacial, cardiac, central nervous system, thymic, and various other abnormalities [104–106]. Female patients of childbearing potential must have at least one or two negative pregnancy tests before starting treatment and practice effective contraception for 1 month prior to, during, and for 1 month after completing therapy.

Long-term treatment with isotretinoin can decrease bone mineral density and cause hyperostosis and osteophytes. However, it is not clear if these effects apply to the short-term treatment of acne with a standard course of isotretinoin [107].

In case of psychological side effects, there is no evidence that there is a causal relationship between mood disturbances such as depression, anxiety, or suicidal ideation and the use of isotretinoin. However, there are many studies demonstrating positive and negative correlation between isotretinoin use and increased risk of depression [108–112]. Nevertheless, given the serious nature of depression and suicidal ideation, close psychological monitoring of patients is recommended.

Before the initiation of isotretinoin therapy, fasting lipids and liver function tests should be checked at baseline, monthly for the first 2 months. If no abnormalities are found and the dose unchanged blood tests are done every 2 months.

8.3. Surgical treatment

Extraction of especially deep and persistent comedos can improve the cosmetic appearance of acne and aid in therapeutic responsiveness to topical comedolytic agents [113]. The keratinous contents of open comedones may be expressed via a comedo extractor. The Schamberg, Unna, and Saalfield types of comedo expressers are most commonly used. Nicking the surface of a closed comedo with an 18-gauge needle or a #11 blade allows easier expression. This procedure should be used in conjunction with a topical retinoid or other comedolytic treatment for maximum benefit. Comedo extraction should not be performed on inflamed comedones or pustules because of the risk of scarring. Light electrocautery, electrofulguration, and cryotherapy can also be effective treatments for comedones.

Photodynamic therapy utilizing topical 5-aminolevulinic acid together with various light sources (e.g., blue, red, intense pulsed) or lasers (e.g., pulsed dye, 635 nm red diode) have been successfully used to treat acne [114]. In addition, blue or intense pulsed light alone and lasers such as the pulsed dye, the 1320 nm neodymium:YAG and especially the 1450 nm diode may be of therapeutic benefit for inflammatory acne.

Intralesional injection of corticosteroid (triamcinolone acetonide 2–5 mg/ml) can quickly improve the appearance and tenderness of deep, inflamed nodules and cysts [115]. Larger cysts may require incision and drainage prior to injection. The maximal amount of corticosteroid used per lesion should not exceed 0.1 ml. The risks of corticosteroid injections include hypopigmentation (particularly in darkly pigmented skin), atrophy, telangiectasias, and needle tract scarring.

Low-concentration chemical peels are also beneficial for the reduction of comedones. The α-hydroxy acids (including glycolic acid), salicylic acid, and trichloroacetic acid are the most common peeling agents. Higher-concentration glycolic acid peels (20–70%, depending on the patient's skin type) and the less predictable phenol peel may also be performed in the office setting. Risks of chemical peels include irritation, pigmentary alteration, and scarring [116].

One of the most distressing consequences of acne vulgaris is scarring. Laser resurfacing (fractional as well as traditional), dermabrasion, and deeper chemical peels can be used in case of scarring [117]. Surgical subscision combined with filler substances is also a commonly used technique in the management of "ice-pick" acne scars. For larger hypertrophic scars, aggregated pitted scars, and sinus tracts, full-thickness surgical excision may result in improved scar placement and a better cosmetic appearance.

http://dx.doi.org/10.5772/65639

Author details

Zekayi Kutlubay[1*], Aysegul Sevim Kecici[2], Burhan Engin[1], Server Serdaroglu[1] and Yalcin Tuzun[1]

*Address all correspondence to: zekayikutlubay@hotmail.com

1 Istanbul University Cerrahpasa Medical Faculty, Department of Dermatology, Istanbul, Turkey

2 Haydarpasa Numune Training and Research Hospital, Department of Dermatology, Istanbul, Turkey

References

[1] Halvorsen JA, Stern RS, Dalgard F, et al. Suicidal ideation, mental health problems, and social impairment are increased in adolescents with acne: a populationbased study. J Invest Dermatol. 2011;131:363–370. DOI: 10.1038/jid.2010.264

[2] Blau S, Kanof NB. Acne: from pimple to pit. N Y J Med. 1965;65:417–424.

[3] Goolamali SK, Andison AC. The origin and use of the word 'acne'. Br J Dermatol. 1977;96:291–294. DOI: 10.1111/j.1365-2133.1977.tb06140

[4] Waisman M. Concepts of acne of the British School of Dermatology prior to 1860. Int J Dermatol. 1983;22:126–129.

[5] Baldwin HE. The interaction between acne vulgaris and the psyche. Cutis. 2002;70:133–139.

[6] Bowe WP, Leyden JJ, Crerand CE, et al. Body dysmorphic disorder symptoms among patients with acne vulgaris. J Am Acad Dermatol. 2007;57:222–230. DOI: 10.1016/j.jaad.2007.03.030

[7] Mackley CL. Body dysmorphic disorder. Dermatol Surg. 2005;33:553–558. DOI: 10.1111/j.1524-4725.2005.31160

[8] Veale D, Boocock A, Gournay K, et al. Body dysmorphic disorder. A survey of fifty cases. Br J Psychiatry. 1996;169:196–201. DOI: 10.1192/bjp.169.2.196

[9] Collier CN, Harper JC, Cafardi JA, et al. The prevalence of acne in adults 20 years and older. J Am Acad Dermatol. 2008;58:5659. DOI: 10.1016/j.jaad.2007.06.045

[10] Thiboutot D, Gollnick H, Bettoli V, et al. New insights into the management of acne: an update from the Global Alliance to Improve Outcomes in Acne group. J Am Acad Dermatol. 2009;60:1–50. DOI: 10.1016/j.jaad.2009.01.019

[11] Oberemok SS, Shalita AR. Acne vulgaris, I: pathogenesis and diagnosis. Cutis. 2002;70:101–105.

[12] Plewig G, Fulton JE, Kligman AM. Cellular dynamics of comedo formation in acne vulgaris. Arch Dermatol Forsch. 1971;242:12–29.

[13] Vowels BR, Yang S, Leyden JJ. Induction of proinflammatory cytokines by a soluble factor of *Propionibacterium acnes*: implications for chronic inflammatory acne. Infect Immun. 1995;63:3158–3165.

[14] Thiboutot D. Hormones and acne: pathophysiology, clinical evaluation, and therapies. Semin Cutan Med Surg. 2001;20:144–153.

[15] Thiboutot D. Acne: hormonal concepts and therapy. Clin Dermatol. 2004;22:419–428. DOI: 10.1016/j.clindermatol.2004.03.010

[16] Thiboutot D. Regulation of human sebaceous glands. J Invest Dermatol. 2004;123:1–12. DOI: 10.1111/j.1523-1747.2004.t01-2

[17] Guy R, Green MR, Kealey T. Modeling acne in vitro. J Invest Dermatol. 1996;106:176–182.

[18] Ghodsi SZ, Orawa H, Zouboulis CC. Prevalence, severity, and severity risk factors of acne in high school pupils: a community-based study. J Invest Dermatol. 2009;129:2136–2141. DOI: 10.1038/jid.2009.47

[19] Powell EW, Beveridge GW. Sebum excretion and sebum composition in adolescent men with and without acne vulgaris. Br J Dermatol. 1970;82:243–249. DOI: 10.1111/j.1365-2133.1970.tb12431

[20] Plewig G, Christophers E. Renewal rate of human sebaceous glands. Acta Dermatovener. 1974;54:177–182.

[21] Cunliffe WJ, Shuster S. Pathogenesis of acne. Lancet. 1969;1:685–687.

[22] Flurh JW, Mao Qiang M, Brown BE, et al. Glycerol regulates stratum corneum hydration in sebaceous gland deficient (Asebia) mice. J Invest Dermatol. 2003;120:728–737. DOI: 10.1046/j.1523-1747.2003.12134

[23] Thiele JJ, Weber SU, Packer L. Sebaceous gland secretion is a major physiologic route of vitamin E delivery to skin. J Invest Dermatol. 1999;113:1006–1010. DOI: 10.1046/j.1523-1747.1999.00794

[24] Gebhart W, Metze D, Jurecka W. Identification of secretory immunoglobulin A in human sweat and sweat glands. J Invest Dermatol. 1989;92:648.

[25] Nakatsuji T, Kao MC, Zhang L, et al. Sebum free fatty acids enhance the innate immune defense of human sebocytes by upregulating beta defensin 2 expression. J Invest Dermatol. 2009;130:985–994. DOI: 10.1038/jid.2009.384

[26] Lee DY, Yamasaki K, Rudsil J, et al. Sebocytes express functional cathelicidin antimicrobial peptides and can act to kill *Propionibacterium acnes*. J Invest Dermatol. 2008;128:1863–1866. DOI: 10.1038/sj.jid.5701235

[27] Lai Y, Gallo RL. AMPed up immunity: how antimicrobial peptides have multiple roles in immune defense. Trends Immunol. 2009;30:131–141. DOI: 10.1016/j.it.2008.12.003

[28] Oeff MK, Seltmann H, Hiroi N, et al. Differential regulation of Toll like receptor and CD14 pathways by retinoids and corticosteroids in human sebocytes. Dermatology. 2006;213:266. DOI: 10.1159/000095056

[29] Gribbon EM, Cunliffe WJ, Holland KT. Interaction of *Propionibacterium acnes* with skin lipids in vitro. J Gen Microbiol. 1993;139:1745–1751.

[30] Ro BI, Dawson TL. The role of sebaceous gland activity and scalp microfloral metabolism in the etiology of seborrheic dermatitis and dandruff. J Investig Dermatol Symp Proc. 2005;10:194–197. DOI: 10.1016/j.cl.2004.03.010

[31] Graham GM, Farrar MD, Cruse Sawyer JE, et al. Proinflammatory cytokine production by human keratinocytes stimulated with *Propionibacterium acnes* and P. acnes GroEL. Br J Dermatol. 2004;150:421–428. DOI: 10.1046/j.1365-2133.2004.05762

[32] Nagy I, Pivarcsi A, Kis K, et al. *Propionibacterium acnes* and lipopolysaccharide induce the expression of antimicrobial peptides and proinflammatory cytokines/chemokines in human sebocytes. Microbes Infect. 2006;8:2195–2205. DOI: 10.1016/j.micinf.2006.04.001

[33] Jeremy AHT, Holland DB, Roberts SG, et al. Inflammatory events are involved in acne lesion initiation. J Invest Dermatol. 2003;121:20–27. DOI: 10.1046/j.1523-1747.2003.12321

[34] Abdel-Fattah NS, Shaheen MA, Ebrahim AA, El Okda ES. Tissue and blood superoxide dismutase activities and malondialdehyde levels in different clinical severities of acne vulgaris. Br J Dermatol. 2008;159:1086–1091. DOI: 10.1111/j.1365-2133.2008.08770

[35] Lauermann FT, Almeida HL Jr, Duquia RP, Souza PR, Breunig J de A. Acne scars in 18-year-old male adolescents: a population-based study of prevalence and associated factors. An Bras Dermatol. 2016;91:291–295. DOI: 10.1590/abd1806-4841.20164405

[36] Holland DB, Jeremy AH, Roberts SG, et al. Inflammation in acne scarring: a comparison of the responses in lesions from patients prone and not prone to scar. Br J Dermatol. 2004;150:72–81. DOI: 10.1111/j.1365-2133.2004.05749

[37] Leyden JJ, McGinley KJ, Mills OH, Kligman AM. Propionibacterium levels in patients with and without acne vulgaris. J Invest Dermatol. 1975;65:382–384. DOI: 10.1111/1523-1747.ep12607634

[38] Kim J, Ochoa MT, Krutzik SR, et al. Activation of toll-like receptor 2 in acne triggers inflammatory cytokine responses. J Immunol. 2002;169:1535–1541. DOI: 10.1159/000087011

[39] Jalian HR, Liu PT, Kanchanapoomi M, et al. All-trans retinoic acid shifts *Propionibacterium acnes*-induced matrix degradation expression profile toward matrix preservation in human monocytes. J Invest Dermatol. 2008;128:2777–2782. DOI: 10.1038/jid.2008.155

[40] Nagy I, Pivarcsi A, Koreck A, et al. Distinct strains of *Propionibacterium acnes* induce selective human beta-defensin-2 and interleukin-8 expression in human keratinocytes through toll-like receptors. J Invest Dermatol. 2005;124:931–938. DOI: 10.1111/j.0022-202X.2005.23705

[41] Sugisaki H, Yamanaka K, Kakeda M, et al. Increased interferon-gamma, interleukin-12p40 and IL-8 production in *Propionibacterium acnes*-treated peripheral blood mononuclear cells from patient with acne vulgaris: host response but not bacterial species is the determinant factor of the disease. J Dermatol Sci. 2009;55:47–52. DOI: 10.1016/j.jdermsci.2009.02.015

[42] Chronnell CM, Ghali LR, Ali RS, et al. Human beta defensin-1 and -2 expression in human pilosebaceous units: upregulation in acne vulgaris lesions. J Invest Dermatol. 2001;117:1120–1125. DOI: 10.1046/j.0022-202x.2001.01569

[43] Nakatsuji T, Kao MC, Zhang L, et al. Sebum free fatty acids enhance the innate immune defense of human sebocytes by upregulating beta-defensin-2 expression. J Invest Dermatol. 2010;130:985–994. DOI: 10.1038/jid.2009.384

[44] Lee DY, Huang CM, Nakatsuji T, et al. Histone H4 is a major component of the antimicrobial action of human sebocytes. J Invest Dermatol. 2009;129:2489–2496. DOI: 10.1038/jid.2009.106

[45] Liu PT, Phan J, Tang D, et al. CD209(+) macrophages mediate host defense against *Propionibacterium acnes*. J Immunol. 2008;180:4919–4923. DOI: 10.4049/jimmunol.180.7.4919

[46] Lucky AW, Biro FM, Huster GA, et al. Acne vulgaris in premenarchal girls. An early sign of puberty associated with rising levels of dehydroepiandrosterone. Arch Dermatol. 1994;130:308–314.

[47] Strauss JS, Pochi PE. Effect of cyclic progestin-estrogen therapy on sebum and acne in women. JAMA. 1964;190:815–819. DOI: 10.1001/jama.1964.03070220021004

[48] Bowe WP, Joshi SS, Shalita AR. Diet and acne. J Am Acad Dermatol. 2010;63:124–141. DOI: 10.1016/j.jaad.2009.07.043

[49] LaRosa CL, Quach KA, Koons K, Kunselman AR, Zhu J, Thiboutot DM, et al. Consumption of dairy in teenagers with and without acne. J Am Acad Dermatol. 2016;75:318–322. DOI: 10.1016/j.jaad.2016.04.030

[50] Capitanio B, Sinagra JL, Bordignon V, et al. Underestimated clinical features of post-adolescent acne. J Am Acad Dermatol. 2010;63:782–788. DOI: 10.1016/j.jaad.2009.11.021

[51] Jansen T, Plewig G. Acne fulminans. Int J Dermatol. 1998;37:254–257. DOI: 10.1046/j.1365-4362.1998.00443

[52] Tan BB, Lear JT, Smith AG. Acne fulminans and erythema nodosum during isotretinoin therapy responding to dapsone. Clin Exp Dermatol. 1997;22:26–27. DOI: 10.1046/j.1365-2230.1997.1830600

[53] Wise CA, Gillum JD, Seideman CE, et al. Mutations in CD2BP1 disrupt binding to PTP PEST and are responsible for PAPA syndrome, an autoinflammatory disorder. Hum Mol Genet. 2002;11:961–969. DOI: 10.1111/j.1600-065X.2008.00747

[54] Friedman SJ, Fox BJ, Albert HL. Solid facial edema as a complication of acne vulgaris: treatment with isotretinoin. J Am Acad Dermatol. 1986;15:286–289. DOI: 10.1016/S0190-9622(86)70168-0

[55] Jungfer B, Jansen T, Przybilla B, Plewig G. Solid persistent facial edema of acne: successful treatment with isotretinoin and ketotifen. Dermatology. 1993;187:34–37. DOI: 10.1159/000247194

[56] Arbegast KD, Braddock SW, Lamberty LF, Sawka AR. Treatment of infantile cystic acne with oral isotretinoin: a case report. Pediatr Dermatol. 1991;8:166–168. DOI: 10.1111/j.1525-1470.1991.tb00311

[57] Beasley JN. Chemistry and metabolism of benzoyl peroxide and other antiacne drugs. Clin Res. 1982;30:698.

[58] Kligman AM, Leyden JJ, Stewart R. New uses for benzoyl peroxide: a broad-spectrum antimicrobial agent. Int J Dermatol. 1977;16:413–417.

[59] Patane AM, Pistillo M. Antimicrobial action of benzoyl peroxide. Ann Sclavo. 1982;24:513–522.

[60] Farmery MR, Jones CE, Eady EA, et al. In vitro activity of azaleic acid, benzoyl peroxide and zinc acetata against antibiotic resistant propionibacteria from acne patients. J Dermatol Treat. 1994;5:63–65. DOI: 10.3109/09546639409084531

[61] Puschmann M. Clinico-experimental studies on the effect of benzoylperoxide. Hautarzt. 1982;33:257–265.

[62] Bojar RA, Holland KT, Cunliffe WJ. The in-vitro antimicrobial effects of azelaic acid upon *Propionibacterium acnes* strain P37. J Antimicrob Chemother. 1991;28:843–853. DOI: 10.1093/jac/28.6.843

[63] Pagnoni A, Kligman AM, Kollias N, et al. Digital flourescence photography can assess the suppressive effect of benzoyl peroxide on *Propionibacterium acnes*. J Am Acad Dermatol. 1999;41:710–716. DOI: 10.1016/S0190-9622(99)70005-8

[64] Fulton JE, Farzad-Bakshandeh A, Bradley S. Studies on the mechanism of action of topical benzoyl peroxide and vitamin A acid in acne vulgaris. J Cutan Pathol. 1974;1:191–200.

[65] Gloor M, Hummel A, Friedrich HC. Experimentelle untersuchungen zur Benzoylperoxidtherapie der acne vulgaris. Z Hautkr. 1975;50:657–663.

[66] Pierard GE, Peirard-Franchimont C, Goffin V. Digital image analysis of microcomedones. Dermatology. 1995;190:99–103.

[67] Gollnick H, Krautheim A. Topical treatment in acne: current status and future aspects. Dermatology. 2003;206:29–36. DOI: 10.1159/000067820

[68] Lassus A. Local treatment of acne. A clinical study and evaluation of the effect of different concentrations of benzoyl peroxide gel. Curr Med Res Opin. 1981;7:370–373.

[69] Bojar RA, Cunliffe WJ, Holland KT. The short-term treatment of acne vulgaris with benzoyl peroxide: effects on the surface and follicular cutaneousmicroflora. Br J Dermatol. 1995;132:204–208.

[70] Del Rosso JQ, Leyden JJ. Status report on antibiotic resistance: implications for the dermatologist. Dermatol Clin. 2007;25:127–132. DOI: 10.1016/j.det.2007.01.001

[71] Del Rosso JQ, Leyden JJ, Thiboutot D, et al. Antibiotic use in acne vulgaris and rosacea: clinical considerations and resistance issues of significance to dermatologist. Cutis. 2008;82:5–12.

[72] Gollnick H, Cunliffe W, Berson D, et al. Management of acne: a report from the global alliance to improve outcomes in acne. J Am Acad Dermatol. 2003;49:1–38. DOI: 10.1067/mjd.2003.618

[73] Levy SB. The challenge of antibiotic resistance. Sci Am. 1998;278:46–53.

[74] Leyden JJ, Del Rosso JQ, Webster GF. Clinical considerations in the treatment of acne vulgaris and other inflammatory skin disorders: focus on antibiotic resistance. Cutis. 2007;79:9–25.

[75] Ross JL, Snelling AM, Carnegie E, et al. Antibiotic resistant acne: lessons from Europe. Br J Dermatol. 2003;148:467–478. DOI: 10.1046/j.1365-2133.2003.05067

[76] Margolis DJ, Bowe WP, Hoffstad O, et al. Antibiotic treatment of acne may be associated with upper respiratory tract infections. Arch Dermatol. 2005;141:1132–1136. DOI:10.1001/archderm.141.9.1132

[77] Levy RM, Huang EY, Rolling D, et al. Effect of antibiotics on the oropharyngeal flora in patients with acne. Arch Dermatol. 2003;139:467–471. DOI: 10.1001/archderm.139.4.467

[78] Simonart T, Dramaix M. Treatment of acne with topical antibiotics: lessons from clinical studies. Br J Dermatol. 2005;153:395–403. DOI: 10.1111/j.1365-2133.2005.06614

[79] Cunliffe WJ, Holland KT. Clinical and laboratory studies on treatment with 20% azelaic acid cream for acne. Acta Derm Venereol. 1989;143:31–34.

[80] Roberts DL, Marshall R, Marks R. Detection of the action of salicylic acid on the normal stratum corneum. Br J Dermatol. 1980;103:191–196. DOI: 10.1111/j.1365-2133.1980.tb06590

[81] Eady EA, Burke BM, Pulling K, et al. The benefit of 2% salicylic acid lotion in acne – a placebo-controlled study. J Dermatol Treat. 1996;7:93–96. DOI: 10.3109/09546639609089537

[82] Shalita AR. Comparison of a salicylic acid cleanser and a benzoyl peroxide wash in the treatment of acne vulgaris. Clin Ther. 1989;11:264–267.

[83] Zander E, Weismann S. Treatment of acne vulgaris with salicylic acid pads. Clin Ther. 1992;14:247–253.

[84] Del Rosso JQ. A status report on the use of subantimicrobial dose doxycycline: a review of the biologic and antimicrobial effects of the tetracyclines. Cutis. 2004;74:118–122.

[85] Eady AE, Cove JH, Layton AM. Is antibiotic resistance in cutaneous propionibacteria clinically relevant? Implications of resistance for acne patients and prescribers. Am J Clin Dermatol. 2003;4:813–831. DOI: 10.2165/00128071-200304120-00002

[86] Ross JI, Snelling AM, Eady EA, et al. Phenotypic and genotypic characterization of antibiotic resistant *Propionibacterium acnes* isolated from acne patients attending dermatologic clinics in Europe, the USA, Japan and Australia. Br J Dermatol. 2001;144:339–346.

[87] Leyden JJ. The evolving role of *Propionibacterium acnes* in acne. Semin Cutan Med Surg. 2001;20:139–143. DOI: 10.1053/sder.2001.28207

[88] Leyden JJ, Wortzman M, Baldwin EK. Antibiotic resistant *Propionibacterium acnes* suppressed by benzoyl peroxide 6% cleanser. Cutis. 2008;82:417–421.

[89] Leyden JJ. A review of the use of combination therapies for the treatment of acne vulgaris. J Am Acad Dermatol. 2003;49:206–210. DOI: 10.1067/S0190-9622(03)01154

[90] Arowojolu A, Gallo M, Lopez L, et al. Combined oral contraceptives for the treatment of acne. Cochrane Database Syst Rev. 2009;3:4425. DOI: 10.1002/14651858

[91] Lidegaard O, Lokkegaard E, Svendsen AL, et al. Hormonal contraception and risk of venous thromboembolism: national follow-up study. BMJ. 2009;339:2890. DOI: 10.1136/bmj.b2890

[92] Trenor CC 3rd, Chung RJ, Michelson AD, et al. Hormonal contraception and thrombotic risk: a multidisciplinary approach. Pediatrics. 2011;127:347–357. DOI: 10.1542/peds.2010-2221

[93] van Hylckama Vlieg A, Helmerhorst FM, Vandenbroucke JP, et al. The venous thrombotic risk of oral contraceptives, effects of oestrogen dose and progestogen type: results of the MEGA case-control study. BMJ. 2009;339:2921. DOI: 10.1136/bmj.b2921

[94] van Wayjen R, van den Ende A. Experience in the long-term treatment of patients with hirsutism and/or acne with cyproterone acetate-containing preparations: efficacy, metabolic and endocrine effects. Exp Clin Endocrinol Diabetes. 1995;103:241–251. DOI: 10.1055/s-0029-1211357

[95] Goodfellow A, Alaghband-Zadeh J, Carter G, et al. Oral spironolactone improves acne vulgaris and reduces sebum excretion. Br J Dermatol. 1984;111:209–214. DOI: 10.1111/j.1365-2133.1984.tb04045

[96] Peck GL, Olsen TG, Yoder FW, et al. Prolonged remissions of cystic and conglobate acne with 13 cis retinoic acid. N Engl J Med. 1979;300:329–333. DOI: 10.1046/j.1365-2230.2002.01094

[97] Khoo KC, Reik D, Colburn WA. Pharmacokinetics of isotretinoin following a single oral dose. J Clin Pharmacol. 1982;22:395–402. DOI: 10.1002/j.1552-4604.1982.tb02692

[98] Colburn WA, Gibson DM, Wiens RE, et al. Food increases the bioavailability of isotretinoin. J Clin Pharmacol. 1983;23:534–539. DOI: 10.1002/j.1552-4604.1983.tb01800

[99] Strauss JS, Stranieri AM. Changes in long term sebum production from isotretinoin therapy. J Am Acad Dermatol. 1982;6:751–756. DOI: 10.1016/S0190-9622(82)80055-8

[100] Strauss JS, Rapini RP, Shalita AR, et al. Isotretinoin therapy for acne: results of a multicenter dose response study. J Am Acad Dermatol. 1984;10:490–496. DOI: 10.1016/S0190-9622(84)80100-0

[101] Azoulay L, Oraichi D, Bérard A. Isotretinoin therapy and the incidence of acne relapse: a nested case control study. Br J Dermatol. 2007;157:1240–1248. DOI: 10.1111/j.1365-2133.2007.08250

[102] Bershad S, Rubinstein A, Paterniti JR, et al. Changes in plasma lipids and lipoproteins during isotretinoin therapy for acne. N Engl J Med. 1985;313:981–985. DOI: 10.1056/NEJM198510173131604

[103] Zane LT, Leyden WA, Marqueling AL, et al. A population based analysis of laboratory abnormalities during isotretinoin therapy for acne vulgaris. Arch Dermatol. 2006;142:1016–1022. DOI: 10.1001/archderm.142.8.1016

[104] Lammer EJ, Chen DT, Hoar RM, et al. Retinoic acid embryopathy. N Engl J Med. 1985;313:837–841. DOI: 10.1056/NEJM198510033131401

[105] Dai WS, LaBraico JM, Stern RS. Epidemiology of isotretinoin exposure during pregnancy. J Am Acad Dermatol. 1992;26:599–606. DOI: 10.1016/0190-9622(92)70088

[106] Lynberg MC, Khoury MJ, Lammer EJ, et al. Sensitivity, specificity, and positive predictive value of multiple malformations in isotretinoin embryopathy surveillance. Teratology. 1990;42:513–519. DOI: 10.1002/tera.1420420508

[107] Lenchik L, Leib ES, Hamdy RC, et al. Executive summary International Society for Clinical Densitometry position development conference Denver, Colorado July 20 22, 2001. J Clin Densitom. 2002;5:1–3. DOI: 10.1385/JCD:7:1:7

[108] Jick SS, Kremers HM, Vasilakis Scaramozza C. Isotretinoin use and risk of depression, psychotic symptoms, suicide, and attempted suicide. Arch Dermatol. 2000;136:1231–1236. DOI: 10.1001/archderm.136.10.1231

[109] Hersom K, Neary MP, Levaux HP, et al. Isotretinoin and antidepressant pharmacotherapy: a prescription sequence symmetry analysis. J Am Acad Dermatol. 2003;49:424–432. DOI: 10.1067/S0190-9622(03)02087-5

[110] Chia CY, Lane W, Chibnall J, et al. Isotretinoin therapy and mood changes in adolescents with moderate to severe acne: a cohort study. Arch Dermatol. 2005;141:557–560. DOI: 10.1001/archderm.141.5.557

[111] Marqueling AL, Zane LT. Depression and suicidal behavior in acne patients treated with isotretinoin: a systematic review. Semin Cutan Med Surg. 2007;26:210–220. DOI: 10.1016/j.sder.2008.03.005

[112] Azoulay L, Blais L, Koren G, et al. Isotretinoin and the risk of depression in patients with acne vulgaris: a case crossover study. J Clin Psychiatry. 2008;69:526–532. DOI: 10.4088/JCP.v69n0403

[113] Lowney ED, Witkowski J, Simons HM, et al. Value of comedo extraction in treatment of acne vulgaris. JAMA. 1964;189:1000–1002. DOI: 10.1001/jama.1964.03070130020005

[114] Santos MA, Belo VG, Santos G. Effectiveness of photodynamic therapy with topical 5 aminolevulinic acid and intense pulsed light versus intense pulsed light alone in the treatment of acne vulgaris: comparative study. Dermatol Surg. 2005;31:910–915. DOI: 10.1111/j.1524-4725.2005.31804

[115] Levine RM, Rasmussen JE. Intralesional corticosteroids in the treatment of nodulocystic acne. Arch Dermatol. 1983;119:480–481. DOI: 10.1001/archderm.1983.01650300034012

[116] Karimipour DJ, Rittie L, Hammerberg C, et al. Molecular analysis of aggressive microdermabrasion in photoaged skin. Arch Dermatol. 2009;145:1114–1122. DOI: 10.1001/archdermatol.2009.231

[117] Elman M, Slatkine M, Harth Y. The effective treatment of acne vulgaris by a high intensity, narrow band 405 420 nm light source. J Cosmet Laser Ther. 2003;5:111–117. DOI: 10.1080/14764170305509

Chapter 3

Pediatric Acne

Bilgen Gencler, Ozge Keseroglu,

Selda Pelin Kartal and Muzeyyen Gonul

Additional information is available at the end of the chapter

http://dx.doi.org/10.5772/66141

Abstract

Acne is a dermatological disorder that can be more commonly seen in adolescents as well as younger patients. The pediatric acne is classified according to the age groups as neonatal acne, infantile acne, mid-childhood acne, and prepubertal acne. The presentation, pathogenesis, differential diagnosis, and treatment of the disease vary in each age group. Early diagnosis is important to prevent the scar formation and determine the underlying abnormalities.

Keywords: neonatal acne, infantile acne, mid-childhood acne, prepubertal acne

1. Introduction

Acne is one of the most common diseases in dermatology practice. Although acne has been known as a disease of the adolescents, it is also observed during the neonatal, infantile, mid-childhood, and prepubertal period. The severity of clinical findings varies mild to moderate in neonates but it could be more severe in different age groups. While the disease usually recovers spontaneously, in some severe scar formation cases, treatment should be needed. The treatment of acne is debate in these age groups, because of the possible adverse effects of the medications. Pediatric acne becomes a greater issue because it has a wide spectrum of differential diagnosis and could be associated with underlying systemic abnormalities [1–3].

2. Classification of pediatric acne

2.1. Neonatal acne

2.1.1. Presentation and pathogenesis

Acne developing in newborns at birth or within 4-6 weeks immediately after birth is called neonatal acne [1]. It is more frequently seen in newborn boys than in girls [2]. The incidence of neonatal acne diagnosed based on the presence of comedone lesions is approximately 20% in newborns [3].

Although the etiopathogenesis is not exactly known, there are debates as to whether they are true acne or not [4]. A positive family history shows that there is role of genetic factors [2]. Sebaceous glands stimulated by maternal and neonatal androgens, increased seborrhea and Malassezia species are also regarded to be responsible from etiology [5]. In addition, there are findings that demonstrate the importance of maternal effects on newborn sebaceous glands. Maternal androgens stimulate sebaceous glands by transplacental transmission instead of transmission by maternal milk [6]. Sebum secreted in large amounts during the neonatal period decreases over time and the sizes of the sebaceous glands gradually decrease towards the end of the sixth month [2]. In particular, the role of enlargement in the zona reticularis of the fetal adrenal gland and the resulting increased production of β-hydroxysteroids have been emphasized. Increased β-hydroxysteroids also cause enlargement in the sebaceous glands, thereby, increasing sebum production. Additionally, β-hydroxysteroids secreted from the neonatal adrenal glands cause the sebaceous glands to become more sensitive to hormones in the future [3]. Luteinizing hormone and testosterone are high in neonatal boys between the sixth and twelfth months. Adrenal androgens are responsible for neonatal acne in both newborn boys and girls. The presence of increased testicular androgens in males confirms why this disease is more frequently seen in boys [2, 3].

Neonatal acne is characterized by inflammatory lesions, such as papules and pustules, in addition to open and closed comedones, and rarely by nodules and cysts [1, 3]. It is most commonly seen in the cheeks and then in the forehead and less frequently in the neck and truncal region [3]. Neonatal acne, which is characterized by self-limiting mild symptoms, rarely continues to the ninth to twelfth months and can transform to infantile acne. In the majority of the patients, there is no underlying disease. Following a detailed history and physical examination, endocrinological abnormalities should be further investigated in the presence of signs of virilization or other abnormal findings [1, 4].

Acneiform eruptions and infectious and noninfectious diseases, which can be sometimes seen during the neonatal period, are involved in the differential diagnosis. In the differential diagnosis, acne venenata infantum, acneiform drug reactions, chloracne, bacterial (*Staphylococcus aureus*, *Listeria monocytogenes*, beta hemolytic group B streptococcus), viral (*Herpes simplex*, *Varicella zoster*, cytomegalovirus), fungal (candidiasis, pityrosporum folliculitis), and parasitic (scabies) infections as infectious causes and erythema toxicum neonatorum, infantile acropustulosis, milia, sebaceous gland hyperplasia, transient neonatal pustular melanosis, and pustular miliaria as noninfectious causes are often considered [5].

2.1.2. *Treatment*

As neonatal acne is a mild and transient condition, it recovers spontaneously within four weeks and three months without scar formation. Rarely, it can persist up to six to twelve months [5]. Topical agents are often beneficial for treatment. The gel, lotion, and solution forms of topical antibiotics containing erythromycin and clindamycin and topical benzoyl peroxide can be used for inflammatory lesions and topical azelaic acid (20% cream) and topical retinoids (tretinoin 0.025-0.05% cream) can be used for comedonal lesions [2, 4]. If systemic treatment is required, an oral antibiotic such as erythromycin should be preferred [7].

The clinical characteristics of neonatal acne are summarized in **Table 1**.

Age at onset	Birth–6 weeks
Clinical presentation	Comedones, inflammatory papules and pustules, nodules, scarring
Differential diagnosis	Neonatal cephalic pustulosis, bacterial-viral-fungal infections, erythema toxicum neonatorum, infantile acropustulosis, milia, sebaceous gland hyperplasia, transient neonatal pustular melanosis, pustular miliaria, chloracne, acne venenata infantum, acneiform drug eruptions
Treatment	Recovers spontaneously without scar formationTopical azelaic acid, topical retinoids, topical antibioticOral antibiotic (erythromycin)

Table 1. Neonatal acne.

2.1.3. *Neonatal cephalic pustulosis*

Neonatal cephalic pustulosis (NCP) is characterized by mild inflammatory papulopustular lesions and is differentiated from neonatal acne by the absence of comedones [1, 8]. In a study including 104 patients, the prevalence of NCP was approximately 25% in neonates [9]. It is thought to be due to the development of lipophilic yeasts in predisposed newborns who have increased sebum production. It has been demonstrated that Malassezia species, in particular, have a role in the etiopathogenesis of NCP [10, 11]. At birth, Malassezia colonization develops, depending on environmental factors, maternal contact, and the characteristics of newborn skin; it gradually increases within the first months of extrauterine life. In particular, *Malassezia sympodialis* and *Malassezia globosa* have a high prevalence. These fungi, which are found in the normal skin flora of infants, likely lead to follicular occlusion in predisposed infants who have increased sebum production. This, in turn, causes acneiform eruptions [8, 10, 12, 13]. However, the presence of negative mycological data in some NCP cases and the absence of NCP development in some culture-positive newborns lead us to believe that different factors also have an effect [1, 5]. There is a debate as to whether it is a hypersensitivity reaction developing against yeast or not [1]. In general, it is characterized by mild, transient lesions in the cheeks, chin, and forehead regions, which restrict themselves within a few weeks. As it is a self-limiting lesion, it does not usually require treatment. However, if needed, topical 2% ketoconazole cream twice daily for 1 week is an appropriate treatment method [4, 8, 14].

2.2. Infantile acne

2.2.1. Presentation and pathogenesis

Infantile acne is a less common occurrence, compared to neonatal acne and it is observed between the first and twelfth months of extrauterine life. However, it can also develop in later periods, such as the 14th and 16th months [4, 15]. Infantile acne is more diffuse, inflamed, and persistent [3]. Similar to neonatal acne, infantile acne is also more common in males [2, 4]. Lesions are typically characterized by open and closed comedones, inflammatory papules and pustules, nodules and less commonly by scar forming cysts [1, 2, 3]. Infantile acne is most frequently seen on cheeks and less commonly seen on the chest and back (**Figure 1**) [1, 2]. Acne conglobata, which has primarily facial involvement and is clinically similar to the adult form, is rarely seen [2]. Infantile acne, particularly conglobate infantile acne, may be associated with severe acne, which is seen during the adolescent period, and there is typically a positive family history of severe acne in these patients [16].

The causes of acne development during the infantile period are not so distinct. The presence of a positive family history emphasizes the role of genetic factors [8]. The general opinion tends toward the presence of sensitivity to the circulating adrenal and gonadal androgens. The release of adrenal androgens decreases close to age 1 and remains silent until the ages of 6-8. Zona reticularis which is the androgen-secreting part of fetal adrenal gland is large in both girls and boys and it gradually gets smaller beginning at age 1, during childhood period [8, 15]. It is thought that high levels of dehydroepiandrosterone (DHEA) and dehydroepiandrosterone sulfate (DHEAS) secreted as a result of the continuation of fetal adrenal gland function after the neonatal period causes acne development by stimulating the sebaceous

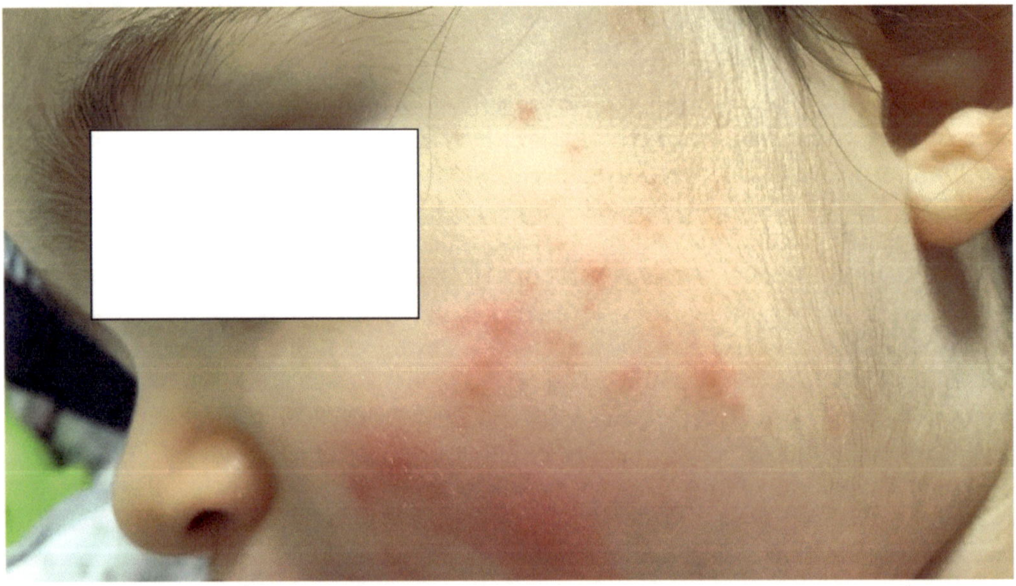

Figure 1. Infantile acne; an 8-month-old girl presented with closed comedones and inflammatory papules and pustules on her cheeks.

http://dx.doi.org/10.5772/66141

glands [4, 8]. While there are high amounts of luteinizing hormone (LH) and testicular androgen production until age one in boys, indeed, there is no testicular androgen production between age one and adrenarche. However, in girls, testosterone levels rapidly decrease at birth or within the first two weeks after birth. Thus, this situation explains why acne is more commonly seen in males [4, 8].

Most infantile acne is not associated with an underlying endocrinological abnormality. However, if the lesions are persistent, severe, and unresponsive to treatment, or if there is a finding of hyperandrogenism in the physical examination of the infant (pubic hair, cliteromegaly, hirsutism, alopecia, accelerated growth, etc.), additional laboratory investigations for underlying abnormalities should be performed [2, 7, 15]. Measurements of bone age, serological tests such as follicle-stimulating hormone (FSH), LH, free and total testosterone, DHEA, DHEAS, 17β-hydroxyprogesterone, prolactin, and adrenocorticotropic hormone (ACTH) stimulation test should be performed [2, 4]. In rapidly developing infantile acne, attention should be given to virilizing tumors [17]. If the tests reveal an abnormality, the infant should be referred to pediatric endocrinology.

In the differential diagnosis, acneiform eruptions developing due to the exposure are present. Acne venenata infantum or pomade acne can be seen due to comedogenic skin care product forms such as pomades, creams, ointments, and oil form that are used by the parents; corticosteroid-induced acne is seen in the perioral, periocular, and infranasal areas due to topical, oral, and inhaler corticosteroids; chloracne is seen in the centrofacial region due to accidental exposure to chlorinated aromatic hydrocarbons. In addition to these conditions, neonatal acne, perioral dermatitis, milia, and miliaria should be also considered in the differential diagnosis [4, 8].

2.2.2. *Treatment*

The course of the disease is variable. While the lesions disappear after one to two years in certain patients, they usually persist and most of the lesions recover after the age of four to five years. Less frequently, they can be active until puberty [3].

Parents of the patient with infantile acne should be warned about the fact that the disease can be persistent and severe acne can relapse during puberty [3]. The treatment of infantile acne is similar to the acne treatment in different age groups. Treatment varies according to the severity of the disease. In mild acne where comedone lesions are dominant, topical retinoids (tretinoin, adapalene) and/or the combination of topical benzoyl peroxide and topical antibiotic (erythromycin) can be used [5, 7, 18, 19]. Oral antibiotics can be used in more inflammatory lesions which are associated with papules, pustules, and nodules. The first choice, erythromycin, can be given in a dose of 125-250 mg, twice daily in this age group; if propionibacterium acne is resistant to erythromycin, trimethoprim 100 mg could be given twice daily [2]. It is necessary to avoid oral tetracycline before age 8, as it could cause damage to the teeth and bones. Intralesional low dose triamcinolone acetonide (2.5 mg/mL), cryotherapy, and short-term topical corticosteroid therapy are options for acne associated with deep nodules and cysts [3, 18, 20]. Oral isotretinoin can be used, if there is no response or if there is scar formation [18, 21, 22]. Oral isotretinoin is approved by the Food and Drug Administration for patients aged 12 and above in the treatment of nodulocystic acne [23]. In the literature, its use in children aged below five, at a dose of 0.36-2 mg/kg/day for 4-6 months, has been found to be effective; however, scar tissue occasionally remains [8, 22]. The optimal cumulative dose of isotretinoin during the infancy is unknown. Its use in young children is slightly more difficult, since it is found in soft gelatin capsules and inactivated by light and oxygen [21]. Thus, it should be opened under dim light and the daily recommended dose should be divided twice daily, by adding to food, such as butter, yogurt, a bread slice with jam, or milk. However, in this way, there is the possibility of inactivation or not taking the drug in recommended doses. Therefore, the capsule can be frozen in a viscous texture and cut in the required doses and given with a delicious food such as a candy bar [18, 21, 22]. This method prevents the wasting of the drug and also facilitates its use by decreasing the poor taste of the drug. Patients should be carefully followed for possible side effects. The most common side effect is dryness of the mucous membranes and the skin [4]. As it may lead to changes in blood counts, liver functions, cholesterol, triglyceride levels, adverse skeletal effects such as calcification of ligaments and tendons, cortical hyperostosis, periosteal thickening, premature epiphyseal closure, decalcification, and possible osteoporosis, laboratory evaluations, and skeletal growth should be followed on regular intervals [8, 21, 24].

The clinical characteristics of infantile acne are summarized in **Table 2**.

Age at onset	**6 weeks–12 months**
Clinical presentation	Comedones, inflammatory papules and pustules, nodules, less commonly by scar forming cysts, acne conglobata
Differential diagnosis	Acne venenata infantum/pomade acne, corticosteroid induced acne, chloracne, neonatal acne, perioral dermatitis, milia, miliaria
Treatment	Topical retinoids, topical benzoyl peroxide, topical antibiotic (erythromycin)Oral antibiotic (erythromycin, trimethoprim sulfamethoxazole)Intralesional low dose triamcinolone acetonide, cryotherapy, short-term topical corticosteroid therapy for nodules and cystsOral isotretinoin for scar formation lesions

Table 2. Infantile acne.

2.3. Mid-childhood acne

2.3.1. Presentation and pathogenesis

Mid-childhood acne is observed between the 1 and 7 years of life [14]. Acne is quite rare during this period. The children in this age group do not secrete significant amounts of adrenal or gonadal androgens. Androgen secretion of adrenals often disappears after the first year of life until age 7 (adrenarche). Then, zona reticularis regains function. Therefore, hyperandrogenism should be investigated at the time of diagnosis [6, 8, 25].

Lesions are characterized by mixed comedones and inflammatory papules and pustules of the face, chest, and back [1].

In addition to premature adrenarche, which is a completely benign event, more severe conditions such as congenital adrenal hyperplasia (CAH), gonadal and adrenal tumors, Cushing's syndrome, central precocious puberty, and exogenous androgen absorption should be excluded [2, 7, 15]. A careful physical examination should be done for the growth chart and the presence of findings related to hormonal abnormality. The bone age could be measured by radiological examination of the left hand or wrist [1, 2]. Laboratory tests such as serum total and free testosterone, DHEA, DHEAS, 17 alpha hydroxyprogesterone, FSH, LH, and prolactin levels should be measured to evaluate hormonal abnormalities [2]. If any abnormality is detected, it should be referred to pediatric endocrinology.

Inflamed keratosis pilaris, which is seen in the cheeks in atopic people, keratin cysts (miliaria), demodicosis, molluscum contagiosum, verruca plana, idiopathic facial aseptic granuloma, pseudoacne of the nasal crease, perioral dermatitis, and angiofibroma should be considered in the differential diagnosis of mid-childhood acne [7, 15, 26, 27]. In the literature, dactinomycin-induced acne has been reported in this age group [28].

2.3.2. *Treatment*

Its treatment depends on the underlying endocrinological abnormality. However, if necessary, topical treatments and oral antibiotics are similar to infantile acne [2, 8].

The clinical characteristics of mid-childhood acne are summarized in **Table 3**.

Age at onset	**1–7 years**
Clinical presentation	Comedones, inflammatory papules and pustules
Differential diagnosis	Inflamed keratosis pilaris, keratin cysts, demodicosis, molluscum contagiosum, verruca plana, idiopathic facial aseptic granuloma, perioral dermatitis, angiofibroma
Treatment	Depends on the underlying abnormalityTopical retinoids, topical benzoyl peroxide, topical antibiotic (erythromycin)Oral antibiotic (erythromycin, trimethoprim)Oral isotretinoin

Table 3. Mid-childhood acne.

2.4. Prepubertal acne

2.4.1. *Presentation and pathogenesis*

Acne, which is observed between the ages of 7 and 11, is called prepubertal acne and its incidence has increased in recent years [15]. Contrary to expectations, acne can occur prior to pubertal signs. There is a genetic predisposition in these patients. An increased early-onset acne can be an initial finding of pubertal development rather than age [2]. Prepubertal acne is a consequence of normal adrenarche, which develops depending on adrenal gland maturation [7]. Acne development in premenarche girls has been reported as 61-71.3% [29, 30]. The most common presentation is comedonal lesions in the center region of the forehead. Inflammatory papules and pustules can be seen in the central of the face and sometimes in the ear concha, chest, and back [1]. Advancing pubertal maturation was found to be correlated with the prevalence and severity of acne in both boys and girls [29, 31]. There are two components of pubertal development. The first component is adrenarche, which is the initiation of androgen synthesis (DHEA, DHEAS) together with the maturation of the adrenal gland at the age of 6-7 years in girls and at the age of 7-8 years in boys. DHEA and DHEAS lead to the development of seborrhea, odor, terminal and sexual hair, and acne. Excessive androgen production could be related to adrenal hyperandrogenism, congenital adrenal hyperplasia, Cushing's disease, 21-hydroxylase deficiency, and androgen-secreting tumors. Furthermore, true puberty, the second component, is the maturation of the ovary and testis under the effect of the hypothalamo-pituitary-adrenal (HPA) axis. Androgen secretion from the gonads is low during this period of life. Excess ovarian androgens can be due to benign and malignant tumors; however, they are most frequently associated with polycystic ovary syndrome (PCOS) [2, 5, 7].

In a 5-year cohort study performed on girls, acne lesions increased with age and maturation was reported. The most common type of lesions was comedone. On the other hand, no ethnic differences were observed. The study revealed that the girls who had severe acne had more comedone and inflammatory lesions beginning from age 10 and 2.5 years before menarche and they had earlier menarche. High levels of serum DHEAS, free and total testosterone suggest that it could be an initiator of severe long-term disease [32].

In general, there is no need to further research prepubertal acne. If there is persistent acne that is unresponsive to treatment or findings suggesting androgen excess are detected, possible endocrinological abnormalities should be suspected. Tanner stages demonstrating pubertal development should be measured, a hand film should be taken for bone age, and serum-free and total testosterone, DHEAS levels and ratio of LH to FSH should be measured [8, 15, 25, 33].

Its differential diagnosis is similar to mid-childhood acne. In addition, the side effects of drugs such as corticosteroids and anticonvulsants, prepubertal hidradenitis suppurativa, adenoma sebaceum, keratosis pilaris, and inflamed keratin cysts should be considered in the differential diagnosis [2, 34–36].

2.4.2. Treatment

Nonetheless, data related to acne medications during the preadolescent period are limited. Most of the acne drugs are approved for age 12 and above. Its treatment is similar to infantile and mid-childhood acne. Topical retinoids (tretinoin 0.04% microsphere gel), benzoyl peroxide, and antibiotics can be used in mild to moderate comedonal and inflammatory acne. Oral antibiotics and oral isotretinoin may also be required in more severe scar forming lesions. As an oral antibiotic, erythromycin and its derivatives, trimethoprim, and cephalexin should be preferred. Tetracycline and its derivatives should be avoided, as these agents may produce dental enamel staining. Oral contraceptives or antiandrogens such as spironolactone can be used for PCOS and low-dose corticosteroids can be used for CAH. However, oral contraceptives should be used carefully due to the risk of premature epiphyseal closure [2, 5, 37].

The clinical characteristics of prepubertal acne are summarized in **Table 4**.

http://dx.doi.org/10.5772/66141

Age at onset	7–11 years
Clinical presentation	Comedones, inflammatory papules and pustules, nodules, cysts
Differential diagnosis	Drug induced acne, prepubertal hidradenitis suppurativa, adenoma sebaceum, keratosis pilaris, inflamed keratin cysts, demodicosis, verruca plana
Treatment	Topical retinoids, topical antibiotics, topical benzoyl peroxideOral antibiotics (erythromycin, trimethoprim, cephalexin)Oral isotretinoinOral contraceptives, antiandrogens, low dose corticosteroids

Table 4. Prepubertal acne.

Author details

Bilgen Gencler*, Ozge Keseroglu, Selda Pelin Kartal and Muzeyyen Gonul

*Address all correspondence to: bilgen16@gmail.com

Department of Dermatology, Ministry of Health Diskapi Yildirim Beyazit Education and Research Hospital, Ankara, Turkey

References

[1] Maroñas-Jiménez L, Krakowski AC. Pediatric acne: clinical patterns and pearls. Dermatol Clin. 2016;**34**:195–202.

[2] Herane MI, Ando I. Acne in infancy and acne genetics. Dermatology. 2003;**206**:24–8.

[3] Jansen T, Burgdorf WH, Plewig G. Pathogenesis and treatment of acne in childhood. Pediatr Dermatol. 1997;**14**:17–21.

[4] Tom WL, Friedlander SF. Acne through the ages: case-based observations through childhood and adolescence. Clin Pediatr. 2008;**47**:639–651.

[5] Antoniou C, Dessinioti C, Stratigos AJ, Katsambas AD. Clinical and therapeutic approach to childhood acne: an update. Pediatr Dermatol. 2009;**26**:373–80.

[6] Zouboulis CC. Acne and sebaceous gland function. Clin Dermatol. 2004;**22:**360-366.

[7] Lucky AW. A review of infantile and pediatric acne. Dermatology. 1998;**196**:95–7.

[8] Cantatore-Francis JL, Glick SA. Childhood acne: evaluation and management. Dermatol Ther. 2006;**19**:202–209.

[9] Ayhan M, Sancak B, Karaduman A, Arikan S, Sahin S. Colonization of neonate skin by Malassezia species: relationship with neonatal cephalic pustulosis. J Am Acad Dermatol. 2007;**57**:1012–1018.

[10] Niamba P, Weill FX, Sarlangue J, Labre'ze C, Couprie B, Taïeh A. Is common neonatal cephalic pustulosis (neonatal acne) triggered by *Malassezia sympodialis*? Arch Dermatol. 1998;**134**:995–998.

[11] Bardazzi F. Transient cephalic neonatal pustulosis. Arch Dermatol. 1997;**133**:528–30.

[12] Bernier V, Weill FX, Hirigoyen V, Elleau C, Feyler A, Labrèze C, Sarlangue J, Chène G, Couprie B, Taïeb A. Skin colonization by Malassezia species in neonates: a prospective study and relationship with neonatal cephalic pustulosis. Arch Dermatol. 2002;**138**:215–218.

[13] Bergman JN, Eichenfield LF. Neonatal acne and cephalic pustulosis: is malassezia the whole story? Arch Dermatol. 2002;**138**:255–257.

[14] Friedlander SF, Baldwin HE, Mancini AJ, Yan AC, Eichenfield LF. The acne continuum: an age-based approach to therapy. Semin Cutan Med Surg 2011;**3**:6–11.

[15] Admani S, Barrio VR. Evaluation and treatment of acne from infancy to preadolescence. Dermatol Ther. 2013;**26**:462–466.

[16] Chew EW, Bingham A, Burrows D: Incidence of acne vulgaris in patients with infantile acne. Clin Exp Dermatol. 1990;**15**:376–377.

[17] Mann MW, Ellis SS, Mallory SB. Infantile acne as the initial sign of an adrenocortical tumor. J Am Acad Dermatol. 2007;**56**:15–8.

[18] Cunliffe WJ, Baron SE, Coulson IH. A clinical and therapeutic study of 29 patients with infantile acne. Br J Dermatol. 2001;**145**:463–6.

[19] Kose O, Koc E, Arca E. Adapalene gel 0.1% in the treatment of infantile acne: an open clinical study. Pediatr Dermatol. 2008;**25**:383–6.

[20] Levine RM, Rasmussen JE. Intralesional corticosteroids in the treatment of nodulocystic acne. Arch Dermatol. 1983;**119**:480–481.

[21] Barnes CJ, Eichenfield LF, Lee J et al. A practical approach for the use of oral isotretinoin for infantile acne. Pediatr Dermatol. 2005;**22**:166–169.

[22] Torrelo A, Pastor MA, Zambrano A. Severe acne infantum successfully treated with isotretinoin. Pediatr Dermatol. 2005;**22**:357–9.

[23] Brecher AR, Orlow SJ. Oral retinoids therapy for dermatologic conditions in children and adolescents. J Am Acad Dermatol. 2003;**49**:171–182.

[24] DiGiovanna JJ. Isotretinoin effects on bone. J Am Acad Dermatol. 2001;**45**:176–82.

[25] Lucky AW. Hormonal correlates of acne and hirsutism. Am J Med. 1995;**98**: 89-94.

[26] Roul S, Léauté-Labrèze C, Boralevi F, Bioulac-Sage P, Maleville J, Taïeb A. Idiopathic aseptic facial granuloma (pyodermite froide du visage): a pediatric entity? Arch Dermatol. 2001;**137**:1253–1255.

[27] Dubus JC, Marguet C, Deschildre A, et al. Réseau de Recherche Clinique en Pneumonologie Pédiatrique. Local side-effects of inhaled corticosteroids in asthmatic children: influence of drug, dose, age, and device. Allergy. 2001;**56**:944–948.

[28] Blatt J, Lee PA. Severe acne and hyperandrogenemia following dactinomycin. Med Pediatr Oncol. 1993;**21**:373–374.

[29] Lucky AW, Biro FM, Huster GA, Leach AD, Morrison JA, Ratterman J. Acne vulgaris in premenarchal girls. An early sign of puberty associated with rising levels of dehydroepiandrosterone. Arch Dermatol. 1994;**130**:308–314.

[30] Rademaker M, Garioch JJ, Simpson MB. Acne in schoolchildren: no longer a concern for dermatologists. BMJ. 1989;**298**:1217–1219.

[31] Lucky AW, Biro FM, Huster GA, Morrison JA, Elder N. Acne vulgaris in early adolescent boys. Correlations with pubertal maturation and age. Arch Dermatol. 1991;**127**:210–216.

[32] Lucky AW, Biro FM, Simbartl LA, Morrison JA, Sorg NW: Predictors of severity of acne vulgaris in young adolescent girls: results of a five year longitudinal study. J Pediatr. 1997;**130**:30–39.

[33] Strauss JS, Krowchuk DP, Leyden JJ et al. Guidelines of care for acne vulgaris management. J Am Acad Dermatol. 2007;**56**:651–663.

[34] Krakowski AC, Eichenfield LF. Pediatric acne: clinical presentations, evaluation, and management. J Drugs Dermatol. 2007;**6**:584–588.

[35] Krowchuk DP. Managing adolescent acne: a guide for pediatricians. Pediatr Rev. 2005;**26**:250–261.

[36] Jozwiak S, Schwartz RA, Janniger CK, Michalowicz R, Chmielik J. Skin lesions in children with tuberous sclerosis complex: their prevalence, natural course, and diagnostic significance. Int J Dermatol. 1998;**37**:911–917.

[37] Yan AC, Baldwin HE, Eichenfield LF, Friedlander SF, Mancini AJ. Approach to pediatric acne treatment: an update. Semin Cutan Med Surg. 2011;**30**:16–21.

Chapter 4

Occupational Acne

Betul Demir and Demet Cicek

Additional information is available at the end of the chapter

http://dx.doi.org/10.5772/64905

Abstract

Occupational and environmental acne is a dermatological disorder associated with industrial exposure. Polyhalogenated hydrocarbons, coal tar and products, petrol, and other physical, chemical, and environmental agents are suggested to play a role in the etiology of occupational acne. The people working in the field of machine, chemistry, and electrical industry are at high risk. The various occupational acne includes chloracne, coal tar, and oil acne. The most common type in clinic is the comedones, and it is also seen as papule, pustule, and cystic lesions. Histopathological examination shows epidermal hyperplasia, while follicular and sebaceous glands are replaced by keratinized epidermal cells. Topical or oral retinoic acids and oral antibiotics could be used in treatment. The improvement in working conditions, taking preventive measures, and education of the workers could eliminate occupational acne as a problem.

Keywords: Chloracne, coal-tar acne, environmental acne, occupational acne, oil acne

1. Introduction

Occupational and environmental acne is a dermatological disorder associated with industrial exposure. Polyhalogenated hydrocarbons, coal tar and products, petrol, and other physical, chemical, and environmental agents are suggested to play a role in the etiology of occupational acne [1]. The people working in the field of machine, chemistry and electrical industry are at high risk [2]. The various occupational acne includes chloracne, coal tar, and oil acne. Chloracne is an acneiform eruption that is observed as a result of intoxication with chlorinated hydrocarbons [3] and clinical signs might be severe [4]. It could also arise due to industrial, agricultural, and environmental contamination and even due to eating contaminated foods [2]. Oils used in the industry such as cutting oils (paraffin/oil mixtures), tars (pitch and creosote), and crude petroleum oil (diesel oil) can cause oil and tar acne. Occupational acne is a type of acne that develops as a result of exposure to insoluble materials causing follicle obstruction. The most common clinical feature is the open and closed comedones, noninflamed nodules, and cystic lesions [5]. Histopathological examination shows epidermal hyperplasia, while follicular and sebaceous glands are replaced by keratinized epidermal cells. [6] In occupational acne, contact should be prevented in individuals working at high risk. In case of contact, the chemical agent should be removed. Topical or oral retinoic acids and oral antibiotics could be used for treatment [7].

2. Classification of occupational acne

2.1. Chloracne

2.1.1. Introduction

Chloracne was first defined by Herxheimer in 1889 [8]. Occupational acne is considered one of the sensitive indicators of systemic intoxication caused by an exposure to certain halogenated aromatic hydrocarbons called chloracnegen. Although the majority of cases with chloracnegen intoxication are associated with occupational exposure, there are also cases with chloracnegen intoxication associated with non-occupational exposure to the industrial wastes and contaminated foods [6].

2.1.2. Etiology

Halogenated aromatic hydrocarbons are the most potent chloracnegen agents [9]. Polychlorinated naphthalenes, polychlorinated biphenyls (PBBs), polychlorinated dibenzofurans (PCDFs), polychlorinated phenols, contaminants of polychlorophenol compounds (especially herbicides), and chlorinated azo- and azoxybenzene are among the chloracnegens [2]. Electrical conductor and insulators, insecticide, fungicide, herbicide, and wood protectors are the agents that cause chloracne [7]. With the introduction of synthetic resins in the 1960s, a high incidence of chloracne after the exposure to polychlorinated naphthalenes and PCBs showed a decline. In later years, the majority of cases exposed to chloracnegens were caused by accidents [10, 11]. The condition has been recently reported in chemical industry workers exposed to chloracne chlorophenols [12, 13] and agricultural workers exposed to pesticides [14].

2,3,7,8-Tetrachlorodibenzo-p-dioxin (TCDD), which is the prototype of polyhalogenated aromatic hydrocarbons is an important cause of chloracne [9]. In the 1970s, chloracne outbreak occurred in a chemical plant in Austria after the exposure of mostly male workers to TCDD, and the workplace was closed for cleaning and reconstruction activities to take place [15]. In 1976, an accident occurred in a chemical plant in Seveso (Italy), known as "ICMESA plant explosion," and 2 kg TCDD was released to the atmosphere, causing chloracne outbreak which mostly affected children [11]. In addition, PCBs and PCDFs are other chloracnegens, and PCBs have been shown to result in direct toxicity by contaminating the cooking oil, and transplacental transmission has also been demonstrated [9]. The largest food pollution of Japan which

http://dx.doi.org/10.5772/64905

occurred in 1968 and currently known as "Yusho" has developed due to the contamination of rice bran oil with polychlorinated hydrocarbons, and it is remembered as an intoxication of a crowd. Although initial analyses failed to detect a chemical substance, biopsy samples obtained from the fat tissues showed deposition of PCBs [16]. In 1979, the incidence of chloracne was reported to be 17.5% in 2000 patients with Yucheng disease (oil disease), which resulted from consuming the food products contaminated by PCBs and PCDFs in Taiwan [17]. Earlier, PCBs have been used frequently as wood preservatives [18].

In modern times, occupational exposure to PCBs often occurs in the fields of construction, paint, ink, adhesive, paper products [19–21], mining, recycling and waste incineration, and hydraulic and transformer systems [22]. Furthermore, PCBs have been detected in plasma and exhaled air in individuals exposed to power transformer oil spilled after an accident during the shipment of the waste products, and these individuals also suffered from acneiform skin lesions [23]. On the other hand, Gawkrodger et al. [24] reported chloracne outbreak in seven chemists working in the pharmaceutical industry exposed to triazoloquinoxaline, a polycyclic halogenated chemical substance, which was not previously reported in association with chloracne. In addition, weed killer containing 2,4-dichloro- and 2,4,5-trichlorophenoxyacetic acid and sodium tetrachlorophenate used for the wood preservatives are the other chloracnegens [9].

2.1.3. Pathogenesis

Although cellular and molecular mechanisms still remain to be elucidated, the major effect is hypoplastic or hyperplastic response of the skin caused by cellular changes triggered by chloracnegens. Epidermis and infundibulum are also involved. Sebaceous and sweat glands lose their secretory functions and are replaced by keratinized cells. According to the epidermal stem cell theory of Panteleyev, chloracnegens activate epidermal stem cells which result in the transformation of the pilosebaceous unit by accelerating the cellular output [3]. TCDD demonstrates its biological effect by binding to cytosolic aryl hydrocarbon receptors. Exposure to TCDD increases keratinocyte proliferation [2].

Genetic studies carried out in patients with chloracne evaluated aryl-hydrocarbon receptor (AhR), transcription, and downstream genes such as CYP1A1, GSTA1, c-fos, and TGF-α expression in the epidermis using the real-time PCR method. These studies showed a high AhR, CYP1A1, GSTA1, and c-fos transactivation in the epidermal tissue associated with long-term exposure to TCDD and dibenzofuran. Therefore, AhR activation has been suggested to play an important role in the pathogenesis of the chloracne pathway and that increased activity might disrupt the normal epidermal cellular proliferation and differentiation [25].

2.1.4. Clinical features

The lesions appear as erythema and edema in the affected areas such as head, neck, malar and retroauricular, and mandibular areas, extremities, axilla, trunk, hip, and scrotum 2–4 weeks after exposure [10] and, then, turn into non-inflammatory black and white comedones and straw-colored cysts, papules (**Figures 1** and **2**) [24], and nodules within a few days. Pustules, non-infectious abscess, and scar formation after healing can be observed in severe cases. In addition, the lesions can relapse [7, 26, 27] and become generalized. Chloracne has a chronic disease course, and the severity of the disease is associated with the exposure dose, potency of the chloracnegen, and individual susceptibility [6]. A correlation has been reported between half-life and body mass index, body fat mass, TCDD mass, and chloracne response [28]. Systemic symptoms and severe chloracne may occur after the TCDD exposure [9]. Additional dermatological findings may also present, such as brownish hyperpigmentation of the nails, hypertrichosis, and hyperpigmentation in the involved areas. Severe cases may exhibit symptoms of systemic intoxication, such as impaired liver functions, porphyria cutanea tarda, and peripheral neuropathy [10], while some cases may suffer from fatigue, anorexia, impotence, hyperlipidemia, anemia, arthritis, and ophthalmopathy [29]. Indeed, diagnostic criteria for Yusho were established after Yusho disaster in Japan, and clinical findings were categorized as subjective, ocular, dermatological manifestations, and overall symptoms. The most important clinical manifestations of this situation have been chloracne and ocular damage [16].

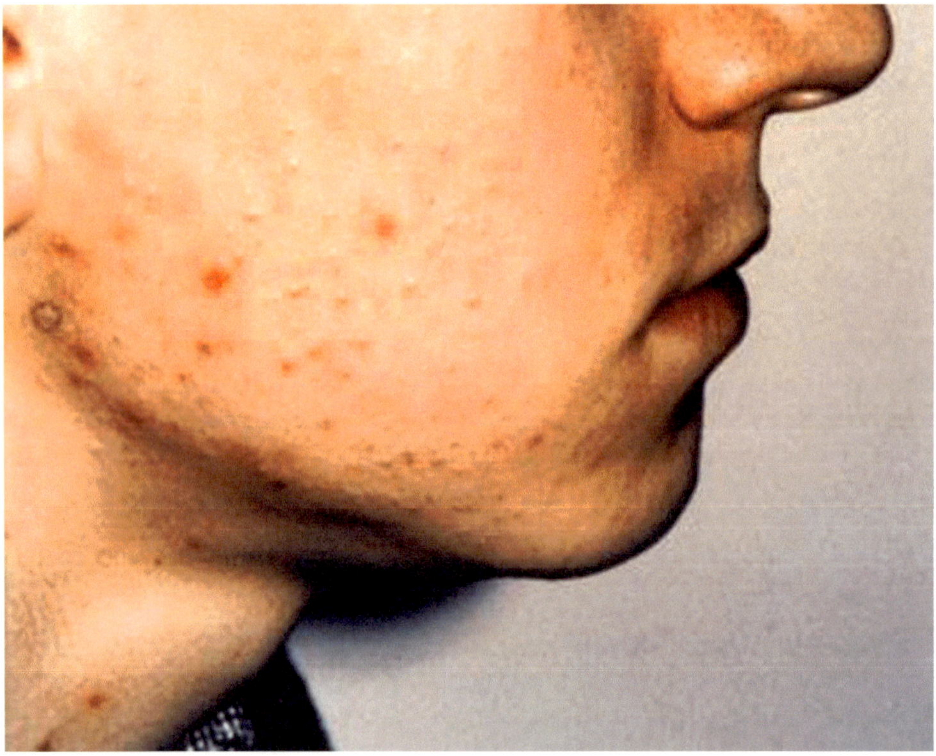

Figure 1. Clinical photograph, showing a combination of small cysts, closed and open comedones, and some inflammatory papules.[1]

[1] Reprinted from Wiley, 161,Gawkrodger DJ, Harris G, Bojar RA. Chloracne in seven organic chemists exposed to novel polycyclic halogenated chemical compounds (triazoloquinoxalines), 939-943, 2009, with permission from John Wiley. (reproduced with permission of the patient).

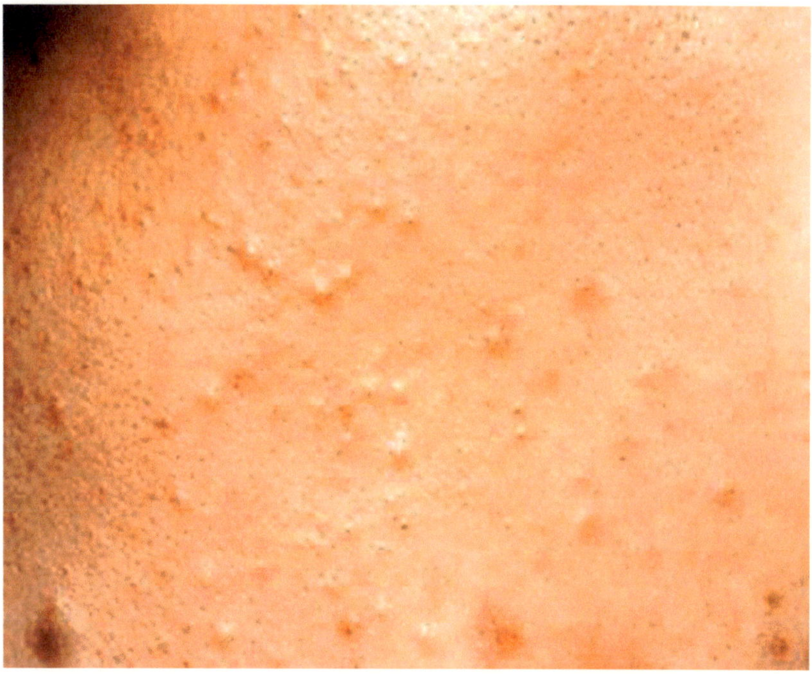

Figure 2. Close up showing small cysts, keratin plugs in pores, and comedones in more detail.[2]

According to the diagnostic criteria revised in 2004, dermatological manifestations were reported as acneiform eruptions and pigmentation (**Table 1**) [30]. It has been suggested that Yucheng disease manifest with dermatological symptoms, such as hyperpigmentation and nail changes, similar to chloracne; however, it may also manifest systemic symptoms such as headache, neuropathy, goiter, arthritis, and anemia [17]. TCDD can stay in the body for many years due to its high lipophilic characteristic and low metabolic rate [31]. Previous studies reported a half-life of 7–11 years [32]. The lesions may persist for 15–30 years after the discontinuation of the chloracnegen exposure [28]. In a study that was conducted in Japan, it was reported that chloracne lesions stay in the body for more than 30 years and are correlated with the blood levels of hydrocarbon [31]. In addition, TCDD was detected in the plasma of the victims 20 years after the Seveso accident [11]. On the other hand, systemic toxicity develops at higher doses than the dose necessary for the development of chloracne. Systemic toxicity is not generally expected in the absence of chloracne [2]. Chloracne is accepted as a sensitive marker of systemic absorption [27]. Hence Geusau et al. [33] detected generalized and severe chloracne lesions together with systemic signs of severe TCDD intoxication and high blood levels of TCDD in one of two female patients who have chloracne together with TCDD intoxication, whereas they have detected moderate facial chloracne in spite of high blood levels of TCDD and systemic signs in the other patient.

[2] Reprinted from Wiley, 161,Gawkrodger DJ, Harris G, Bojar RA. Chloracne in seven organic chemists exposed to novel polycyclic halogenated chemical compounds (triazoloquinoxalines), 939-943, 2009, with permission from John Wiley. (reproduced with permission of the patient).

The diagnostic criteria for Yusho have been revised according to some changes in the symptoms and signs, as well as advances in analytical techniques. The diagnostic criteria for Yusho were revised on October 26, 1972. A supplement was added to the diagnostic criteria on June 14, 1976, and the concentration of polychlorinated quarterphenyls (PCQs) in the blood was added to the diagnostic criteria on June 16, 1981. The concentration of 2,3,4,7,8-pentachlorodibenzofuran (2,3,4,7,8-PeCDF) was added to the diagnostic criteria on September 29, 2004.

Conditions of the incident

- Proof that Kanemi® rice bran oil contaminated with PCBs was ingested.
- There are also some cases in which PCB is transferred from mothers with Yusho to their children.
- Familial occurrence is also seen in many cases.

Important manifestations

1. Acneiform eruptions

Black comedones seen on the face, buttocks, and other intertriginous sites; comedones with inflammatory manifestations; and subcutaneous cysts with atheroma-like contents that tend to suppurate.

2. Pigmentation

Pigmentation of the face, palpebral conjunctivae, and nails of both the fingers and the toes (including babies).

3. Hypersecretion by the meibomian glands.

4. Unusual composition and concentration of PCBs in the blood.

5. Unusual concentration of PCQs in the blood (reference 1).

6. Unusual concentration of 2,3,4,7,8-PeCDF in the blood (reference 2).

Symptoms and signs

1. Subjective symptoms

- A feeling of lassitude
- A feeling of heaviness in the head or headache
- Paresthesia of the limbs (abnormal sensation)
- Increased eye discharge
- Cough and sputum
- Inconsistent abdominal pain
- Altered menstruation

2. Objective manifestations

- Manifestations of bronchitis
- Deformation of the nails
- Bursitis
- Increased neutral fat in the serum
- Serum γ-glutamyl transpeptidase (γ-GTP)

- Decrease of serum bilirubin
- Neonatal small-for-date baby
- Growth retardation and dental abnormality (retarded eruption of permanent teeth)

Reference 1.

The following conclusions have been made in regard to the concentration of PCQs in the blood:

1. ≥0.1 ppb: an abnormally high concentration
2. 0.03–0.09 ppb: the boundary between high and normal concentrations
3. ≤0.02 ppb (detection limit): normal concentration

Reference 2.

The following conclusions have been made in regard to the concentration of 2,3,4,7,8-PeCDF in the blood:

1. ≥50 pg/g lipids: an abnormally high concentration
2. 30–50 pg/g lipids: slightly high concentration
3. ≤30 pg/g lipids: normal concentration

Both age and sex of patients should also be considered.

Notes:

- With reference to the above-mentioned conditions of the incident, symptoms, and manifestations, and taking into account the age of the examinees and the temporal progress of their illness, a diagnosis is comprehensively made.
- These diagnostic criteria are to be used to determine whether a patient is affected by Yusho, but they do not necessarily relate to its severity.
- In regard to the abnormal properties of PCBs and the concentrations of PCBs and 2,3,4,7,8-PeCDF in the blood, regional differences as well as the patient's occupation should also be considered.
- Measurements should be performed by inspection agencies recognized by the Study Group of Yusho, at which quality control is carried out.

Table 1. Diagnostic criteria for Yusho (2004)[3].

2.1.5. Pathology

Histopathologically, hyperplasia in outer root sheath keratinocytes and the sebaceous canal is the first sign. Hyperplastic outer root sheath and hyperkeratinized dilated follicle structure are observed in the proximal part of the infundibulum of the involved hair follicles. Dilated infundibulum is filled with keratinized cells and comedones consisting of sebum. Sebaceous glands have disappeared or they have become quite small. Then the wall of the hair follicles gets thinner and abscess formation develops due to rupture toward dermis (**Figure 3**).

[3]. Reprinted from Elsevier, 82, Mitoma C, Uchi H, Tsukimori K, Yamada H, Akahane M, Imamura T, Utani A, Furue M, Yusho and its latest findings-A review in studies conducted by the Yusho Group, 41-48, 2015, with permission from Elsevier.

Furthermore, TCDD has been suggested to be a factor irritating directly the follicular wall and determining atypical keratinization and squamous metaplasia in the follicle epithelium. The involution of the sebaceous glands is not a direct chemical effect, but rather a condition secondary to the follicular obstruction [2]. Hyperpigmentation due to increased melanin production throughout the epidermis and epithelial basal layer of infundibulum has been reported [34]. From the perspective of dermatopathology, chloracne must be differentiated from acne vulgaris, nodular elastosis accompanied by cysts and comedones (Favre-Racouchot syndrome), acne rosacea, pilar keratosis, lichen planopilaris, chronic discoid lupus erythematosus due to loss of sebaceous glands, and hyperpigmentation in the stratum corneum [35].

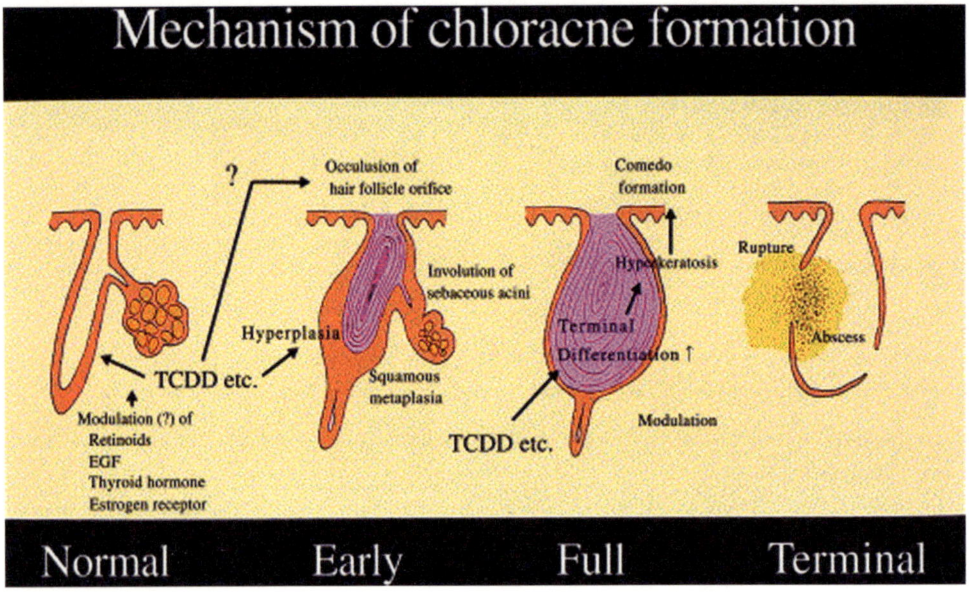

Figure 3. Mechanism of chloracne.[4]

2.1.6. Treatment

Chloracne may resolve gradually after the discontinuation of the chloracnegen exposure. It often weakly responds to acne medications, such as retinoic acid and antibiotics [10]. Corticosteroids, dermabrasion, and electrodessication may yield success to a certain extent. However, chloracne is resistant to therapy, and therefore, protection is of utmost importance [6]. Earlier studies attempted to prevent the chloracnegen exposure and facilitate the elimination from the body. A study evaluated the fecal excretion of chloracnegen using a synthetic dietary fat substitute called olestra [36]. Another study demonstrated 30-fold higher excretion of chloracnegen with the use of olestra diet and calorie restriction [37].

[4] Reprinted from Elsevier, 32, Yamamoto O, Tokura Y. Photocontact dermatitis and chloracne: two major occupational and environmental skin diseases induced by different actions of halogenated chemicals, 85-94, 2003, with permission from Elsevier.

2.2. Coal-tar acne

2.2.1. Introduction

It is a form of acne due to the obstruction of sebaceous glands by the mixture of coal tar and keratin products. In a study investigating the frequency of occupational dermatosis in Greece, coal-tar acne was detected at a rate of 23% in workers exposed to coal tar [38].

2.2.2. Etiology

Coal tar is a fatty fluid that is dark brown-nearly black in color, heavier than water, with a naphthalene-like odor and a sharp burning taste. This is a by-product that is formed as a result of distillation of hazardous parts of coal. Creosote, coal tar pitch, crude naphthalene, and anthracene oils are by-products of the coal tar, which are produced from the crude coal tar. The exposure to the coal tar occurs through the respiratory and gastrointestinal tract and the skin [39]. Coal tar was first described by Becker and Serle in 1681 and its use in dermatological disorders was described by Fishel in 1894 and Goeckerman in 1925 [40]. Coal tar has anti-inflammatory, antimicrobial, antipruritic, and cytostatic effects. Thus, for many decades it has been used as a therapeutic agent in skin diseases, such as psoriasis, and dermatitis [41]. Coal tar is also found in the cleansing bars, creams, gels, lotions, ointments, shampoo, and topical solutions and suspensions [39]. On the other hand, occupation exposure is more prevalent than the therapeutic use and environmental contamination [41]. Coal tar has a wide range of utility in the industry and consumer products. It is used as fuel in open-hearth furnaces and furnaces in the steel industry, as a filling material ingredient of surface coating formulations, and as a modifying agent ingredient of epoxy-resin surface coatings [39]. Coal tar exposure usually occurs in the workers working in the aluminum production, iron-steel foundry, coal tar refinery, road paving, roof insulation, pavement seal coat, and wood surfaces painting [41]. Pitch and creosote is the cause of acne in canal and road construction workers [42].

2.2.3. Pathogenesis

Keratin production and accumulation of fatty fluid causes an obstruction of the sebaceous glands and comedone formation [4, 41].

2.2.4. Clinical features

Clinically it is observed as multiple open comedones in the malar regions of face. The absence of inflammatory papules and pustules and big yellow cysts helps to distinguish coal-tar acne from oil acne and chloracne. It is found in extensor surfaces of the arm and thigh. The relationship between coal tar and periorbital comedone formation was investigated and the incidence of periorbital comedone was found to be high in people exposed to coal tar [1]. Under the experimental conditions, crude coal tar was reported to show a higher inflammatory activity in white-skinned people, compared to dark-skinned individuals [42].

2.2.5. Pathology

There are widened follicular openings with keratin plugs and there are no inflammatory infiltrates [1].

2.2.6. Treatment

Cold tar workers were recommended avoiding hazardous doses of exposure, wearing protective work clothes, receiving training on how to keep their outwear clean with frequent changing, using cleansers at the work places, working equipped with shower facilities and ventilation systems, and undergoing regular health check-ups. The response to therapy was reported to be higher than in chloracne [4, 41].

2.3. Oil acne

2.3.1. Introduction

Oil acne is the most common type of occupational acne [5]. Oil acne generally develops in people exposed to oil circuit breaker. It is due to oil circuit breaker and grease oil, which are used to lubricate machines and which contains a great amount of insoluble mineral oil [1].

2.3.2. Etiology

It has been reported in people working in prefabricated panel production and automobile industry. Moreover, it may be seen in ready-mixed concrete workers [43–45], engine drivers, roofers, and coal tar workers [10]. Oil mist exposure has also been considered a cause of industrial disease, and cases with systemic toxicity and oil acne have been reported to be associated with the oil mist exposure [46]. Actors (applying stage make-up), fast food workers (McDonald 's acne), and workers applying the facemask for prolonged periods as part of their jobs are at a high risk [10]. Acneiform eruptions have been reported more commonly in marine engineers, compared to other seaman due to the use of solvents or diesel fuel as hand cleanser and these lesions were reported to be oil acne [47]. Impure paraffin oil mixtures are the most widely available acnegen chemical agents with a varying degree of acnegen capacity, and they are commonly used in the engineering industry [43]. Brilliantine also shows similar effects due to their impure paraffin content [48]. Concentrated mineral oil is an emulsion of water in oil containing additives and water. Organic substrates and water constitute an environment for the microbial growth. Bacterial endotoxins are, therefore, commonly detected in the metal-working fluids. In a study investigating the exposure to biological agents in the metal-working industry in Poland, oil acne on the skin was reported [49].

2.3.3. Pathogenesis

Exposure to solvent and grease oil causes mechanical obstruction of pilosebaceous glands and development of oil acne [50].

2.3.4. Clinical features

The typical clinical findings are comedones and inflammatory lesions in the dorsum of hand and extensor surfaces of the arm [1]. Clinical presentation, lesions often involve the arms and thighs, depending on the contact of the oily clothing [10]. Of note, males are more commonly affected than females. This can be attributed to the fact that males are more vulnerable to the development of acne [43]. Comedones and cysts associated with the use of brilliantine can be found in the retroauricular area, unless rinsed thoroughly [48].

2.3.5. Treatment

Previous studies reported favorable effects of systemic tetracycline for 3 months in the treatment of oil acne [51]. Isotretinoin is also known to play a role in the treatment of oil acne [52]. Avoiding contact is also one of the prevention methods. [1] Additional protective measures may be also required, such as changing cloths and showering on a daily basis. Improved engineering control with a more emphasis on personal hygiene, there has been a decline in the prevalence of oil acne, compared to the previous years [10].

3. Conclusion

When the literature was reviewed, it was observed that occupational acne is a severe health problem. The improvement in working conditions, taking preventive measures, and education of the workers could eliminate occupational acne as a problem.

Acknowledgements

We thank 'NOVA Language Services' for the English language edition.

Author details

Betul Demir* and Demet Cicek

*Address all correspondence to: drbkaraca@yahoo.com

Department of Dermatology, Firat University Hospital, Elazig, Turkey

References

[1] Adams BB, Chetty VB, Mutasim DF. Periorbital comedones and their relationship to pitch tar: a cross-sectional analysis and a review of the literature. J Am Acad Dermatol. 2000;42:624-627. DOI:10.1067/mjd.2000.101600

[2] Yamamoto O, Tokura Y. Photocontact dermatitis and chloracne: two major occupational and environmental skin diseases induced by different actions of halogenated chemicals. J Dermatol Sci. 2003;32:85-94. DOI: 10.1016/S0923-1811(03)00097-5

[3] Panteleyev AA, Bickers DR. Dioxin-induced chloracne—reconstructing the cellular and molecular mechanisms of a classic environmental disease. Exp Dermatol. 2006;15:705-730. DOI: 10.1111/j.1600-0625.2006.00476.x

[4] Ancona AA. Occupational acne. Occup Med 1986;1:229-243.

[5] Friedmann PS, Wilkinson M. Occupational Dermatoses. In: Bolognia JL, Jorizzo JL, Rapini RP, editors. Dermatology. 2nd ed. New York: Mosby; 2008. p. 231-242.

[6] Ju Q, Zouboulis CC, Xia L. Environmental pollution and acne: Chloracne. Dermatoendocrinol. 2009;1:125-128.

[7] Zaenglein AL, Thiboutot DM. Acne Vulgaris. In: Bolognia JL, Jorizzo JL, Rapini RP, editors. Dermatology. 2nd ed. New York: Mosby; 2008. p. 495-508.

[8] Herxheimer K. Uber chloracne. Munch Med Wochenschr. 1899;46:278.

[9] Rycroft RJG. Occupational Dermatoses. In: Champion RH, Burton JL, Burns DA, Breathnach SM, editors. Rook/Wilkinson/Ebling Textbook of Dermatology. 6th ed. Oxford: Blackwell; 1998. p. 861-881.

[10] Adams RM. Occupational Skin Disease. In: Freedberg IM, Eisen AZ, Wolff K, Austen KF, Goldsmith LA, Katz SI, Fitzpatrick TB, editors. Fitzpatrick's Dermatology in General Medicine. 5th ed. New York: McGraw-Hill; 1999. p. 1609-1632.

[11] Baccarelli A, Pesatori AC, Consonni D, Mocarelli P, Patterson DG Jr, Caporaso NE, Bertazzi PA, Landi MT. Health status and plasma dioxin levels in chloracne cases 20 years after the Seveso, Italy accident. Br J Dermatol. 2005;152:459-465. DOI: 10.1111/j.1365-2133.2005.06444.x

[12] Collins JJ, Budinsky RA, Burns CJ, Lamparski LL, Carson ML, Martin GD, Wilken M. Serum dioxin levels in former chlorophenol workers. J Expo Anal Environ Epidemiol. 2006;16:76-84. DOI:10.1038/sj.jea.7500439

[13] Violante FS, Milani S, Malenchini G, Barbieri A. Reply to the comments by Coenraads and Tang 'Chloracne due to o-dichlorobenzene in a laboratory worker', Contact Dermatitis. 2005:52:108. 2005;53:65. DOI: 10.1111/j.0105-1873.2005.00633.x

[14] Cellini A, Offidani A. An epidemiological study on cutaneous diseases of agricultural workers authorized to use pesticides. Dermatology. 1994;189:129-132.

[15] Neuberger M, Rappe C, Bergek S, Cai H, Hansson M, Jäger R, Kundi M, Lim CK, Wingfors H, Smith AG. Persistent health effects of dioxin contamination in herbicide production. Environ Res. 1999;81:206-214. DOI: 10.1006/enrs.1999.3983

[16] Yoshimura T. Yusho in Japan. Ind Health. 2003;41:139-148. DOI: 10.2486/indhealth.41.139

[17] Guo YL, Yu ML, Hsu CC, Rogan WJ. Chloracne, goiter, arthritis and anemia after polychlorinated biphenyl poisoning: 14-year follow-up of the Taiwan Yucheng cohort. Environ Health Perspect. 1999;107:715-719. DOI: 10.2307/3434656

[18] Hryhorczuk DO, Wallace WH, Persky V, Furner S, Webster JR Jr, Oleske D, Haselhorst B, Ellefson R, Zugerman C. A morbidity study of former pentachlorophenol-production workers. Environ Health Perspect. 1998;106:401-408. DOI: 10.1289/ehp.98106401

[19] Robson M, Melymuk L, Csiszar SA, Giang A, Diamond ML, Helm PA. Continuing sources of PCBs: the significance of building sealants. Environ Int. 2010;36:513. DOI: 10.1016/j.envint.2010.03.009

[20] Herrick RF, Meeker JD, Hauser R, Altshul L, Weymouth GA. Serum PCB levels and congener profiles among US construction workers. Environ Health. 2007;6:25. DOI: 10.1186/1476-069X-6-25

[21] Selden A, Lundholm C, Johansson N, Wingfors H. Polychlorinated biphenyls (PCB), thyroid hormones and cytokines in construction workers removing old elastic sealants. Int Arch Occup Environ Health. 2008;82:99-106. DOI 10.1007/s00420-008-0313-5

[22] Breivik K, Gioia R, Chakraborty P, Zhang G, Jones KC. Are reductions in industrial organic contaminants emissions in rich countries achieved partly by export of toxic wastes? Environ Sci Technol. 2011;45:9154-9160. DOI: 10.1021/es202320c

[23] Budnik LT, Wegner R, Rogall U, Baur X. Accidental exposure to polychlorinated biphenyls (PCB) in waste cargo after heavy seas. Global waste transport as a source of PCB exposure. Int Arch Occup Environ Health. 2014;87:125-135. DOI: 10.1007/s00420-012-0841-x

[24] Gawkrodger DJ, Harris G, Bojar RA. Chloracne in seven organic chemists exposed to novel polycyclic halogenated chemical compounds (triazoloquinoxalines). Br J Dermatol. 2009;161:939-943. DOI: 10.1111/j.1365-2133.2009.09302.x.

[25] Tang NJ, Liu J, Coenraads PJ, Dong L, Zhao LJ, Ma SW, Chen X, Zhang CM, Ma XM, Wei WG, Zhang P, Bai ZP. Expression of AhR, CYP1A1, GSTA1, c-fos and TGF-alpha in skin lesions from dioxin-exposed humans with chloracne. Toxicol Lett. 2008;177:182-187. DOI:10.1016/j.toxlet.2008.01.011

[26] Zugerman C. Chloracne. Clinical manifestations and etiology. Dermatol Clin. 1990;8:209-213.

[27] McDonagh AJ, Gawkrodger DJ, Walker AE. Chloracne—study of an outbreak with new clinical observations. Clin Exp Dermatol. 1993;18:523-525. DOI: 10.1111/j.1365-2230.1993.tb01021.x

[28] Kerger BD, Leung HW, Scott P, Paustenbach DJ, Needham LL, Patterson DG Jr, Gerthoux PM, Mocarelli P. Age- and concentration-dependent elimination half-life of 2,3,7,8-tetrachlorodibenzo-p-dioxin in Seveso children. Environ Health Perspect. 2006; 114:1596-1602. DOI: 10.1289/ehp.8884

[29] Pelclová D, Urban P, Preiss J, Lukás E, Fenclová Z, Navrátil T, Dubská Z, Senholdová Z. Adverse health effects in humans exposed to 2,3,7,8-tetrachlorodibenzo-p-dioxin (TCDD). Rev Environ Health. 2006;21:119-138.

[30] Mitoma C, Uchi H, Tsukimori K, Yamada H, Akahane M, Imamura T, Utani A, Furue M. Yusho and its latest findings—A review in studies conducted by the Yusho Group. Environ Int. 2015;82:41-48. DOI: 10.1016/j.envint.2015.05.004.

[31] Imamura T, Kanagawa Y, Matsumoto S, Tajima B, Uenotsuchi T, Shibata S, Furue M. Relationship between clinical features and blood levels of pentachlorodibenzofuran in patients with Yusho Environ. Toxicology. 2007;22:124-131. DOI: 10.1002/tox.20251

[32] Wolfe WH, Michalek JE, Miner JC, Pirkle JL, Caudill SP, Patterson DG Jr, Needham LL. Determinants of TCDD half-life in veterans of operation ranch hand. J Toxicol Environ Health. 1994;41:481-488. DOI:10.1080/15287399409531858

[33] Geusau A, Abraham K, Geissler K, Sator MO, Stingl G, Tschachler E. Severe 2,3,7,8-tetrachlorodibenzo-p-dioxin (TCDD) intoxication: clinical and laboratory effects. Environ Health Perspect. 2001;109:865-869. DOI: 10.2307/3454832

[34] Pastor MA, Carrasco L, Izquierdo MJ, Fariña MC, Martín L, Renedo G, Requena L. Chloracne: histopathologic findings in one case. J Cutan Pathol. 2002;29:193-199. DOI: 10.1034/j.1600-0560.2002.290401.x

[35] Passarini B, Infusino SD, Kasapi E. Chloracne: still cause for concern. Dermatology. 2010;221:63-70. DOI: 10.1159/000290694

[36] Geusau A, Tschachler E, Meixner M, Sandermann S, Päpke O, Wolf C, Valic E, Stingl G, McLachlan M. Olestra increases faecal excretion of 2,3,7,8-tetrachlorodibenzo-p-dioxin. Lancet. 1999;354:1266-1267. DOI: 10.1016/S0140-6736(99)04271-3

[37] Redgrave TG, Wallace P, Jandacek RJ, Tso P. Treatment with a dietary fat substitute decreased Arochlor 1254 contamination in an obese diabetic male. J Nutr Biochem. 2005;16:383-384. DOI: 10.1016/j.jnutbio.2004.12.014

[38] Zorba E, Karpouzis A, Zorbas A, Bazas T, Zorbas S, Alexopoulos E, Zorbas I, Kouskoukis K, Konstandinidis T. Occupational dermatoses by type of work in Greece. Saf Health Work. 2013;4:142-148. DOI: 10.1016/j.shaw.2013.06.001

[39] National Toxicology Program. Coal tars and coal-tar pitches. Rep Carcinog. 2011;12:111-113. Available from: http://ntp.niehs.nih.gov/go/roc13

[40] Thami G, Sarkar R. Coal tar: past, present and future. Clin Exp Dermatol. 2002;27:99-103. DOI: 10.1046/j.1365-2230.2002.00995.x

[41] Moustafa GA, Xanthopoulou E, Riza E, Linos A. Skin disease after occupational dermal exposure to coal tar: a review of the scientific literature. Int J Dermatol. 2015;54:868-879. DOI: 10.1111/ijd.12903

[42] Kaidbey KH, Kligman AM. A human model of coal tar acne. Arch Dermatol. 1974;109:212-215. DOI:10.1001/archderm.1974.01630020028006.

[43] Farkas J. Oil acne from mineral oil among workers making prefabricated concrete panels. Contact Dermatitis. 1982;8:141. DOI: 10.1111/j.1600-0536.1982.tb04167.x

[44] Santarius-Kaczur D. Oil-induced acne in workers in the automobile industry. Med Pr. 1984;35:309-311.

[45] Upreti RK, Das M, Shanker R. Dermal exposure to kerosene. Vet Hum Toxicol. 1989;31:16-20.

[46] Karube H, Aizawa Y, Nakamura K, Maeda A, Hashimoto K, Takata T. Oil mist exposure in industrial health—a review. Sangyo Eiseigaku Zasshi. 1995;37:113-122.

[47] Svendsen K, Hilt B. Skin disorders in ship's engineers exposed to oils and solvents. Contact Dermatitis. 1997;36:216-220. DOI: 10.1111/j.1600-0536.1997.tb00273.x

[48] Plewig G, Fulton JE, Kligman AM. Pomade acne. Arch Dermatol. 1970;101:580-584. DOI:10.1001/archderm.1970.04000050084011.

[49] Cyprowski M, Kozajda A, Zielińska-Jankiewicz K, Szadkowska-Stańczyk I. Harmful impact of biological agents released at metalworking. Med Pr. 2006;57:139-147.

[50] Kokelj F. Occupational acne. Clin Dermatol. 1992;10:213-217.

[51] Czernielewski A, Skwarczyńska-Banyś E. Oral treatment of acne vulgaris and oil acne with tetracycline. Dermatologica. 1982;165:62-65.

[52] Finkelstein E, Lazarov A, Cagnano M, Halevy S. Oil acne: successful treatment with isotretinoin. J Am Acad Dermatol. 1994;30:491-492.

Chapter 5

Drug-Induced Acneiform Eruptions

Emin Özlü and Ayşe Serap Karadağ

Additional information is available at the end of the chapter

http://dx.doi.org/10.5772/65634

Abstract

Acne vulgaris is a chronic skin disease that develops as a result of inflammation of the pilosebaceous unit and its clinical course is accompanied by comedones, papules, pustules, and nodules. A different group of disease, which is clinically similar to acne vulgaris but with a different etiopathogenesis, is called "acneiform eruptions." In clinical practice, acneiform eruptions are generally the answer of the question "What is it if it is not an acne?" Although there are many subgroups of acneiform eruptions, drugs are common cause of acneiform eruptions, and this clinical picture is called "drug-induced acneiform eruptions." There are many drugs related to drug-induced acneiform eruptions. Discontinuation of the responsible drug is generally sufficient in treatment.

Keywords: acne, cutaneous toxicities, drug-induced acneiform eruptions, papule, pustule

1. Introduction

Acne vulgaris (AV) is a common skin disorder, which affects almost 85% of individuals at least once during life time. Although AV pathogenesis is not clearly understood yet, increased sebum production, androgenic hormones, ductal hypercornification, abnormal follicular keratinization, colonization of *Propionibacterium acnes* (*P. acnes*), inflammation, and genetic predisposition have been suggested to enhance acne development [1]. Hormone-dependent juvenile acne is a more frequent subgroup, whereas mechanical and drug-induced acne, which are particularly encountered during adulthood, are associated with the drug use with specific underlying etiologies [2]. Acneiform drug eruptions represent a sudden-onset clinical presentation, where the comedones are not observed [3]. In addition, several drugs are known to be associated with drug-induced acneiform eruptions [2]. In particular, the development of new target-specific molecules in the field of oncology, such as epidermal growth factor receptor inhibitors (EGFRIs), has caused a significant increase in the incidence of drug-induced acneiform eruptions [2, 3] (**Table 1**).

Hormones
Oral, inhaled and topical corticosteroids
Corticotropin (ACTH)
Androgens and anabolic steroids
Hormonal contraceptives
Other hormones
- thyroid-stimulating hormone, danazol

Neuropsychotherapeutic drugs
Tricyclic antidepressants
- amineptine, maprotiline, imipramine
Lithium
Antiepileptic drugs
- hydantoin, lamotrigine, valproate
Antipsychotics
- aripiprazole
Selective serotonin reuptake inhibitors

Vitamins
Vitamins B1, B6, B12

Cytostatic drugs
Dactinomycin (actinomycin D)
Azathioprine, thiourea, thiouracil

Immunomodulating molecules
Cyclosporine
Sirolimus
Others
- topical tacrolimus, topical pimecrolimus

Antituberculosis drugs
Isoniazid
Rifampin (rifampicin)
Ethionamide

Halogens
Iodine
Bromine
Chlorine
Others: halothane gas, lithium

Miscellaneous
Dantrolene
Quinidine
Antiretroviral therapy

Targeted therapies
Epidermal growth factor receptor inhibitors (EGFR inhibitors)
- erlotinib, gefitinib, imatinib
Epidermal growth factor receptor monoclonal antibodies
- cetuximab, panitimumab
TNFa inhibitors
- lenalidomide
- infliximab
- adalimumab
G-CSF
- vemurafenib
VEGF inhibitor
- bevacizumab

http://dx.doi.org/10.5772/65634

Proteasome inhibitor	
- bortezomib	
Histone deacetylase inhibitor	
- vorinostat	

EGF, epidermal growth factor; **TNFa**, tumor necrosis factor-a; **VEGF**, vascular endothelial growth factor; **G-CSF**, granulocymte colony-stimulating factor.

Table 1. Drugs involved with acneiform eruptions [2, 3].

This section focuses on the clinical and differential characteristics of drug-induced acneiform eruptions, drugs which may lead to this clinical presentation, and available treatment options in the light of the current literature data.

2. Clinical characteristics

Drug-induced acneiform eruptions may occur during childhood, adolescence, and adulthood. Lesions typically appear as monomorphic inflammatory papules and pustules without comedones or cysts. Papulopustular lesions usually involve on face, neck, chest, and upper back and can be extended beyond the seborrheic regions. Although its clinical course varies between patients, it often has a rapid onset without a previous history of AV. Papulopustular lesions may develop weeks, months, or even years after the exposure of the causative drug, and lesions may continue developing after the discontinuation of the drug [1].

3. Diagnosis and differential diagnosis

Diagnosis of drug induced acneiform eruptions is not based on any specific criteria. There are some clue signs that may be helpful to differentiate this clinical presentation from other common skin disorders. The sudden onset and monomorphic character of the lesions, absence of comedones in general, the presence of lesions in regions where acne vulgaris is not commonly present, the development of lesions at any age, and the presence of a history of drug use were

Drug-induced acneiform eruption	Acne vulgaris
Monomorphic lesions, lacking comedones, and cysts	Polymorphic lesions (mixture of comedones, papules, pustules, and nodules)
Extension beyond seborrheic areas to include arms, trunk, lower back, and genitalia	Localized primarily on seborrheic areas such as the face and neck and, less commonly, on the upper back, chest, and arms
Unusual age of onset (>30 years)	Commonly affects adolescents and young adults
Resistant to conventional acne therapy	Improves with conventional acne therapy
Onset after drug initiation, improvement after drug withdrawal, or reoccurrence after drug reintroduction	No causative relationship to drug therapy

Table 2. Drug-induced eruption versus acne vulgaris [1, 3].

the supportive findings and clues in the diagnosis. Clues, which may be helpful to differentiate drug-induced acneiform eruptions from idiopathic AV, are summarized in [1, 3] (**Table 2**). Cases that represent a diagnostic challenge should be extensively questioned with respect to medication history. Temporal relationship between the medication use and symptom development is very important [1].

4. Causative drugs

4.1. Hormones

4.1.1. Corticosteroids and corticotropin (ACTH)

Acneiform eruptions induced by the use of systemic corticosteroid therapy were first reported in 1950s [4]. Exposure to oral [5], intravenous [6], topical [7], or inhaled steroids [8] may result in or exacerbate acne. Development of acneiform eruptions was also reported during corticotropin therapy [4]. Perioral dermatitis is a form of acneiform eruption which may develop due to the use of highly potent corticosteroids [9]. During topical corticosteroid therapy, lesions may not become erythematous due to anti-inflammatory effects [10]. Although lesions usually begin to develop within 2–4 weeks after the administration of oral or topical therapy, they can also occur months after therapy. Dose, treatment duration, and individual factors may significantly affect the clinical presentation [2].

4.1.2. Androgens and anabolic steroids

Androgens are known to cause adolescent acne by increasing sebum production. In addition, anabolic steroids and synthetic hormones, which have androgenic activities, also show similar effects on the sebaceous glands [11]. In a prospective study, Fyrand et al. reported an increase in acne incidence among puberty-aged men who were administered injectable testosterones [12]. Moreover, acne incidence was also found to be higher among young athletes who used anabolic-androgenic steroids to increase their muscle mass [13].

4.1.3. Hormonal contraceptives

Hormonal contraceptive agents may induce or exacerbate acne [2]. A previous study demonstrated that 26.8% of women who used contraceptive etonogestrel implants developed acne [14]. Additionally, women who were placed a levonorgestrel-releasing intrauterine device developed inflammatory papular lesions 1–3 months after the procedure [15].

4.1.4. Other hormones

Danazole is an antigonadotropic agent used for the treatment of hereditary angioedema and endometriosis. Development of nodulocystic acneiform eruptions was previously reported in a woman receiving danazole therapy for endometriosis [16]. Thyroid hormones may also rarely result in acneiform eruptions [17].

4.2. Neuropsychotherapeutic drugs

4.2.1. Tricyclic antidepressants

Amineptine is one of the non-halogenated tricyclic antidepressants [3]. Amineptine may result in fast-onset acneiform eruptions consisting of macrocysts, microcysts, and comedones, months or even years after the initiation of therapy. Severity of the disease is associated with the dose and duration of therapy [1]. Amineptine and its products were found in serum, urine, and skin lesions, and histological examinations showed that this drug may result in keratinizing syringometaplasia in neutrophilic eccrine hidradenitis and eccrine glands [18]. Tricyclic antidepressants such as maprotiline [19] and imipramine [20] are also known to cause acneiform eruptions.

4.2.2. Lithium

Lithium may cause fast-onset inflammatory lesions on face, axilla, groin, arms, and buttocks. Lithium-induced acneiform eruptions are more frequent among men and those who are allergic to lithium [21]. No direct relation was shown between dose and severity of acne [2].

4.2.3. Antiepileptic drugs

Several antiepileptic agents were associated with drug-induced acneiform eruptions [22]. Phenytoin [23], phenobarbital [22], lamotrigine [24], and valproate [25] are among the most common culprits. Phenytoin is known to cross the placenta and cause acneiform eruptions, hypertrichosis, and gingival hyperplasia [26].

4.2.4. Aripiprazole

Aripiprazole is a quinolone-derivative antipsychotic drug reported to induce papulopustular acneiform eruptions in a patient 10 days after the initiation of therapy [27].

4.2.5. Selective serotonin reuptake inhibitors

All selective serotonin reuptake inhibitors may cause acneiform eruptions on the face, chest, and back regions [28].

4.3. Vitamins B1, B6 and B12

Acneiform eruptions characterized by monomorphic inflammatory papulopustular lesions localized on the face, neck, upper back, and chest may develop after the B12 injection therapy (**Figure 1**). The reason underlying this is not clearly known; however, the lesions rapidly disappear after discontinuation of therapy [29]. Several pharmaceutical preparations also involve B1 (thiamine) and B6 (pyridoxine) vitamins in addition to B12; however, the role of these vitamins in acne development is still controversial [30].

4.4. Cytostatic drugs

4.4.1. Dactinomycin (actinomycin D)

Dactinomycin, which is a cytostatic agent used for the treatment of solid tumors, is associated with acneiform eruptions. It has been suggested that dactinomycin induces acneiform eruptions through its androgenic characteristics and due to its tricyclic chemical structure [1].

4.4.2. Other cytostatic drugs

Although rare, the development of acneiform eruptions has been reported upon the use of azathioprine, thiourea, and thiouracil; however, the evidences are still limited [17, 31].

4.5. Immunomodulating molecules

4.5.1. Cyclosporine

Cyclosporine is an agent with immunosuppressive activity and it is used after organ transplantations and for the treatment of psoriasis and atopic dermatitis. As it is a highly lipophilic

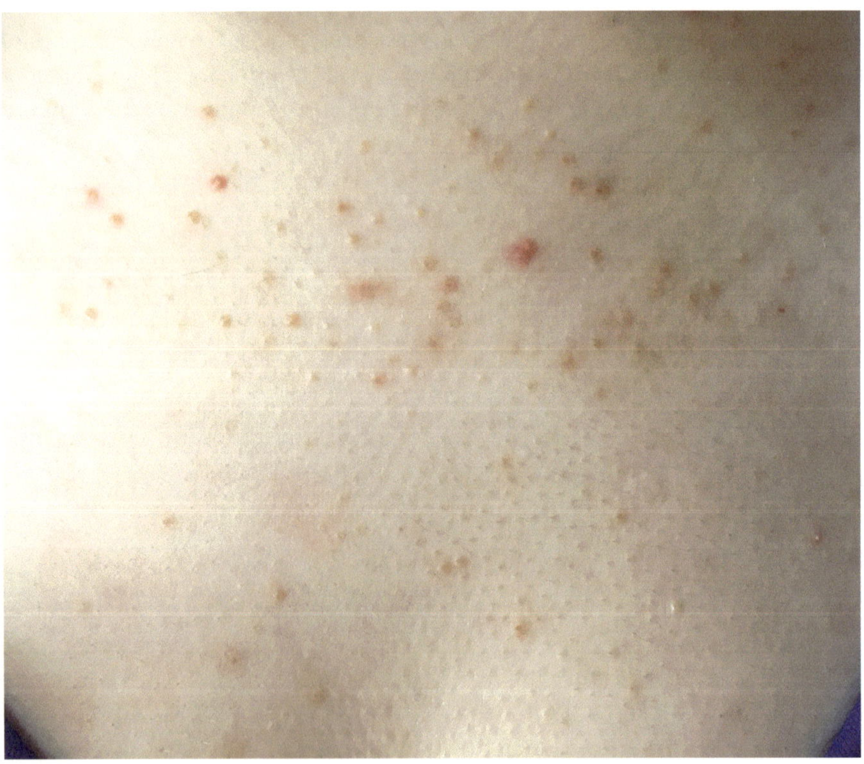

Figure 1. Inflammatory papules and pustules on the chest after B12 injection treatment.

compound, it can potentially be eliminated through the sebaceous glands. Therefore, cyclosporine may induce acneiform eruptions by affecting the pilosebaceous follicle structures and functions [31].

4.5.2. Sirolimus

Sirolimus, which is an immunosuppressive agent used after organ transplantation, can result in acneiform eruptions [32]. Sirolimus is believed to exert toxic effects on the follicles and alter the sebum production and synthesis of epidermal growth factor (EGF) and testosterone [33]. In a prospective French study, acneiform eruptions were reported to develop in 46% of 80 patients who received sirolimus therapy after renal transplantation [34].

4.5.3. Other immunosuppressants

Tacrolimus is a macrolide-derivative agent with T-cell-specific immunosuppressive activity which blocks calcineurin-dependent-signaling pathway [3]. There are case reports indicating that topical tacrolimus [33] and pimecrolimus [35] may result in facial acne.

4.6. Antituberculosis drugs

4.6.1. Isoniazid

Isoniazid (INH) is a drug used for the treatment and prophylaxis of tuberculosis. It has been suggested that INH more easily results in acneiform eruptions in patients with slow acetylating phenotypes [3]. Previously, it was reported that acneiform eruptions might develop even 18 months after the initiation of INH therapy and disappear after the discontinuation of therapy [36].

4.6.2. Rifampin

Rifampin was associated with chronic papular acneiform eruption on face, neck, and shoulders, developing 5 weeks after the treatment onset [37].

4.6.3. Ethionamide

Ethionamide is an agent used for the treatment of tuberculosis and is associated with the development of acneiform eruptions [38].

4.7. Halogens

Iodide, bromide, and chloride are salt-containing drugs which result in iododerma, bromoderma, and chloracne, respectively. It has been suggested that these drugs induce acneiform eruptions, as they are eliminated via the sebaceous glands [1].

4.7.1. Iodine

Iododerma refers to the skin eruptions with different clinical presentations caused by oral, parenteral, or topical iodine administration. Lesions may be papular, pustular, or vesicular;

however, lesions in erythematous, urticarial, froncular, carbuncular, bullous, vegetating, or ulcerating pattern can also develop. Lesions beginning at the seborrheic region may extend to the whole body [2]. Although its pathogenesis is unclear, a suggested hypothesis includes cell-mediated immune reaction, inflammatory mechanism, and idiosyncratic reactions [39]. Discontinuation of iodine therapy is usually sufficient for symptom recovery, whoever the use of topical or systemic steroids may become necessary in severe cases [1].

4.7.2. Bromine

Although bromoderma is defined as skin eruption induced by bromide intoxication, it is not frequent at the present. Currently, several drugs with sedative, anti-epileptic, spasmolytic, and expectorant activities contain bromide [40]. Bromoderma clinically resembles iododerma and its diagnosis can be confirmed by increased serum and urine levels of bromide [41].

4.7.3. Chlorine

Acneiform eruptions may develop due to skin exposure to various industrial chemicals such as chlorine and its products. These chlorinated hydrocarbons result in the presentation of chloracne, characterized by cysts, pustule, folliculitis, and comedones [42]. Lesions usually develop at malar, postauricular, axillary, and genital regions, but may extend further [43]. Chloracne treatment is challenging and the lesions may continue developing for a long time, despite avoiding exposure to chloracnegens [44].

4.7.4. Other agents

Halothane is a halogenated anesthetic gas which may result in the development of acneiform eruptions hours after the exposure of the administering health-care personnel [45].

Lithium was reported to cause halogenoderma-like eruptions in two cases in the literature [46].

4.8. Miscellaneous drugs

Dantrolene is a muscle relaxant used for the treatment of spasticity. Dantrolene-induced acne consists of blackheads, comedones, cysts, pustules, and abscesses, and the lesions particularly localize at the regions exposed to chronic trauma, friction, and pressure. Lesions may develop 6 months to 4 years after the treatment onset [1].

Quinidine [47] and antiretroviral therapy [48] were also reported to cause acneiform eruptions.

4.9. Targeted therapies

Targeted therapies refer to a special group of medicines interacting with specific key molecules that play roles in the pathophysiology of inflammatory and tumoral diseases. This group of therapeutic agents includes tyrosine kinase inhibitors such as gefitinib, erlotinib, and imatinib, monoclonal antibodies such as cetuximab, panitumumab, and infliximab, soluble

http://dx.doi.org/10.5772/65634

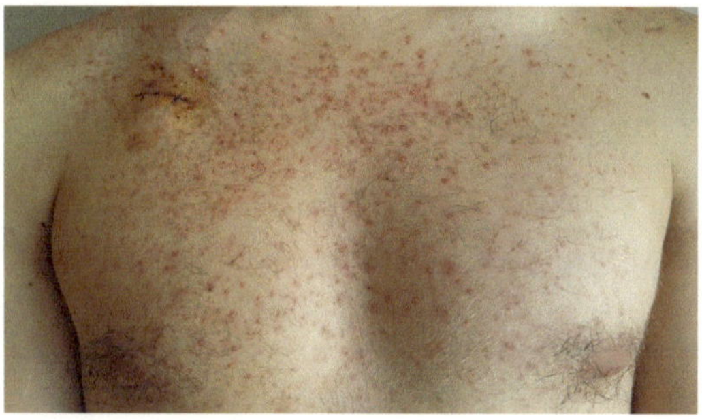

Figure 2. Severe acneiform eruption on the chest during therapy with panitimumab for metastatic colon cancer.

antibodies such as etanercept, transcription modulators such as vorinostat, and proteosome inhibitors such as bortezomib [2].

Epidermal growth factor receptor (EGFR) inhibitors are chemotherapeutic agents used for the treatment of specific cancer types. Rapidly developing acneiform eruption has been a hallmark of EGFR inhibitor therapy [49]. Based on previously published series, 60–100% of patients receiving EGFR inhibitor therapy develop acneiform eruptions [49–52]. Monoclonal antibodies targeting EGFR, such as panitimumab, may also cause acneiform eruptions (**Figure 2**). Patients with a previous history of adolescent acne or folliculitis are more prone to acneiform eruptions and lesions commonly develop after the first cycle of therapy. Inflamed papules and pustules, accompanied by itching in seborrheic regions, are characteristic findings [3]. The development of acneiform eruptions after the EGFR inhibitor therapy was suggested to be a prognostic factor indicating good treatment response [53]. Incidence and severity of acneiform eruption are dose-dependent. Tetracycline derivatives may be used to control severe lesions [3].

Tumor necrosis factor (TNF) inhibitors are particularly used for the treatment of autoimmune disorders and they may also induce acneiform eruptions. Among this class of drugs, infliximab was the agent most frequently associated with acneiform eruptions [54]. The development of acneiform eruptions was also reported in a male patient receiving adalimumab therapy due to Crohn's disease [55]. In addition, lenalidomide, a thalidomide derivative, was demonstrated to be associated with acneiform eruptions due to its anti-TNF activity [56].

5. Treatment

Drug-induced acneiform eruptions are usually well tolerated. The most important step of treatment is identification of the causative drug and discontinuation of treatment, whenever possible. Conventional acne therapy may be used, if the treatment cannot be discontinued; however, treatment resistance is a common concern. Oral antibiotics such as doxycycline can be used in moderate and severe cases. In more severe cases, oral isotretinoin may also be used under close monitoring and by avoiding potential drug interactions [1].

6. Conclusion

Drug-induced acneiform eruptions are frequently seen side effects, and it is difficult to prevent them. It should be kept in mind that many drugs could cause drug-induced acneiform eruptions in clinical practice, and it is important to obtain a detailed history of drug use in suspected cases for appropriate follow-up and treatment approach.

Author details

Emin Özlü[1] and Ayşe Serap Karadağ[2]*

*Address all correspondence to: karadagaserap@gmail.com

1 Department of Dermatology, Kayseri Research and Training Hospital, Kayseri, Turkey

2 Department of Dermatology, School of Medicine, Istanbul Medeniyet University, Istanbul, Turkey

References

[1] Christopher P Schiavo, Carol W Stanford. Acne and Drug Reactions. In: John C Hall, Brian J Hall, eds. Cutaneous Drug Eruptions Diagnosis, Histopathology and Therapy. 1st ed. Springer-Verlag, London, 2015; pp. 157–166. doi: 10.1007/978-1-4471-6729-7_15.

[2] Du Thanh A, Kluger N, Bensalleh H, et al. Drug-induced acneiform eruption. Am J Clin Dermatol. 2011;12(4):233–45. doi: 10.2165/11588900-000000000-00000.

[3] Ha K Do, Navid E, Wolverton ES. Drug Induced Acneiform Eruptions. In: Zeichner Joshua A, ed. Acneiform Eruptions in Dermatology. 1st ed. New York, NY: Springer-Verlag 2014; pp. 389–404. doi 10.1007/978-1-4614-8344-1_54.

[4] Brunner MJ, Riddell Jr JM, Best WR. Cutaneous side effects of ACTH cortisone and pregnenolone therapy. J Invest Dermatol. 1951;16:205–10. PMID: 14841382

[5] Clementson B, Smidt AC. Periorificial dermatitis due to systemic corticosteroids in children: report of two cases. Pediatric Dermatol. 2012;29:331–2. doi: 10.1111/j.1525-1470.2011.01651.x. Epub 2011 Nov 28.

[6] Fung MA, Berger TG. A prospective study of acute-onset steroid acne associated with administration of intravenous corticosteroids. Dermatology. 2000;200:43–4. doi: 18314

[7] Plewig G, Kligman AM. Induction of acne by topical steroids. Arch Dermatol Forsch. 1973;247:29–52. PMID: 4270567

[8] Monk B, Cunliffe WJ, Layton AM, et al. Acne induced by inhaled corticosteroids. Clin Exp Dermatol. 1993;18:148–50. PMID: 8481992

[9] Cohen HJ. Perioral dermatitis. J Am Acad Dermatol. 1981;4:739–40. PMID: 6453885

[10] Wells K, Brodell RT. Topical corticosteroid "addiction". A cause of perioral dermatitis. Postgrad Med. 1993;93:225–30. PMID: 8460079

[11] Scott III MJ, Scott AM. Effects of anabolic-androgenic steroids on the pilosebaceous unit. Cutis. 1992;50:113–6. PMID: 1387354

[12] Fyrand O, Fiskaadal HJ, Trygstad O. Acne in pubertal boys undergoing treatment with androgens. Acta Derm Venereol. 1992;72:148–9. PMID: 1350406

[13] Melnik B, Jansen T, Grabbe S. Abuse of anabolic-androgenic steroids and bodybuilding acne: an underestimated health problem. J Dtsch Dermatol Ges. 2007;5:110–7. doi: 10.1111/j.1610-0387.2007.06176.x

[14] Yildizbas B, Sahin HG, Kolusari A, et al. Side effects and acceptability of Implanon: a pilot study conducted in eastern Turkey. Eur J Contracept Reprod Health Care 2007;12:248–52. doi: 10.1080/13625180701442228

[15] Ilse JR, Greenberg HL, Bennett DD. Levonorgestrel-releasing intrauterine system and new- onset acne. Cutis. 2008;82:158. PMID: 18792549

[16] Greenberg RD. Acne vulgaris associated with antigonadotropic (Danazol) therapy. Cutis. 1979;24:431–3. PMID: 159808

[17] Bedane C, Souyri N. Induced acne. Ann Dermatol Venereol 1990;117:53–8. PMID: 2138865

[18] Huet P, Dandurand M, Joujoux JM, et al. Acne induced by amineptin: adnexal toxiderma. Ann Dermatol Venereol 1996;123:817–20. PMID: 9636770

[19] Ponte CD. Maprotiline induced acne. Am J Psychiatry 1982;139:141. PMID: 6459743

[20] Ossofsky J. Amenorrhea in endogenous depression. Int Pharmacopsychiatry 1974;9:100–8. PMID: 4850494

[21] Yeung CK, Chan HH. Cutaneous adverse effects of lithium: epidemiology and management. Am J Clin Dermatol 2004;5:3–8. PMID: 14979738

[22] Hesse S, Berbis P, Lafforgue P, et al. Acne and enthesiopathy during anti-epileptic treatment. Ann Dermatol Venereol. 1992;119:655–8. PMID: 1285592

[23] Jenkins RB, Ratner AC. Diphenylhydantoin and acne. New Engl J Med. 1972;287:148. doi: 10.1056/NEJM197207202870314

[24] Nielsen JN, Licht RW, Fogh K. Two cases of acneiform eruption associated with lamotrigine. J Clin Psychiatry. 2004;65:1720–2. PMID: 15641879

[25] Joffe H, Cohen LS, Suppes T, et al. Valproate is associated with new-onset oligoamenorrhea with hyperandrogenism in women with bipolar disorder. Biol Psychiatry. 2006;59:1078–86. doi: 10.1016/j.biopsych.2005.10.017

[26] Norris JF, Cunliffe WJ. Phenytoin-induced gum hypertrophy improved by isotretinoin. Int J Dermatol. 1987;26:602–3. PMID: 2965113

[27] Mishra B, Praharaj SK, Prakash R, et al. Aripiprazole-induced acneiform eruption. Gen Hosp Psychiatry 2008;30:479–81. doi: 10.1016/j.genhosppsych.2008.02.004. Epub 2008 Jul 23

[28] Warnock JK, Morris DW. Adverse cutaneous reactions to antidepressants. Am J Clin Dermatol 2002;3:329–39. PMID: 12069639

[29] Dupre′ A, Albarel N, Bonafe JL, et al. Vitamin B-12 induced acnes. Cutis 1979;24:210–1. PMID: 157854

[30] Sheretz EF. Acneiform eruption due to 'megadose' vitamins B6 and B12. Cutis 1991;48:119–20. PMID: 1834437

[31] Schmoeckel C, von Liebe V. Acneiform exanthema caused by azathioprine [in German]. Hautarzt 1983;34:413–5. PMID: 6225752

[32] Fidan K, Kandur Y, Sozen H, et al. How often do we face side effects of sirolimus in pediatric renal transplantation? Transplant Proc. 2013;45:185–9. doi: 10.1016/j.transproceed.2012.08.005.

[33] Bakos L, Bakos RM. Focal acne during topical tacrolimus therapy for vitiligo. Arch Dermatol. 2007;143:1223–4. doi: 10.1001/archderm.143.9.1223

[34] Mahe′ E, Morelon E, Lechaton S, et al. Cutaneous adverse events in renal transplant recipients receiving sirolimus-based therapy. Transplantation 2005;79:476–82. PMID: 15729175

[35] Li JC, Xu AE. Facial acne during topical pimecrolimus therapy for vitiligo. Clin Exp Dermatol 2009;34: e489–90. doi: 10.1111/j.1365-2230.2009.03556.x.

[36] Oliwiecki S, Burton JL. Severe acne due to isoniazid. Clin Exp Dermatol 1988;13:283–4. PMID: 2977579

[37] Nwokolo U. Acneiform lesions in combined rifampicin treatment in Africans [letter]. Br Med J 1974;3:473. PMID: 4137745

[38] Levantine A, Almeyda J. Cutaneous reactions to antituberculosis drugs. Br J Dermatol 1972;86:651–5. PMID: 4114691

[39] Inman P. Proceedings: iododerma. Br J Dermatol 1974;91:709–11. PMID: 4451645

[40] Maffeis L, Musolino MC, Cambiaghi S. Single-plaque vegetating bromoderma. J Am Acad Dermatol 2008;58:682–4. doi: 10.1016/j.jaad.2007.08.011.

[41] Arditti J, Follana J, Bonerandi JJ, et al. Bromide vegetating skin diseases after treatment by a bromocalcic specialty. Eur J Toxicol Environ Hyg 1976;9:59–63. PMID: 1253832

[42] Plewig G, Jansen T. Acneiform dermatoses. Dermatology. 1998;196:102–7. PMID: 9557242

[43] Fisher AA. Drug eruptions in geriatric patients. Cutis. 1976;18:402–9. PMID: 138570

[44] Webster GF. Pustular drug reactions. Clin Dermatol. 1993;11:541–3. PMID: 8124644

[45] Soper LE, Vitez TS, Weinberg D. Metabolism of halogenated anaesthetic agents as a possible cause of acneiform eruptions. Anaesth Analg 1973;52:125–7. PMID: 4265185

[46] Alagheband M, Engineer L. Lithium and halogenoderma. Arch Dermatol 2000;136:126–7. PMID: 10632224

[47] Burkhart CG. Quinidine-induced acne. Arch Dermatol 1981;117:603–4. PMID: 6456697

[48] Scott C, Staughton RC, Bunker CJ, et al. Acne vulgaris and acne rosacea as part of immune reconstitution disease in HIV-1 infected patients starting antiretroviral therapy. Int J STD AIDS 2008;19:493–5. doi: 10.1258/ijsa.2008.008026.

[49] Jacot W, Bessis D, Jorda E, et al. Acneiform eruption induced by epidermal growth factor receptor inhibitors in patients with solid tumours. Br J Dermatol. 2004;151:238–41. doi: 10.1111/j.1365-2133.2004.06026.x

[50] Harding J, Burtness B. Cetuximab: an epidermal growth factor receptor chimeric human-murine monoclonal antibody. Drugs Today 2005;41:107–27. doi: 10.1358/dot.2005.41.2.882662

[51] Hannoud S, Rixe O, Bloch J, et al. Skin signs associated with epidermal growth factor inhibitors. Ann Dermatol Venereol 2006;133:239–42. PMID: 16800173

[52] Segaert S, Van Custem E. Clinical signs, pathophysiology and management of skin toxicity during therapy with epidermal growth factor receptor inhibitors. Ann Oncol 2005;16:1425–33. doi: 10.1093/annonc/mdi279

[53] Journagan S, Obadiah J. An acneiform eruption due to erlotinib: prognostic implications and management. J Am Acad Dermatol. 2006;54:358–60. doi: 10.1016/j.jaad.2005.08.033.

[54] Sladden MJ, Clarke PJ, Mitchell B. Infliximab-induced acne: report of a third case. Br J Dermatol. 2008;158:172. doi: 10.1111/j.1365-2133.2007.08172.x

[55] Fernandez-Crehuet P, Luiz Villaverde R. Acneiform eruption as a probable paradoxical reaction to adalimumab. Int J Dermatol. 2015 Aug;54(8):e306–8. doi: 10.1111/ijd.12416

[56] Michot C, Guillot B, Dereure O. Lenalidomide-induced acute acneiform folliculitis of the head and neck: not only the anti-EGF receptor agents. Dermatology 2010;220:49–50. doi: 10.1159/000258050

Chapter 6

Acneiform Eruptions and Pregnancy

Aslı Feride Kaptanoglu and Didem Mullaaziz

Additional information is available at the end of the chapter

http://dx.doi.org/10.5772/67015

Abstract

Acne and acneiform eruptions during pregnancy need special attention. The physician should be aware of the special condition of a pregnant patient. Acne treatments may aim to prevent worsening, secondary infections, scarring and lowering self-esteem of the mother. However, the treatment of acne and acneiform eruptions are not easy to treat during pregnancy. First, because many cosmetics and procedures are not tested on pregnant patients and it is impossible to predict the possible consequences of the procedures on fetus, many women quit cosmetic procedures during pregnancy. Second, the underlying conditions such as hormonal influx and immunosuppression continue. Third, the medications for acne have limitations due to the lack of evidence of safety during pregnancy. Here, a acneiform eruptions during pregnancy, including acne vulgaris, acne rosacea, perioral dermatitis, and hidradenitis suppurativa, are reviewed focusing on these points and each of them is evaluated by clinical presentation, differential diagnosis and treatment options focusing on maternal and fetal safety.

Keywords: acne, acneiform eruptions, sebaceous gland, pregnancy, treatment

1. Introduction

Pregnancy is one of the most "special periods" for a woman. Changes in the endocrine and immune systems and in the metabolism will result in an overall change in body, including skin. Although some of these changes may be physiologic, pregnant women are more careful, meticulous and concerned about their body. As the skin changes can easily be observed by naked eye, this additional problem helps to increase anxiety and lower their self-esteem. During pregnancy, acne can have psychological effects. Even very small changes draw attention and raise questions related to the medical concerns for the baby. Moreover, pregnant women can be anxious and depressed because of their health, self-image, cosmetic problems and limitations on treatments.

Some of the metabolic changes may also trigger sebaceous and eccrine glands to produce acneiform eruptions. Acneiform eruptions are follicular eruptions characterized by papules and pustules resembling acne. Diagnosis of acne is usually done clinically. However, differential diagnosis of acneiform eruptions during pregnancy should be done carefully and mostly depends on exclusion. Typically acne has predilection sites such as face, neck, chest, and back [1]. Papular and pustular lesions appearing on this sites are generally considered as "acne" which can be a misdiagnose. Moreover, during pregnancy acne rosacea, perioral dermatitis, hidradenitis suppurativa, Fox-Fordyce disease, pruritic folliculitis of pregnancy may be seen in different clinical presentations. So, differential diagnosis of acneiform eruptions should not be underestimated. Gynecologists and family physicians also should be aware of "acne-like" eruptions and consult a dermatologist [2].

Acne and acneiform eruptions during pregnancy also need treatments to prevent worsening, secondary infections, scarring, and lowering self esteem of the mother. However, the treatment of acne and acneiform eruptions are not easy to treat in this life period. First, as many cosmetics and procedures are not tested on pregnant patients and impossible to predict the possible consequences of the procedures on fetus, many women quit cosmetic procedures during that period [3]. Second, the underlying conditions such as hormonal influx and immunosuppression continue. Third, the medications for acne have limitations due to the lack of evidence of safety during pregnancy.

Here in this chapter we will make a close look to acneiform eruptions during pregnancy period including acne vulgaris, acne rosacea, perioral dermatitis, and hidradenitis suppurativa. Each of these diseases will be evaluated by clinical presentation, differential diagnosis and treatment options focusing on maternal and fetal safety.

2. Hormonal changes during pregnancy

In the pregnant women subsequent hormonal changes which are unique for that period appear. The placenta is a fantastic hormone factory that produces large amounts of hCG, relaxin, oestradiol, progesterone and human chorionic somato mammatrophin (hCS or human placental lactogen, hPL). Estrogen production from the placenta as well as the ovary increases gradually from the second month of pregnancy until term. Also, placental progesterone rises to a peak during the fifth month of pregnancy. Moreover, the placenta is a source of human chorionic gonadotropin, which increases during the first trimester and decreases dramatically with the elevation of estrogen and progesterone. The hPL is synthesised from the 4 week of gestation. The hPL stimulates maternal lipolysis and inhibits insulin effects, causing hyperglycaemia [2].

During pregnancy some other hormonal changes occur as well. The anterior pituitary gland increases in weight by more than two-fold during pregnancy with a concomitant increase in gonadotropin hormone secretion. The production and secretion of adrenal cortex hormones are increased in addition to the adrenal hypertrophy. The typical hormonal changes and immunity in pregnancy cause a shift in maternal immune function from cell mediated (helper T 1 [TH1] cytokine production) to humoral (helper T 2 [TH2] cytokine production). Moreover, the activity of sebaceous and eccrine glands is increased and apocrine gland activity is decreased. So, all these physiologic changes may influence the course of inflammatory and glandular skin disease during gestation [4].

3. Acne in pregnancy

Acne vulgaris is a chronic inflammatory disorder clinically presenting with comedones, papules, pustules and cysts. The course of acne in pregnancy is unpredictable and severity shows variations [4, 5]. In the majority, pregnancy has a beneficial effect on the activity of acne, and often improves in the first trimester. This is suggested to be related with the sebosuppressive effect of estrogens [5]. In a small number of cases, there is a flare-up of acne requiring active intervention, especially if scarring is a threat. Ratzer reported 58% improvement and 29% reporting worsening of acne during pregnancy [6]. In another study, improvement of acne by 41% in pregnant women was reported [7].

The increase in sebaceous gland activity, especially during the third trimester, results in an aggrevation of acne which is most upsetting at this time. Other clinical findings are post inflammatory pigment alterations and flare of truncal acne [2]. Some women experience new-onset acne, such as acne conglobata, in the postpartum period ("postgestational acne") [4, 8].

Hyperandrogenism in pregnancy is rare and can develop in any trimester. The signs and symptoms are similar as the non pregnant women and may present as acne and hirsutism. The most common ovarian pathologies that present during pregnancy and which lead to hyperandrogenic states are hyperreactio luteinalis (HL) and pregnancy luteoma (PL) whereas ovarian tumors and adrenal pathologies are very rare. Although spontaneous regression occurs in the post-partum period in the vast majority of cases, such cases with a clue of androgen excess should be re-evaluated by means of underlying pathologies and fetal virilisation [9].

Acne cosmetica and pregnancy: sunscreens are commonly used in pregnancy to treat or prevent melasma. Pregnant women are adviced and prefer to use inorganic sun blockers such as zinc oxide, titanium dioxide, iron oxide, talc, and calamine which are generally safer than their organic counterparts due to their nontoxic, stable properties and absence of systemic absorption. But these formulations are thick pastes that promote comedogenesis [10, 11]. So, pregnant women may experience extensive acne problem while trying to prevent melasma.

Treatment of acne in pregnancy is challenging as most drugs are contraindicated or considered unsafe [12]. The Food and Drug Administration (FDA) has five established categories to indicate potential teratogenicity of a medication when used by patients during pregnancy. FDA categories are shown as **Table 1**.

The treatment of acne during pregnancy depends on its type and severity. Unfortunately, there are no "evidence" level studies to support the clinical efficacy of any acne treatment during pregnancy or lactation [13]. The available reports are mainly observational studies and often with small samples sizes. There are pregnancy-exposure registries that collect data

Category	
A	Well-controlled studies in humans show no risk to the fetus
B	No well controlled studies have been conducted in humans, animal studies show no risk to the fetus
C	No well controlled studies have been conducted in humans; animal studies have demonstrated an adverse effect on the fetus
D	Evidence of human risk to the fetus exists; however benefits may outweigh risks in certain situations
X	Controlled studies in animals or humans demonstrate fetal abnormalities; the risk in pregnant women clearly outweighs any possible benefit

Table 1. FDA categories for drug use during pregnancy.

on the use of certain medications in pregnancy. However, there are no relevant registries for "acne" treatments [14]. Although there is no evidence-based recommendations about acne treatment during pregnancy, it should depend on acne type, severity and in its impact on quality of life. The goal of treatment and expectations of patient should be determined based on risk/benefit ratio and should rely on relief of symptoms rather than total clearance.

There are many oral and topical medications for the treatment of acne. Some of the patients might be using one or more of these treatments before conception. It is not always very easy while deciding to stop or not therapy because the evidence to guide this clinical question is not relevant. The half-life of medications and FDA categories may be a key to answer these questions.

3.1. Systemic treatments

For severe acne, systemic treatments may be needed to avoid scarring. There are only few options available for the safe management of acne in pregnancy. Isotretinoin, which is the mainstay of treatment for severe and nodulocystic acne, is contraindicated in pregnancy. Hormonal treatments (anti-androgens, spironalacton) also should be avoided for its effects on fetus. Some of the oral antibiotics are safe during pregnancy and can be used.

3.1.1. Isotretinoin

Systemic retinoids are important treatments in women with moderate to severe acne, but must be avoided during pregnancy due to teratogenicity. Isotretinoin, is FDA pregnancy category X. Its association with increased risk of spontaneous abortion, retinoid embryopathy which is specific with facial and palatal defects, micrognathia, cardiovascular defects, and developmental problems of the central nervous system and thymus have been reported [15, 16]. Both isotretinoin and its metabolite are thought to be teratogenic. The half-life of isotretinoin is 10–20 h and its metabolite (4-oxo-isotretinoin) between 17 and 50 h. General recommendation is five times this half-life would be enough to allow levels of the drug to return to negligible levels. So, a washout period (one month between completely discontinuing isotretinoin – beginning attempts to conceive a pregnancy) will be needed [13]. Similarly, conception one menstrual cycle after completely stopping isotretinoin is advised in a published guideline [17]. But on the contrary, many cases of unwanted pregnancies and relevant abortuses have been reported all over the world [18]. This indicates that there is still insufficient control of isotretinoin associated with pregnancy. So pregnant women with acne should be questioned in detail about the total dosing, the time of last dose of isotretinoin and in case of a suspicion, prenatal diagnostic research should be provided.

3.1.2. Antibiotics

In non-pregnant patients oral antibiotics are commonly prescribed as a second-line therapy for acne and the most commonly used are tetracyclines: doxycycline, oxytetracycline, lymecycline, minocycline, and tetracycline [19]. Penicillins, macrolides, and cephalosporins are thought to have the best safety profile in pregnancy with erythromycin the oral antibiotic most commonly used for acne in pregnancy [18]. But tetracyclines should not be used during pregnancy, as use in the second and third trimester can cause discoloration of teeth and bones [20].

During pregnancy, erythromycin should be the first choice in case of a necessity [21]. As it is used in pregnancy to treat other infections, there is quite satisfactory data coming from these retrospective studies of pregnancy outcomes. Its usage in combination with a topical preparation is recommended to avoid bacterial resistance [14, 22]. Only, erythromycin estolate is not recommended in pregnancy because of potential risk of reversible hepatotoxicity which is rarely reported with other ester forms. The common side effect of erythromycin is gastrointestinal dyspepsy and rarely increasing serum levels of medications metabolized by cytochrome p450 enzymes [20].

Another macrolide antibiotic that can be used for treatment of acne in pregnancy is oral azithromycin. It has efficacy against *Propionibacterium acnes* and anti-inflammatory actions and in a study comparing the efficacy of azithromycin with doxycycline, azithromycin was found to be as effective as doxycycline. The longer half-life of 68 h also can be advantage as a single daily dose [23]. Also a new macrolide antibiotic, roxithromycin is shown to be effective on acne lesions with similar safety with erythromycin, has a better side effect profile and less frequently associated with bacterial resistance. The only disadvantage is being expensive [24].

Oral clindamycin is also considered to be effective and safe for use in pregnancy but due to one serious potential side effect it is rarely used. Disturbance of gastrointestinal flora by this agent can cause pseudo-membranous colitis. Diarrhea is also a common side effect [25].

3.1.3. Hormonal treatment

Hormonal therapy includes oral contraceptive pills (OCP) and androgen receptor blockers such as cyproterone acetate and spironolactone which are particularly useful in the treatment of acne linked to hyperandrogenism. However, these anti androgenic treatments are not suggested to be used during pregnancy because of the risk of hypospadias and feminization of a male fetus [26]. Also, higher incidence of Down syndrome has been reported with use of OCPs in early pregnancy [27].

3.1.4. Zinc

Oral zinc salt preparations have historically been shown to be effective in reducing the severity of mild and moderate inflammatory acne vulgaris when either used alone or in combination with another acne treatment [28]. Zinc sulfate (N) and zinc gluconate (N) have been shown to be effective in the treatment of acne vulgaris at elemental doses of 30–150 mg daily [29]. It is shown that elemental zinc has no harm at doses below 75 mg/day to the growing fetus [30]. There is huge literature data on the use of zinc salts in lactation, but no adverse effects have been reported thus far.

3.2. Topical treatments

Topical medications are first line therapies for acne [31]. Most of the pregnant women prefer staying on the safe zone rather than aesthetic targets. Also, both patients and physicians prefer topical treatments only to avoid possible side effects especially on fetus [32].

Proper cleansing is an important step in acne treatment, also in pregnancy. Twice daily washing with a gentle cleanser followed by a topical preparation should be the first step. Mechanical comedo removal can be performed with a comedone extractor in comedonal forms.

3.2.1. Azelaic acid

It is a dicarboxylic acid with antimicrobial, anti-inflammatory and comedolitic properties. Also, being a competitive inhibitor of thyrosinase it decreases pigmentation. This effect on pigmentation could be used as an advantage when tendency to pigmentation is increased in pregnancy. It is generally well tolerated with a transient burning sensation but has no phototoxic or photoallergic potential. Azelaic acid is pregnancy category B, with no known fetal effects. Studies indicate that using high oral doses in animals do not cause teratogenic effects in the offspring, but there are no controlled studies in humans. It is also present in milk, rye, barley, and wheat. So azelaic acid can be a good choice for topical acne treatment in pregnancy [31].

3.2.2. Benzoyl peroxide

Benzoyl peroxide (BP) is one of the most common topical preparations with varying concentrations of 2.5–10%. There are many forms of BP such as cream, lotion, gel, wash, and pledgets. BP is a powerful antimicrobial agent. By decreasing the hydrolysis of triglycerides and generation of reactive oxygen species within the follicle, it has bactericidal effect. Moreover, bacterial resistance does not develop against that antimicrobial agent. That makes it an ideal combination for topical or systemic antibiotic therapy. But it is in FDA category C should be used during pregnancy on a limited area and only if needed [32].

3.2.3. Salicylic acid

Salicyclic acid is a comedolytic and anti inflammatory agent which is commonly found in many over the counter and prescription acne preparations. It is FDA pregnancy category C. Although there are no human studies on topical salicylic acid usage during pregnancy, there is no report of teratogenicity as well. It is usage may be limited with facial washes or cleansers to avoid long exposure and systemic absorption during pregnancy [31].

3.2.4. Glycolic acid

Glycolic acid is an alpha-hydroxy acid with keratolytic effect and used in the treatment of mild, comedogenic, and noninflammatory acne by its comedolytic effect. It also reduces sebum production [33]. There is no FDA pregnancy category assigned for glycolic acid but glycolic acid peels have been used extensively, and apparently safely in pregnancy [31].

3.2.5. Sulfacetamide with sulfur compounds

Sulfacetamide is a bacteriostatic agent that inhibits bacterial growth via inhibition of dihydropteroate synthetase with additional anti-inflammatory action from additional sulfur compounds [34]. Sulfur has been used for many years for treating pregnant women suffering from scabies with sulfur-containing ointments on a whole body surface with no adverse results. Although elemental sulfur, typically compounded in cream or ointment form, is considered safe in pregnancy; there are minimal data about safety of sulfacetamide during pregnancy.

3.2.6. Topical antibiotics

Many topical antibiotics can be used in the treatment of acne for their effect on *P. acnes*. In general, if a systemic antibiotic is considered safe in pregnancy, its topical formulation is also deemed safe. Topical agents are often added to oral antibiotics because of synergistic effects [13]. Erythromycin and clindamycin are the most commonly used topical antibiotics for acne. Both erythromycin and clindamycin are category B. They have bactericidal effect on *P. acnes*, reduce pro-inflammatory free fatty acids and have anti-inflammatory effect. However, antibiotic resistance to *P. acnes* is a very frequent problem. Results of many studies denote combination of these antibiotics with different concentrations of BP are suggested to overcome this problem [31].

Metronidazole is also an antiinflammatory, immunosuppressive, and antimicrobial properties. In a study, 2% metronidazole gel was shown to be effective for moderate acne vulgaris [35]. It is in FDA pregnancy categorize B. Also, an investigation of metronidazole usage during pregnancy revealed no association with preterm birth, low birth weight, or congenital anomalies [36].

Tetracyclines are also commonly used topical acne preparations in non-pregnant patients. Even though they have a broad-spectrum bacteriostatic activity, their use in pregnancy is not suggested as they cross the placenta and bind strongly to calcium ions. After the 16th week of pregnancy, these can result in deciduous teeth discoloration and bone growth inhibition [20].

3.2.7. Topical retinoids

Topical retinoids are commonly used in acne treatment especially in comedogenic and inflammatory forms as they have anti-comedonegic, anti-inflammatory effects and normalize desquamation of the follicular epithelium. Three topical retinoids are currently available: adapalene, tretinoin, and tazarotene. Adapalene and tretinoin are pregnancy category C while tazarotene is category X. Tazoretene cannot be used in pregnancy. However, the data about the systemic absorption and teratogenity of adapalene and tretinoin are limited. There are case reports describing retinoid embryopathy, specifically ear, cerebral, and cardiac malformations in infants who were exposed to retinoids in utero, due to maternal topical tretinoin usage [37–41]. But some other studies did not reveal a significantly increased risk associated with topical tretinoin [42–44]. In one retrospective case control study of 235 pregnant women exposed to topical retinoids in the first trimester (including adapalene, tretinoin, tazarotene, and retinol) were evaluated for fetal embryopathy and were compared with 444 controls. No significant difference was reported between the groups regarding the rate of spontaneous abortion, minor or major birth defects; including retinoid teratogenity [45]. However, study authors concluded that topical retinoids could not be safely recommended for use during pregnancy because of the inferred risk based on safety data associated with systemic retinoid medications. Still, topical retinoids cannot be advised for use during pregnancy [32].

3.3. Phototherapy and lasers

Various forms of phototherapy and lasers are under investigation for their use in treating acne vulgaris and some of them have already been FDA approved for the treatment of some forms of acne. As ultraviolet light has been reported to be beneficial by most of the patients, studies focused on mechanisms and using light as a treatment option [31]. Both visible and laser light are effective treatments for acne. Visible light and many lasers target porphyrins endogenously produced by *P. acnes*. Laser and light therapies have few if any side effects and appear to be safe during pregnancy. Ultimately, combining laser and light with topical therapy may well become the mainstay of acne treatment [46].

The main devices used for acne treatments are lasers (pulse dye lasers (PDL), potassium titanyl phosphate lasers (KTP), infrared diode lasers) and intense pulsed light systems (IPL), broad-spectrum of visible light sources (blue light, blue-red light), and photodynamic therapy (PDT). The supposed mechanisms of action for optical treatments are photothermal heating of sebaceous glands and photochemical inactivation of *P. acnes*, which produces coproporphyrins and protoporphyrins. Moreover, photoimmunological reactions may possibly contribute to improve acne [47].

Narrowband-ultraviolet B phototherapy (NB-UVB) has been reported as a treatment for acne in pregnancy with its local immunosuppressive effects on skin. In one case report, a successful treatment with NBUVB treatment of acne vulgaris in a woman who was 5 months pregnant was reported [48]. The data regarding the safety of NBUVB treatment in pregnant women comes from its use in pregnant psoriasis patients. But recently it has been shown that patients with high cumulative NBUVB doses have a decrease in serum folic acid levels [49]. This finding is especially important for the pregnant women as they usually need folic acid supplementation to prevent neural tube defects. During treatment period dermatologists should be aware of the folic acid levels, check regularly and cooperate with the obstetrician of the patient.

4. Rosacea in pregnancy

Acne Rosacea is a chronic inflammatory condition of the facial skin affecting the blood vessels and pilosebaceous units. Patients usually present with red papules pustules on the face in addition to complaints of flushing, blushing, and sensitivity of skin [50]. It may manifest as papules and pustules as well as other forms such as centrofacial distribution of blushing and telangiectasia (erythematotelangiectatic rosacea), phymatous changes, or ocular rosacea [4].

Similar to acne, the course of rosacea in pregnancy is unpredictable. There are a limited number of case studies related with the course of rosacea during pregnancy. But, as there are reports about rosacea fulminans in pregnancy, it should be taken into consideration by means of prognosis. Rosacea fulminans is a rare and severe subtype of rosacea that is characterized by the sudden onset of severe facial inflammation consisting of numerous pustules, cystic swellings and coalescing sinuses. Three cases of RF in pregnancy were reported with differing obstetric outcomes: an intrauterine death, a termination of pregnancy, and a normal vaginal delivery [51]. Rosacea fulminans is the only indication for topical or systemic corticosteroids in the treatment of rosacea [52]. One case of RF in pregnancy successfully treatment with systemic azithromycin and topical metronidazole [53]. Another patient with RF in pregnancy presented with severe ocular disease culminating in ocular perforation [54]. A case of pregnant woman who had rosacea fulminans during the first trimester presented and treated with conventional therapeutic approaches with systemic corticosteroids were associated with clear improvement within 2 months, and subsequently only 0.75% metronidazole topical cream was used during the second trimester [55]. One patient with rosacea fulminans in pregnancy was complicated by stillbirth [56].

Generally the treatment of rosacea during pregnancy relies the avoiding triggering factors such as sun exposure, wind, physical irritation, anxiety and spicy food, as so as in the non pregnants. In pregnancy, general safety precautions are the same with acne medications. Azelaic acid and topical antibiotics, including metronidazole, clindamycin, and erythromycin, may be used for treating papulopustular rosacea. In the erythematotelangiectatic form light based therapies such as lasers can be used [57]. But a delay in their use is suggested as the condition may improve spontaneously after delivery [4].

5. Perioral dermatitis in pregnancy

Perioral dermatitis is also should be differentiated from acne vulgaris. It is an acneiform eruption of unknown etiology. Fluorinated topical corticosteroids, contact dermatitis, and over moisturization of skin were implicated in the etiology. Clinical appearance is papulopustular lesions as clusters localizing periorally (on the chin or nasolabial folds, but not on the vermilion border of the lips) with an erythematous base [58]. There are few data about the perioral dermatitis in pregnancy. Yang et al. emphasizes flares to have been noted, but not as a regular finding [4]. Treatment with topical and oral agents is the same as that of acne vulgaris or rosacea.

6. Hidradenitis suppurativa in pregnancy

Hidradenitis suppurativa/acne inversa (HS) is a chronic, inflammatory, recurrent and debilitating skin disease of the terminal follicular epithelium caused by occlusion and rupture of follicular units with subsequent inflammation of the apocrine glands [4]. It is destructive in nature and manifests as painful inflammatory nodules and sterile abscesses located in hair and apocrine gland-bearing skin creases in the axilla; groin or perineum, buttocks, and/or breast [59]. The disease often progresses with the formation of draining sinus tracts and due to subcutaneous extension with induration, destruction of skin appendages, and subsequent scarring [2, 60]. The etiology of the disease seems to be multifactorial and is only fragmentarily understood. The role of hormones in HS remains unclear, but the female predominance, typical onset of the disease after puberty, observation of premenstrual flares, and improvement during pregnancy and the traditionally described resolution after menopause suggest a hormonal/metabolic background [61, 62]. However, as some patients experience improvement and some other worsening in pregnancy. A typical relationship between HS and pregnancy has not been confirmed. A literature review presents two cases of women who had improvement or remission of their disease during pregnancy with some rebound symptoms postpartum supporting this hormonal effect [63]. The condition is associated with hyperandrogenism and often is accompanied by acne, hirsutism, and irregular menses. The reported positive effects of antiandrogen therapy supports a possible role of androgens [64]. Another study showed no evidence of biochemical hyperandrogenism in HS, noting both persistence and primary development of the disease in the postmenopausal state [65]. Findings, therefore, remain inconsistent. Obesity contributes significantly to HS pathogenesis; diabetes, dyslipidemia, the metabolic syndrome, and polycystic ovarian syndrome are among the commonest comorbidities. More studies are required to clarify a potential hormonal dysregulation in HS [61].

One of the first staging systems for HS was proposed by Hurley (**Table 2**). Hurley separated patients into three groups based largely on the presence and extent of cicatrization and sinuses [66].

Management of HS includes emotional support, given the debilitating nature of the disease; counseling to wear loose fitting clothing to avoid aggravating the areas. For patients with Hurley stage I, antibiotics are a good first-line therapy. The same oral antibiotics mentioned for acne as well as oral clindamycin can help during pregnancy and provide antiinflammatory effects. Limited lesions can be injected with corticosteroids, and flares can be addressed with short courses of oral or intramuscular corticosteroids. Patients with Hurley stage II,

Hurley stage	Extent of disease in tissue
I	Abscess formation (single or multiple) without sinus tracts and cicatrization
II	One or more widely separated recurrent abscesses with tract formation and scars
III	Multiple interconnected tracts and abscesses throughout an entire area

Table 2. Hurley staging system for hidradenitis suppurativa.

long-term immunosuppressive therapy or surgical therapies, such as limited excisions or the laying open of sinus tracts, may be helpful. Patients with Hurley stage III may have such debilitating disease that only surgery can adequately address their symptoms. Wide excision of all the patients' affected tissue and the underlying sinus tracts is the most effective treatment for these patients [67]. The use of TNF-α inhibitors in pregnancy remains controversial, and biologic medications should be used only if benefit greatly outweighs the risks and all other treatment options have been exhausted [68].

Author details

Asli Feride Kaptanoglu[1]* and Didem Mullaaziz[2]

*Address all correspondence to: dr.aslikaptanoglu@gmail.com

1 Marmara University Medical Faculty, Department of Dermatology and Venereology, İstanbul, Turkey

2 Department of Dermatology and Venereology, Near East University, Lefkoşe, North Cyprus

References

[1] Schaller M, Plewig G. Structure and function of eccrine, apocrine, apoeccrine and sebaceous glands. In: Dermatology. Bolognia JL, Jorizzo JL, Rapini RP (eds). Edinburgh: Mosby; 2003. pp. 525–86.

[2] Lowenstein EB, Lowenstein EJ. Glandular changes. In: Text Atlas of Obstetric Dermatology. Kroumpouzos G (ed). Philadelphia, PA: Lippincott Williams & Wilkins; 2013. pp. 47–56.

[3] Durmazlar SPK, Eskioğlu F. Cosmetic procedures in pregnancy: review. Turkiye Klinikleri J Med Sci. 2008;28(6):942–6

[4] Yang CS, Teeple M, Muglia J, Robinson-Bostom L. Inflammatory and glandular skin disease in pregnancy. Clin Dermatol. 2016;34(3):335–43.

[5] Chien AL, Qi J, Rainer B, Sachs DL, Helfrich YR. Treatment of acne in pregnancy. J Am Board Fam Med. 2016;29(2):254–62.

[6] Ratzer MA. The influence of marriage, pregnancy and childbirth on acne vulgaris. Br J Dermatol. 1964;76:165–8.

[7] Shaw JC, White LE. Persistent acne in adult women. Arch Dermatol. 2001;137:1252–3.

[8] Van Pelt HP, Juhlin L. Acne conglobata after pregnancy. Acta Derm Venereol. 1999;79:169.

[9] Das G, Eligar VS, Govindan J, Rees DA. Late presentation of hyperandrogenism in pregnancy: clinical features and differential diagnosis. Endocrinol Diabetes Metab Case Rep. 2013;2013:130048. doi:10.1530/EDM-13-0048.

[10] Moloney FJ, Collins S, Gillian MM. Sunscreens: safety, efficacy and appropriate use. Am J Clin Dermatol. 2002;3:185–91.

[11] Palm MD, O'Donoghue MN. Update on photoprotection. Dermatol Ther. 2007;20:360–76.

[12] Kubba R, Bajaj AK, Thappa DM, Sharma R, Vedamurthy M, Dhar S, Criton S. Acne in pregnancy. Indian J Dermatol Venereol Leprol. 2009;75(suppl 1):59.

[13] Pugashetti R, Shinkai K. Treatment of acne vulgaris in pregnant patients. Dermatol Ther. 2013;26:302–11.

[14] US Food and Drug Administration. List of pregnancy exposure registries [online]. http://www.fda.gov/scienceresearch/specialtopics/womenshealthresearch/ucm134848.htm (Accessed September 27, 2016)

[15] Meredith FM, Ormerod AD. The management of acne vulgaris in pregnancy. Am J Clin Dermatol. 2013;14:351–8.

[16] Loureiro KD, Kao KK, Jones KL, et al. Minor malformations characteristic of the retinoic acid embryopathy and other birth outcomes in children of women exposed to topical tretinoin during early pregnancy. Am J Med Genet. 2005;136(2):117–21.

[17] Dai WS, Hsu MA, Itri LM. Safety of pregnancy after discontinuation of isotretinoin. Arch Dermatol. 1989;125:362–5.

[18] Ozyurt S, Kaptanoglu AF. Systemic isotretinoin treatment and pregnancy: a longitudinal cohort study from Turkey. Eurasian J Med. 2015;47(3):179–83.

[19] Dreno B, Bettoli V, Ochsendorf F, et al. European recommendations on the use of oral antibiotics for acne. Eur J Dermatol. 2004;14:391–9.

[20] Padberg S. Anti-infective agents. In: Drugs During Pregnancy and Lactation: Treatment Options and Risk Assessment. Schaefer C, Peters P, Miller RK, et al. (eds). 3rd ed. Munich: Elsevier; 2015. pp. 116–62.

[21] Hernandez S, Werler MM, Walker AM, et al. Folic acid antagonists during pregnancy and the risk of birth defects. N Engl J Med. 2000;343:1608–14.

[22] Romøren M, Lindbæk M, Nordeng H. Pregnancy outcome after gestational exposure to erythromycin: a population-based register study from Norway. Br J Clin Pharmacol. 2012;74:1053–62.

[23] Kus S, Yucelten D, Aytug A. Comparison of efficacy of azithromycin vs. doxycycline in the treatment of acne vulgaris. Clin Exp Dermatol. 2005;30(3):215–20.

[24] Hayashi N, Kawashima M. Efficacy of oral antibiotics on acne vulgaris and their effects on quality of life: a multicenter randomized controlled trial using minocycline, roxithromycin and faropenem. J Dermatol. 2011;38(2):111–9.

[25] Tedesco FJ, Barton RW, Alpers DH. Clindamycin-associated colitis: a prospective study. Ann Intern Med. 1974;81:429–33

[26] Kong YL, Tey HL. Treatment of acne vulgaris during pregnancy and lactation. Drugs. 2013;73(8):779–87.

[27] Martinez-Frıas ML, Bermejo E, Rodrıguez-Pinilla E, et al. Periconceptional exposure to contraceptive pills and risk for Down syndrome. J Perinatol. 2001;21(5):288–92.

[28] James KA, Burkhart CN, Morrell DS. Emerging drugs for acne. Expert Opin Emerg Drugs. 2009;14(4):649–59.

[29] Katsambas A, Dessinioti C. New and emerging treatments in dermatology: acne. Dermatol Ther. 2008;21(2):86–95 (Review).

[30] Dreno B, Blouin E. Acne, pregnant women and zinc salts: a literature review. Ann Dermatol Venereol. 2008;135(1):27–33.

[31] Zaenglein AL, Graber E, Thiboutot DM, Strauss JS. Acne vulgaris and acneiform eruptions. In: Fitzpatricks Dermatology in General medicine. Wolff K, Goldsmith LA, Ktaz SI, Gilchrest BA, Paller AS, Lefell DJ (eds). 7th ed. Mc Graw Hill, New York. pp. 690–712.

[32] Horev L. How to treat acne in pregnant women?. Curr Derm Rep. 2014;3:135–40

[33] Kaminaka C, Uede M, Matsunaka H, Furukawa F, Yamomoto Y. Clinical evaluation of glycolic acid chemical peeling in patients with acne vulgaris: a randomized, double-blind, placebo-controlled, split-face comparative study. Dermatol Surg. 2014;40(3):314–22.

[34] Kalla G, Garg A, Kachhawa D. Chemical peeling. Glycolic acid versus trichloroacetic acid in melasma. Indian J Dermatol Venereol Leprol. 2001;67:82–4.

[35] Mays RM, Gordon RA, Wilson JM, et al. New antibiotic therapies for acne and rosacea. Dermatol Ther. 2012;25:23–37.

[36] Khodaeiani E, Fouladi RF, Yousefi N, Amirnia M, Babaeinejad S, Shokri J. Efficacy of 2% metronidazole gel in moderate acne vulgaris. Indian J Dermatol. 2012;57(4):279–81.

[37] Koss CA, Baras DC, Lane SD, Aubry R, Marcus M, Markowitz LE, et al. Investigation of metronidazole use during pregnancy and adverse birth outcomes. Antimicrob Agents Chemother. 2012;56(9):4800–5.

[38] Camera G, Pregliasco P. Ear malformation in baby born to mother using tretinoin cream. Lancet. 1992;339(8794):687.

[39] Colley SM, Walpole I, Fabian VA, et al. Topical tretinoin and fetal malformations. Med J Aust. 1998;168(9):467.

[40] Lipson AH, Collins F, Webster WS. Multiple congenital defects associated with maternal use of topical tretinoin. Lancet. 1993;341(8856):1352–3.

[41] Navarre-Belhassen C, Blanchet P, Hillaire-Buys D, et al. Multiple congenital malformations associated with topical tretinoin. Ann Pharmacother. 1998;32(4):505–6.

[42] Selcen D, Seidman S, Nigro MA. Otocerebral anomalies associated with topical tretinoin use. Brain Dev. 2000;22(4):218–20.

[43] Jick SS, Terris BZ, Jick H. First trimester topical tretinoin and congenital disorders. Lancet. 1993;341(8854):1181–2.

[44] Shapiro L, Pastuszak A, Curto G, et al. Safety of first-trimester exposure to topical tretinoin: prospective cohort study. Lancet. 1997;350(9085):1143–4.

[45] Panchaud A, Csajka C, Merlob P, et al. Pregnancy outcome following exposure to topical retinoids: a multicenter prospective study. J Clin Pharmacol. 2012;42:1844–51.

[46] Nestor MS, Swenson N, Macri A. Physical modalities (devices) in the management of acne. Dermatol Clin. 2016;34(2):215–23.

[47] Haedersdal M, Togsverd-Bo K, Wulf HC. Evidence-based review of lasers, light sources and photodynamic therapy in the treatment of acne vulgaris. Eur Acad Dermatol Venereol. 2008;22(3):267–78.

[48] Zeichner J. Narrowband UVB phototherapy for the treatment of acne vulgaris during pregnancy. Arch Dermatol. 2011;147:537–9.

[49] El-Saie LT, Rabie AR, Kamel MI, et al. Effect of narrowband ultraviolet B phototherapy on serum folic acid levels in patients with psoriasis. Lasers Med Sci. 2011;26(4):481–5.

[50] Culp B, Scheinfeld N. Rosacea: a review. P T. 2009;34:38–45.

[51] Jarrett R, Gonsalves R, Anstey AV. Differing obstetric outcomes of rosacea fulminans in pregnancy: report of three cases with review of pathogenesis and management. Clin Exp Dermatol. 2010;35(8):888–91

[52] Jansen T, Plewig G, Kligman AM. Diagnosis and treatment of rosacea fulminans. Dermatology. 1994;188:251–4.

[53] Fuentelsaz V, Ara M, Corredera C, Lezcano V, Juberias P, Carapeto FJ. Rosacea fulminans in pregnancy: successful treatment with azithromycin. Clin Exp Dermatol. 2011;36(6):674–6.

[54] de Morais e Silva FA, Bonassi M, Steiner D, da Cunha TV. Rosacea fulminans in pregnancy with ocular perforation. J Dtsch Dermatol Ges. 2011;9(7):542–3.

[55] Ferahbas A, Utas S, Mistik S, Uksal U, Peker D. Rosacea fulminans in pregnancy: case report and review of the literature. Am J Clin Dermatol. 2006;7(2):141–4.

[56] Lewis VJ, Holme SA, Wright A, Anstey AV. Rosacea fulminans in pregnancy. Br J Dermatol. 2004;151(4):917–9.

[57] Van Zuuren EJ, Fedorowicz Z, Carter B, van der Linden MMD, Charland L. Interventions for rosacea. Cochrane Database Syst Rev. 2015;4:CD003262.

[58] Malik R, Quirk CJ. Topical applications and perioral dermatitis. Australas J Dermatol. 2000;41:34–8.

[59] Smith HS, Chao JD, Teitelbaum J. Painful hidradenitis suppurativa. Clin J Pain. 2010; 26(5):435–44.

[60] Oumeish OY, Al-Fouzan AW. Miscellaneous diseases affected by pregnancy. Clin Dermatol. 2006;24(2):113–7.

[61] Karagiannidis I, Nikolakis G, Zouboulis CC. Endocrinologic aspects of hidradenitis suppurativa. Dermatol Clin. 2016;34(1):45–9.

[62] Yu CC, Cook MG. Hidradenitis suppurativa: a disease of follicular epithelium, rather than apocrine glands. Br J Dermatol. 1990;122:763–9.

[63] Cornbleet T. Pregnancy and apocrine diseases: hidradenitis, Fox-Fordyce disease. Arch Dermatol Syph. 1952;65:12–9.

[64] Mortimer PS, Dawber RP, Gales MA, et al. Mediation of hidradenitis suppurativa by androgens. Br Med J (Clind Res Ed). 1986;292:245–8.

[65] Barth JH, Layton AM, Cunliffe WJ. Endocrine factors in pre- and postmenopausal women with hidradenitis suppurativa. Br J Dermatol. 1996;134:1057–9.

[66] Hurley H. Dermatologic surgery, principles and practice. New York: Marcel Dekker; 1989.

[67] Alikhan A, Lynch PJ, Eisen DB. Hidradenitis suppurativa: a comprehensive review. J Am Acad Dermatol. 2009;60(4):539–61.

[68] Gupta AK, Studholme C. Adalimumab (Humira) for the treatment of hidradenitis suppurativa. Skin Therapy Lett. 2016;21(4):1–4.

Chapter 7

Acneiform Papulopustular Eruptions in Behçet's Disease

Sevgi Akarsu and Işıl Kamberoğlu

Additional information is available at the end of the chapter

http://dx.doi.org/10.5772/65732

Abstract

Behcet's disease (BD) is a multisystemic inflammatory vasculitic disorder which diagnosed by clinical criteria because of the lack of specific laboratory test and/or pathognomonic histopathological findings. The most frequent diagnostic criteria of this disease are mucocutaneous lesions, appearing at the disease onset or during the course, usually begin before significant organ dysfunction. According to BD International Study Group Criteria, one of the five criteria is dermatologic findings including pseudofolliculitis, acneiform nodules or papulopustular lesions (PPL) diagnosed by clinician in postadolescent patients. In some case reports and clinical studies, the PPL of BD are also denoted as Behcet's pustulosis, folliculitis, acneiform eruptions and pseudofolliculitis. Owing to implementation of follicular lesions in these criteria, there may be difficulties in the distinction between most of the PPL of BD and the other acneiform eruptions/nonspecific follicular lesions (e.g., acne vulgaris, bacterial folliculitis, steroid acne). Certainly, clinicians should distinguish these patterns for accurate diagnosis. Although earlier studies involve numerous quandaries regarding the diagnostic histopathologic pattern of BD (e.g., whether to include vasculitis or nonspecific folliculitis), it was reported recently that the determination of vasculitic changes in histopathological and direct immunofluorescence results might be useful in the differential diagnosis of patients suspected to have BD.

Keywords: Behcet's disease, acneiform eruption, papulopustular lesion, pseudofolliculitis

1. Introduction

Acneiform eruptions have a broad clinical spectrum, where they differ via lesion location and morphology. Certainly, clinicians should distinguish these patterns for accurate diagnosis. One of the differential diagnoses in acneiform papulopustular lesions (PPL) is Behcet's disease (BD), and it should have been firstly recognized, particularly around the Silk Route region [1, 2].

BD is a multisystemic vasculitic disorder that is characterized by recurrent oral aphthous ulcerations, genital ulcerations, mucocutaneous manifestations, uveitis, and a positive pathergy test. Additionally, later studies showed that the vasculitic pattern has shown articular, gastrointestinal, urogenital, neurological, pulmonary, and cardiac involvement. This disease has a chronic course with unpredictable exacerbations and remissions [1, 3, 4].

In 1937, Prof. Dr. Hulusi Behcet (1889–1948), who was a great scientist and the first professor in Turkey, diagnosed this disease as a trisymptom complex consisting of aphthous ulcerations, genital ulcerations, and ocular involvement. In the ancient literature, some authors named the disease as Adamantiades-Behcet disease. Adamantiades was an ophthalmologist who insisted on "relapsing iritis with hypopyon" in BD. Prof. Dr. Hulusi Behcet insisted on a complex multisystemic synonym, not only ocular involvement. As an honor to Turkish Medical history, the disease was renamed as "Maladie de Behcet," as it is known today [5].

BD is mainly distributed along the Silk Route region, with higher prevalence in the Mediterranean, the Middle East, and the Far East countries. Turkey has the highest prevalence, with about 80–370 cases per 10^5 population. This disease usually begins around the third or fourth decade of life. Globally, female and male distribution rates are equal. Although, if we want to categorize by geographical areas, BD shows male predominance in some Middle Eastern and Mediterranean countries and female predominance in Japan and Korea. Male predominance and young onset usually have worse prognosis [1, 6].

The etiology of BD has not yet been fully elucidated, but the strongest genetic susceptibility is HLAB51 or HLAB5. It has been demonstrated that in some studies, herpes simplex virus and streptococcus sanguinis/pyogenes activate innate and adaptive immunity so that a neutrophilic vasculitic reaction occurs. Additionally, some authors reported that interleukin (IL)-23 and IL-12 share p40 subunits and induce the IL17 pathway. Induced IL-17 and T-helper 17 levels activate oral ulcerations, genital ulcerations, and articular involvements [1, 7].

2. Diagnosis/classification criteria for BD

Due to a lack of distinctive diagnostic laboratory tests, the diagnosis of BD is based on certain clinical criteria. From onset of the disease, diagnosis time has taken approximately 8 years. Based on that, several criteria have been established during the years, all consist of three major criteria, including oral ulceration, genital ulceration, and eye lesions [1, 8, 9].

First of all, in 1969, Mason and Barnes identified major criteria (oral ulceration, genital ulceration, eye lesions, skin lesions) and minor criteria (gastrointestinal lesions, thrombophlebitis, cardiovascular lesions, arthritis, central nervous system lesions, family history), and then suggested that to make the diagnosis of BD, a minimum of three major, or two major and two minor criteria were required [10]. After that, in 1972, the Behcet's Disease Research Committee of Japan answered with a different set of criteria more suitable for their population. In order to get a new point of view, O'Duffy [11] published another criteria in 1974 for Japanese national criteria [12].

In 1990, criteria that were later accepted worldwide were developed by an International Study Group at the fourth International Conference on BD in London. The most specific and sensitive

Major criteria	BD diagnosis	Minor criteria
Recurrent oral ulceration	Major criteria plus any two of the minor criteria	**Recurrent genital ulceration**
Minor aphthous, major aphthous, or herpetiform ulceration observed by physician or patient recurring at least three times in one 12-month period		Aphthous ulceration or scarring observed by physician or patient
		Eye lesions
		Anterior uveitis, posterior uveitis, cells in the vitreous on slit-lamp examination; or retinal vasculitis observed by ophthalmologist
		Skin lesions
		Erythema nodosum observed by the physician or patient; pseudofolliculitis or papulopustular lesions; or acneiform nodules observed by physician in postadolescent patients not on corticosteroid treatment
		Pathergy test
		Test interpreted as positive by physician at 24–48 hours

Table 1. International Study Group diagnostic criteria of Behcet's diseasexs.

guide that clinicians have used globally for years is demonstrated in **Table 1**. To make BD diagnosis, the presence of major and two minor criteria is considered to be adequate [13].

Lastly, International Criteria for Behcet's Disease was also renewed in 2010, which is occasionally prevalent in Iran. In this point score system, the criteria (ocular lesions, genital aphthous ulcerations, and oral aphthous ulcerations, each of them 2 points; skin lesions, neurological manifestations, vascular manifestations, and positive pathergy test, each of them 1 point; and scoring ≤4 indicates BD) should not be seen as a part of universal agreement but also have chance to criticize the sensitive ones [8].

Among the many quandaries, the International Study Group criteria and the International Criteria for Behcet's Disease were configured in different cohorts. Davatchi et al. analyzed Iranian BD patients by using the International Study Group criteria versus International Criteria for Behcet's Disease. These authors found that International Criteria for Behcet's Disease sensitivity was 98.2% (78.1% with International Study Group criteria), the specificity was 95.6% (98.8% with International Study Group criteria), and the accuracy was 97.3% (85.5% with International Study Group criteria) [14]. Moreover, Leonardo and McNeil mentioned that the International Criteria for Behcet's disease has higher sensitivity and less specificity due to the fact that they evaluated data from 27 countries. They also said that those studies emphasized that International Criteria for Behcet's Disease can be an easier tool for diagnosis but also may cause overdiagnosis [6].

3. Clinical features of BD

As we mentioned before, the constant diagnostic feature of BD is oral ulcerations. Additionally, other factors occasionally depend on the dermatologist. Thus, mucocutaneous lesions are a "hallmark of the disease." Oral ulcerations are the most common manifestation, followed by genital ulcerations, mucocutaneous lesions, skin pathergy reaction, and articular and ocular involvement [1, 9].

Recurrent oral aphthous ulcerations are the most common and significant criteria in diagnosis, constituting "fingerprint" of BD. They are characterized by painful ulcerations in non-keratinized mucous membranes such as lips, tongue, gingiva, buccal mucosa or vestibulum. Typically, oral aphthous ulcerations have recurred at least three times over a 1-year period. On the onset of the lesion, slightly elevated erythematous area with a vesiculopustular lesion that changed to an ulceration with well-defined borders and greyish yellow necrotic base in 24–48 hours. Oral ulcerations can be divided into three types: minor, major, and herpetiform. Major and herpetiform types may cause scarring formation [9, 15].

Genital ulcerations are the second most common clinical finding and are similar to oral ulcerations. Mostly, it begins with fragile papule or nodule, after that becomes ulceration area. They are usually located in labia minor, labia major, and vagina for women, and penis and scrotum in men. They are seen as deeper lesions and also heal slowly with scarring. The patients also have fistulas between urethra and bladder that may cause dyspareunia, severe pain, and difficulty of urination [1, 2, 9].

The most common type of mucocutaneous features is PPL. In addition, these lesions may occasionally occur following erythema nodosum-like lesions, superficial thrombophlebitis, skin pathergy test, extragenital ulceration, and Sweet's syndrome-like lesions. Subungual infarctions, hemorrhagic bullae, furuncles, abscesses and acral purpuric papulonodular lesions and also pyoderma gangrenosum-like lesions, erythema multiforme-like lesions, pernio-like cutaneous lesions, Henoch-Schsönlein purpura and bullous necrotizing vasculitis can also be seen in some case reports of BD [1, 9, 15].

4. PPL in BD

In some case reports and clinical studies, the PPL of BD are also denoted as Behcet's pustulosis, folliculitis, acneiform eruptions, and pseudofolliculitis. Clinicians may find papules, pustules, nodules, and also comedones in some BD patients [16–20]. It usually starts as a papule with erythematous base that changes to a pustule in 24–48 hours (**Figure 1**). The PPL of BD mainly stay on the trunk and extremities, except for the palms and soles, where there is a surplus sebum production and hair follicle, but also similar to acne vulgaris they have been occasionally seen on the face. As a point of view, pustules are common in both diseases but microbiological specimens are not similar so that it could be a clue for differential diagnosis [7, 21].

Since BD is a neutrophilic dermatosis, histopathologic findings of PPL include neutrophilic vasculitis and both of the lymphocytic and leukocytoclastic types in late onset, together. However, some authors found only perifollicular and perivascular mononuclear, or neutrophilic infiltrations in PPL of BD; they could not detect vasculitis [22–27].

BD is an autoinflammatory disease that is qualified by primary dysfunction of the innate and adaptive immune system such as neutrophil hyper-reactivity and T-lymphocytes hypersensitivity to some antigens. In some research studies, increased cytokine and chemokine

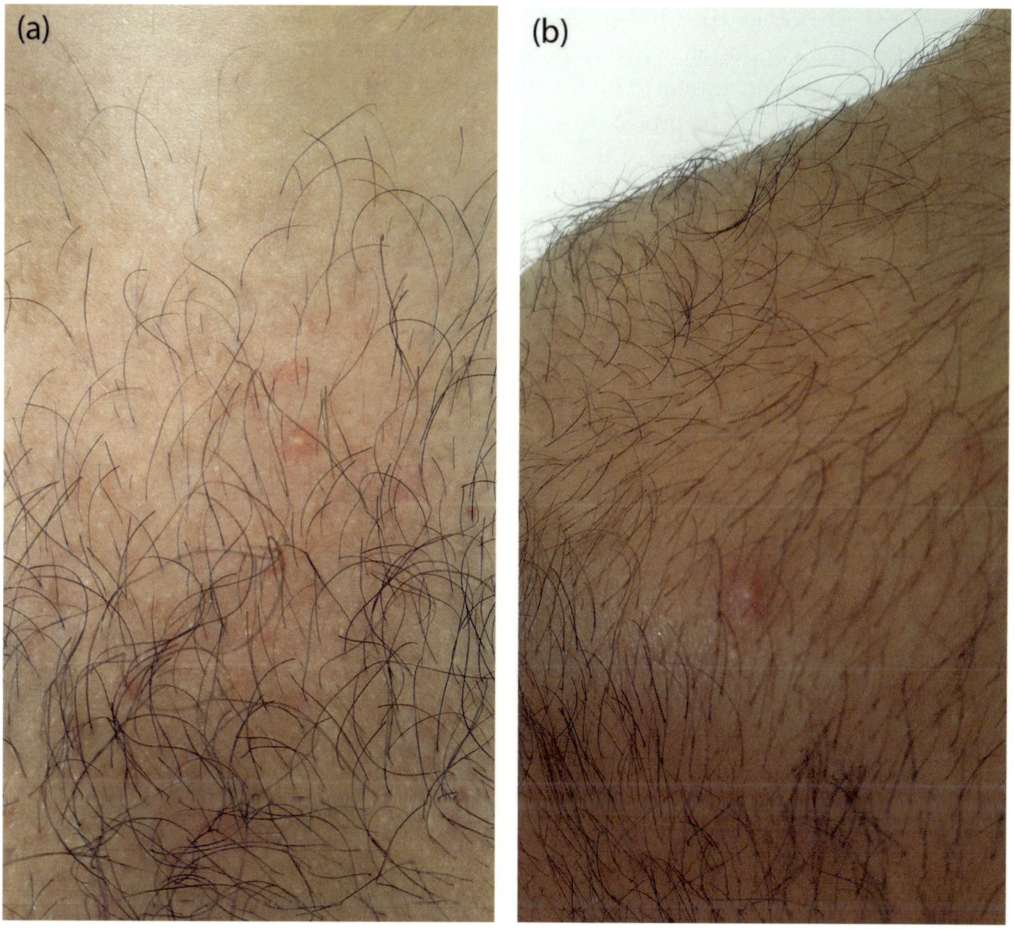

Figure 1. (a) Erythematous papulopustular lesions on chest region (upper trunk) and (b) erythematous papulopustular lesions on pectoral region (upper trunk).

levels are also found in blood samples. Nonetheless, the mechanism underlying these skin lesions remained elusive. Furthermore, investigations have continued during years in order to explain the immunological mechanism. In the beginning in adaptive immune system, cytotoxic T-lymphocytes have been demonstrated as significant effector cells in BD. Cytotoxic T-lymphocytes have been expressed granulysin, which is a cytolytic granule protein. Yamasaki et al. investigated granulysin levels in mucocutaneous lesions of BD by ELISA technique. They found strong expression of granulysin levels in CD4+ and CD8+ T-lymphocytes infiltrating acne-like eruptions. As a result, they suspect that granulysin positive cytotoxic T-lymphocytes may have a significant role in the pathogenetic mechanism for acneiform eruptions [28]. At genetic levels, it is known to have common associations with higher HLA B51 subtypes. Park et al. determined the association of a certain polymorphism (C438T) of the *SUMO4* gene with HLA B51 positive BD patients in Korea. Small ubiquitin-like modifier has been referred as SUMO4 that downregulate the transcription activity of nuclear factor–kappa B. They found that the C438T polymorphism in the *SUMO4* gene is associated with a significantly increased risk of PPL in HLA-B51-positive BD patients [29]. Moreover, Demirseren et al. configured out the association between the subtypes of HLA-B51. Much interesting data are HLA-B5109 subtype was found to be less frequent in patients with PPL in BD. Thus, the HLA-B5109 subtype could be protective against acneiform eruptions [30]. Finally, Cho et al. detected the immunophenotypes of the common BD-related skin lesions and evaluated the expression of cytokines and composition of the infiltrating cells. In PPL, neutrophils were the most commonly infiltrated type and followed by CD8+ T cells, despite the fact that it was not found as statistically significant. Also, percentage of CD8+ T cells was significantly more than FoxP3.These authors recognized that IL-4 levels were also higher than the interferon (IFN) levels so that the adaptive immune system plays a major role in PPL [31].

4.1. Frequency of PPL in BD

In the diagnosis of BD, the primary aim is to find early diagnostic clues to prevent systemic involvement. For dermatologists, PPL has significant role in these diagnostic criteria. According to International Study Group, data of the chosen patients demonstrated as sensitivity and specificity of these lesions were 70% and 76%, respectively [13]. However, the sensitivity and specificity of PPL were found to be 96% and 11% by Alpsoy et al., so it depends on the experience of the clinician. They suggested that PPL is very sensitive but not specific, so the location of lesions is more important for differentiation from other diseases [22].

Based on a literature review, it may be said that the frequencies of PPL in BD patients range from 12% to 96%, varying greatly from country to country, as demonstrated in **Table 2**. [14, 16–20, 22, 29, 30, 32–46]. There are many studies consisting BD patients in Turkey, which is one of the most common country in terms of BD frequency varying between 39.6% and 75% [22, 30, 34–37, 41, 42]. National-based surveys were evaluated to understand the global pattern of the disease. Some authors analyzed five nationwide surveys of BD in Iran with 5059 patients, Japan with 3316 patients, China with 1996 patients, Korea with 1527 patients, and Germany with 590 patients. It was shown that PPL have varying proportion in terms of incidence in different regions, such as 62% in Germany, 57% in Iran, and 31% in China. These results were interpreted to mean that immigrations have changed the value of the Silk Route Region pattern [47].

The evaluation and differentiation of PPL in 65 patients were considered by Hamdan et al.; they found that 49 patients (55.7%) had PPL, including 25 (28.4%) with acneiform lesions, 17 (19.3%) with pseudofolliculitis, 4 (4.4%) with pustular eruptions, and 3 (3.3%) with nonspecific subcutaneous nodules and rashes. According to this point of view, acneiform lesions are the most common type of PPL so clinicians should take special care to distinguish them from acne vulgaris [16]. According to some previous studies, male patients have more frequent PPL than females and their prognosis was worse [17–20, 29, 35, 36, 39, 41, 43, 46]. Bonitsis et al. [43] has already clarified these results via a meta-analysis study of a German population. Some authors speculated that the main reason of provoking PPL in males may be related with testosterone levels. Durusoy et al. [48] indicated that androgens may play a role at least in the formation of PPL and disease activity in patients with BD.

References	Country of study (year)	No. of patients	Frequency of acneiform lesions in BD (%) (different terms used in literature)	Comparisons according to certain variables
Alpsoy et al. [22]	Turkey (–1998)	50	PPL: 96%	–
Zouboulis et al. [32]	Germany (1990–2000)	347	PPL: 53%	–
Shahram et al. [33]	Iran (–2001)	4704	PPL: 62%	–
Azizlerli et al. [34]	Turkey (–2003)	101	PF: 39.6%	Male vs female: 55% vs 45%
Tursen et al. [35]	Turkey (1976–98)	2313	PPL: 54%	Male vs female: 56.1% vs 43.9%*
Hamdan et al. [16]	Lebanon (1977–2005)	90	PPL: 55.7% (28.4% with acneiform lesions, 19.3% with PF, 4.4% with pustular eruptions, 3.3% with nonspecific subcutaneous nodules and rashes)	Male vs female: 59.1% vs 45.5%
Houman et al. [17]	Tunisia (1987–2006)	260	PF: 70.4%	Male vs female: 75.5% vs 58.3%* Ocular lesions (+) vs (–): 69.8% vs 71.6% BD-DVT (+) vs (–): 70.9% vs 70.5% BD Neuro (+) vs (–): 61.9% vs 73.6%
Alpsoy et al. [36]	Turkey (2007)	661	PPL: 55.4%	Male vs female: 62% vs 44.3%*
Alli et al. [37]	Turkey (2001–2004)	213	PPL: 56%	Male vs female: 63.5% vs 49.5%*
Arida et al. [18]	Greece (2000–2008)	142	PF: 44.4%	Male vs female: 61.3% vs 22.6%*
Vaiopoulos et al. [19]	Greece (1991–2007)	202	PF: 1.5% as onset sign, 5.9% as second symptom	Male vs female: 57.1% vs 21.9%*
Davatchi et al. [14]	Iran (1975–2010)	6500	PF: 54.5%	Age groups: <21: 57.0%, 21–40: 54.9%, 41–60: 40.4%, >60: 63.6%
Oliveira et al. [20]	Brazil (2011)	60	PPL: 23.3%, acne-like lesions: 6.7%	Male vs female: 40.7 vs 9.1%*
Park et al. [29]	Korea (2012)	83	PPL: 56.6%	HLA-B51 (+) vs (–):35.7 vs 67.3%*
Singal et al. [38]	India (1997–2011)	29	PPL and acneiform lesions: 31%	
Hamzaoui et al. [39]	Tunisian (1989–2009)	430	PF: 74.4%	Age < 20: 84%, age > 40: 63.2%*
Sula et al. [40]	Southeastern Turkey (2005–2009)	132	PPL: 74.2%	Male vs female: 76.7 vs 72.3%
Balta et al. [41]	Turkey (–2014)	521	PPL: 61.0%	Male vs female: 71.4 vs 52.6%*
Ugurlu et al. [42]	Turkey (2001–2012)	368	PPL: 75.0%	Male vs female: 80.7 vs 68.4%
Bonitsis et al. [43]	Germany (1990–2012)	747	PPL: 46.6%, PF: 47.2%	PPL: Male vs female: 50.6 vs 41.1%*PF: Male vs female: 52.2 vs 40.1% *

References	Country of study (year)	No. of patients	Frequency of acneiform lesions in BD (%) (different terms used in literature)	Comparisons according to certain variables
Ndiaye et al. [44]	Senegal (2015)	50	PF: 30%, acneiform papules:12%	
Fatemi et al. [45]	Iran (2010–2015)	2312	PF: 7.2% (in 430 patients with musculoskeletal manifestations)	Patients with arthritic attacks: 84% * Patients with no arthritic attacks: 16%
Demirseren et al. [30]	Turkey (2014)	51	PPL: 64.7%	
Davatchi et al. [46]	Iran (1975–2014)	6075	PF: 53.2%	Male vs Female: 60 vs 44.4% *

PPL, Papulopustular lesions; PF, Pseudofolliculitis; DVT: Deep vein thrombosis.
*Statistically significant ($p < 0.05$).

Table 2. Frequency of acneiform papulopustular lesions related to Behcet's disease in different ethnic groups.

One study focused on the relationship between age and the frequency of diagnostic criteria. In this study, Hamzaoui et al. separated patients into two groups who were less than 20 years old and more than 40 years old. It was found that cutaneous involvement and pseudofolliculitis were significantly more common in younger age group. However, joint involvements in the older group were more frequent, which is controversial regarding the frequent association between PPL and arthritis [39].

4.2. PPL accompanied by some clinical features in BD

Clinicians should suspect some clinical findings that frequently accompany PPL to facilitate a correct diagnosis. Of these situations, the most known is arthritis. Diri et al. determined acneiform eruptions and relationship of arthritis and BD through evaluating four groups consisting of 44 BD patients with arthritis, 42 BD patients without arthritis, 21 patients with active rheumatoid arthritis and 33 healthy volunteers. They reported that only the BD with arthritis group had significantly higher PPL. As a conclusion, arthritis and acneiform lesions may have same pathogenesis so that they occasionally appear together [49]. Moreover, Karaca et al. argued that PPL and arthritis have an inherited pathogenesis. Likewise, they found BD appears as cluster in familial BD constantly. They also suggested a mechanism that works on the same bacterial pathway responsible for this association [50]. Calgüneri et al. [51] also manifested that prophylactic penicillin treatment alleviated both acneiform eruptions and arthritis attacks. In another study, Fatemi et al. investigated articular involvement in BD. They emphasized that PPL was higher during episodes of arthritis, and in episodic attacks, only the presence of PPL as an extra-articular involvement was statistically meaningful [45].

The pathergy test had been researched as another entity. Arida et al. found positive correlation between pathergy test and folliculitis only in male patients [18]. The acronym SAPHO was defined as synovitis, acne, pustulosis, hyperostosis, and osteitis. Due to a lack of research SAPHO overlaps clinically with BD remains to be elucidated. Caravatti et al. published a case report in which the patient met all diagnostic criteria of both SAPHO and BD. This study shows that similar arthritis mechanism occurs between BD and SAPHO and also both of them consist of acne-like eruptions [52]. Due to necessity of further investigation, Yabe et al. reported two case reports and compared with other studies in literature. They manifested that SAPHO syndrome and BD referred as seronegative arthropathies and also SAPHO could be clinical overlap of BD [53]. However, Alli et al. could not find a statistically significant relationship between arthritis and PPL in SAPHO syndrome [37]. Thus, there is a need for to work harder in order to elucidate similar mechanisms.

4.3. Comparison of the PPL characteristics between BD and acne vulgaris/acneiform disorders

PPL of BD can easily be confused with the acneiform papular and pustular lesions of acne vulgaris. As everyone knows, typical acne vulgaris usually begins around first and second decades and is easily diagnosed. However, both diseases can occur in patients aged 20–40. As how importance is the early diagnosis for BD, clinicians should focus on their main differentiation [54].

The PPL of BD patients are mainly known as sterile pustules, but some authors suggest that they contain a different type of bacteria than acne vulgaris lesions [7, 21]. Hatemi et al. studied 58 BD patients and 37 acne patients, and obtained the culture of pustules. They suggested that *Staphylococcus aureus* and *Prevotella* spp. were significantly more common in pustules from BD patients, and coagulase-negative staphylococci in pustules from acne patients. Prevotella spp. was not cultured from the acne pustules. BD pustules thus have different types of bacteria, which results in a different pathogenesis [21].

BD is a neutrophilic dermatosis that is commonly based on vasculitic disorders, but acne vulgaris is a hyperfunction of sebaceous glands under hormonal control. PPL in BD has been observed mainly in the lower extremities and trunk, but acne vulgaris has been observed mainly in face, chest, and back. Alpsoy et al. researched on 100 patients (50 patients with BD, 79 cases for control group including 21 patients with acne vulgaris) and consequently, it was found that the frequency of PPL in BD patients was 96% and the most common location was the trunk, whereas in the control group the frequency of PPL was 89% and the most common location was the face. The total numbers of PPL on the trunk, upper and lower extremities, and genitalia were higher in patients with BD than in controls [22]. Kutlubay et al. observed that papules and folliculitis on the back and the lower extremities in BD were higher than acne vulgaris group [27]. Prior clinical studies in literature comparing locations, types and numbers of PPL lesions between BD and acne vulgaris are summarized in **Table 3**.

As mentioned before, PPL of BD were evaluated using the International Study Group Criteria due to their 70% sensitivity and 76% specificity [13]. Davatchi et al. [46] determined that BD has dome-shaped pustule, not a sharp pustule like acne vulgaris. However, both of them resembled follicular lesions so that arguments continue about whether or not histopathological differentiation must be necessary via lesional skin biopsy for differential diagnosis. In the literature, there are some histopathological investigation studies of PPL in BD patients. As a result of these studies, there are numerous quandaries about the diagnostic histopathologic patterns

References	No. of patients	Location, type and mean number of PPL
Alpsoy et al. [22]	50 BD/21 AV	Face: 2.6 ± 2.8 in BD/7.5 ± 5.6* in AV; Neck: 1.0 ± 1.4 in BD/2.3 ± 1.9* in AV; Mean total number: 18.8 ± 15.9 in BD/28.3 ± 23.4* in AV
Kutlubay et al. [27]	58 BD/31 AV	Face/papule: 4.41 ± 4.47 in BD/11.8 ± 13.4* in AV; Face/pustule: 1.55 ± 2.07 in BD/5.75 ± 5.1* in AV; Face/comedone: 9.79 ± 14.8 in BD/42.5 ± 43.7* in AV; Back/papule: 8.73 ± 7.13* in BD/5.62 ± 5.77 in AV; Back/folliculitis: 0.58 ± 1.92* only in BD Lower extremity/folliculitis: 1.64 ± 3.47* only in BD

AV, acne vulgaris; BD, Behcet's disease; PPL, papulopustular lesions.
*Statistically significant ($p < 0.05$).

Table 3. Clinical studies comparing locations, types and numbers of papulopustular lesions between Behcet's disease and acne vulgaris.

and regarding whether to include vasculitis or nonspecific folliculitis [23, 27, 55]. Comparison data of the histopathological and direct immunofluorescence findings of PPL between BD and other acneiform lesions consisting of acne vulgaris and folliculitis are summarized in **Table 4**.

When considering the histopathological findings of PPL in BD, Ergun et al. took samples, which were chosen as only fresh pustules from the legs and arms of 17 patients with BD and 6 patients with acne vulgaris. Only 12% patients with BD revealed perivascular involvement without leucocytoclastic vasculitis and results stated that there was no differentiation between acne vulgaris and BD by histopathological evidence. They argued that there is no need to con-

References	Benchmarking acne vulgaris with PPL in BD	No. of patients	Histopathological findings	Direct immunofluorescence findings
Alpsoy et al. [55]	PPL vs normal-appearing skin	17 BD	LV: 64.7% lesional/ 11.8% nonlesional; Pustule: 17.6% lesional; LympV: 5.9% lesional/ 11.8% non-lesional; Mixed: 5.9% lesional/ 17.6% non-lesional; MNC: 5.9% lesional/ 17.6% non-lesional; PMN: 5.9% lesional/ 5.9% non-lesional;	IR on vessels: 70.9% lesional/ 23.5% non-lesional; IgM: 52.9% lesional/ 17.6% non-lesional; IgG: 35.3% lesional; 11.8% non-lesional; C3: 41.2% lesional; 17.6% non-lesional Fibrin: 47.1% lesional; 17.6 non-lesional
Ergun et al. [23]	PPL of BD vs AV	17 BD, 6 AV	**In epidermis** (intraepidermal pustule: 47.1% BD; spongiosis: 35.3% BD/16.7% AV; exocytosis: 11.8% BD; necrotic keratinocytes: 5.9% BD) **In follicle epithelium** (plugging: 58.9% BD/ 100% AV; rupture: 23.5% BD/16.7% AV; necrotic keratinocytes or epithelial necrosis: 11.8% BD/33.3% AV) **In dermis** (endothelial swelling: 23.5% BD/33.3% AV; nuclear dust: 17.6% BD/16.7% AV) **Eccrine** glands (41.2% BD/33.3% AV)	–

References	Benchmarking acne vulgaris with PPL in BD	No. of patients	Histopathological findings	Direct immunofluorescence findings
Boyvat et al. [24]	Specific vessel-based PPL vs nonspecific follicular lesions	20 (23 PPL)	LV: 13.04%; Perivascular infiltration: 21.7%; Perivascular and interstitial infiltration: 8.7%; Perifollicular and perivascular infiltration: 39.1%; Perifollicular inflammation only: 17.4%	–
İlknur et al. [25]	PPL of BD vs folliculitis/AV	18 BD 16 control PPL (11 folliculitis, 5 AV)	Pattern I: vasculitis (lymphocytic or leucocytoclastic) 27.8% BD/ 0% control group; Pattern II: folliculitis and/or perifolliculitis 16.7% BD/ 50% control group; Pattern III: superficial and/or deep perivascular and/or interstitial dermatitis 22.2% BD/ 18.8% control group	IR depositions on vessels; In 22.2% of BD patients (16.7% in pattern I, 5.6% in pattern II; in pattern I; 5.6% IgG, IgM, C3 and fibrinogen as quadruple conjugate, 5.6% C3 and fibrinogen as double conjugate, 5.6% only C3)/In 18.7% of control groups (6.2% in pattern I, 12.4% in pattern II)
Kalkan et al. [26]	PPL of BD vs AV	42 BD, 21 AV	LV: 6.7% in BD*; LympV: 7.1% BD; Superficial perivascular and/ or interstitial infiltration: 35.7% BD/38.1% AV; superficial and deep perivascular and/or interstitial infiltration: 28.6% BD/19.0% AV; Folliculitis or perifolliculitis: 11.9%, BD/42.9% AV*	–
Kutlubay et al. [27]	PPL of BD vs AV	58 BD, 31 AV	PNL infiltration without folliculitis: 1.7% BD/1.6% AV; Mononuclear infiltration without folliculitis: 0.8% BD/4.8% AV; Folliculitis/perifolliculitis: 85.3% BD,83.9% AV; LV:12.1% BD/9.7% AV; Comedone formation: 39.6% BD/64.5% AV; Intrafollicular abscess formation: 62.1% BD/61.3% AV; Presence of microorganisms, etc: 13.8% BD/14.5% AV	–

AV, acne vulgaris; BD, Behcet's disease; PPL, papulopustular lesions; LV, leucocytoclastic vasculitis; LympV, lymphocytic vasculitis; MNC, mononuclear cells; PMN, polymorphonuclear cells; Mixed, mixed cell infiltration; IR, Immunoreactant.
*statistically significant ($p < 0.05$).

Table 4. Histopathological and direct immunofluorescence findings for papulopustular lesions in Behcet's disease.

firm PPL of BD with biopsies [23]. Moreover, Chun et al. [55] also agreed on this hypothesis based on their research. More recently, Kutlubay et al. analyzed punch biopsy samples from 58 BD and 31 acne vulgaris patients by two blinded pathologist. Both of them found vasculitis in the same patients in 7% of BD and 3% of acne vulgaris patients. Follicle-based pathology was detected in totally 87.6% (78/89 patients) and 82% (73/89 patients) in both the BD and AV groups by both pathologists; controversially vessel-based pathology was rarely observed, 9% (10/89 patients) in both the BD and AV groups [27]. Therefore, they also claimed that there is no pathological difference between BD and acne vulgaris such as vasculitis.

On the other hand, Ilknur et al. evaluated the follicular and nonfollicular lesions from 18 patients with BD and from 16 patients (11 with bacterial folliculitis, 5 with acne vulgaris) as a control group. They manifested that only the useful pattern for BD diagnosis was vasculitic changes which were not found in control group. The strength of this research is histopathological specimens were analyzed by two different pathologists for the first time, so the results were made with a consensus [25]. According to the study of Boyvat et al., the clinical features cannot be distinguishable for a BD diagnosis, but biopsy specimens must include vessel-based neutrophilic reactions [24]. In another study, Kalkan et al. [26] found that 16.7% leukocytoclastic vasculitis and 7.1% lymphocytic vasculitis were present in BD patients although any vasculitic finding was not found in acne vulgaris patients. Furthermore, arguments still continue to clarify the exact pattern of PPL in BD. More assessments are needed to investigate.

If histopathological findings cannot provide any benefit for BD diagnosis, we may use immuno his to chemical techniques as an additional diagnostic test. In 2003, Alpsoy et al. evaluated 17 patients whose biopsies had taken from lesional and non lesional skin parts to study via immunological tools. The polyclonal antibodies including IgA, IgG, IgM, C3, and fibrin were measured, IgM deposition of thelesional skin was significantly higher than non lesional skin (52.9% and 17.6%, respectively); despite of that, there were no statistically significant differences in terms of IgG, C3, and fibrin deposits on the vessels [55]. Subsequently, Ilknur et al. investigated the direct immunofluorescence results of 18 patients with BD and 16 control patients in order to evaluate any deposition of immunoreactants on dermal blood vessels. They found no significant difference between the groups [25].

4.4. Management of PPL in BD

BD has now become a treatable disease, although it is not yet curable. The choice of treatment is based on clinical features and the severity of the disease. Main treatment approach should be prevention of the severe organ damage. Recent guidelines could not establish a standard therapy for mucocutaneous lesions. A wide spectrum of agents can be used successfully to heal and prevent the formation of new lesions. As our study specifies the PPL management, first-line treatment is topical ones such as corticosteroid or combination with corticosteroid and antibiotics. To support antibiotic use, it is reported that like *Prevotella* spp. and *Staphylococcus aureus* have been cultured in PPL. Although benzathin penicillin is the most commonly used one, minocycline is more effective than benzathin penicillin in reducing of lesions. The systemic approach to BD treatment consists mainly of corticosteroids and colchicine. Corticosteroids are effective choices in almost all mucocutaneous lesions. They can be combined with other drugs such as colchicine, IFN-a or azathioprine. Guidelines recommend that corticosteroid administration begins with 40–60 mg/d for 1–2 weeks and tapers the dosage over 4 weeks. However, this therapy has limitations due to its long-term side effects [57–59]. Corticosteroid treatment has been also a potent trigger for acne and referred as steroid acne. Clinicians have to keep in mind that acneiform papulopustular eruptions in BD may also appear as a result of steroid treatment. It is also important to know that steroid acne have some similarities and differences between Behcet's pseudofolliculitis. Similarly, both of them mostly stay in trunk and extremities rather than face. At the same time, PPL in BD may arise as papules, pustules, and comedones at different stages of development. However, steroid acne usually stays as small folliculitis at the same stage in the proper area where the corticoid therapy is applied and it usually appears 2 weeks after the therapy has begun. Both of them resembled in neutrophilic involvement in the lesions but BD also has the vasculitic pattern. If the distinction can be made between true PPL and steroid acne in BD, management of the acneiform eruptions in these patients would be different and reasonable [60].

Colchicine is the one of the strongest medications for BD. Colchicine inhibits the chemotactic activity and decreases the tumor necrosis factor-α, leukotrien-B4, cyclooxygenase-2 activity, and prostoglandin-E2 levels. Mainly, it is approached in erythema nodosum and arthritis treatment for female patients. Colchicine combined with benzathine penicillin increases the potency of the therapy. The lack of evidence in the efficacy of colchicine for treatment of mucocutaneous lesions could be related to relative lack of inappropriate researches. Moreover, IFN-a and etanercept treatment has been reported to decrease PPL frequency. Alternative therapy (dapson) has shown a significant capacity to diminish PPL. For severe lesions, azathioprine, pentoxifylline and thalidomide have demonstrated beneficial effects [57–59].

5. Conclusion

According to the International Study Group criteria for BD diagnosis, skin lesions are restricted to erythema nodosum-like lesions, pseudofolliculitis, papulopustular lesions, and acneiform nodules. These lesions excepting erythema nodosum-like lesions are nonspecific and clinically confused with other acneiform papulopustular eruptions (e.g., acne vulgaris, bacterial folliculitis, steroid acne). Although earlier studies involve numerous quandaries regarding the diagnostic histopathologic pattern of BD (e.g., whether to include vasculitis or nonspecific folliculitis), it was reported recently that the determination of vasculitic changes in histopathological and direct immunofluorescence results might be useful in the differential diagnosis of patients suspected to have BD.

Author details

Sevgi Akarsu* and Işıl Kamberoğlu

*Address all correspondence to: sevgi.akarsu@deu.edu.tr

1 Department of Dermatology and Venereology, Faculty of Medicine, Dokuz Eylul University, Izmir, Turkey

References

[1] Alpsoy E. Behçet's disease: A comprehensive review with a focus on epidemiology, etiology and clinical features, and management of mucocutaneous lesions. J Dermatol. 2016 Jun;**43**(6):620-32. doi: 10.1111/1346-8138.13381. Epub 2016 Apr 14

[2] Davatchi F, Shahram F, Chams-Davatchi C, Shams H, Nadji A, Akhlaghi M, Faezi T, Sadeghi Abdollahi B. How to deal with Behcet's disease in daily practice. Int J Rheum Dis. 2010;**13**:105–116.

[3] Mat MC, Sevim A, Fresko I, Tüzün Y. Behçet's disease as a systemic disease. Clin Dermatol. 2014;**32**:435–442. DOI: 10.1016/j.clindermatol.2013.11.012.

[4] Kartal Durmazlar SP. Venous Thrombosis in Behcet's Disease. In: Ertugrul Okuyan, editor. Venous Thrombosis - Principles and Practice. InTech; 2012. pp. 43–54. Publisher: InTech, Chapters published January 05, 2012 under CC BY 3.0license

[5] Kartal Durmazlar SP, Akgül A. Prof. Dr. Hulusi Behçet: An eponym who is referred to. Turkiye Klinikleri J Med Sci. 2015;**35**: 57–59.

[6] Leonardo NM, McNeil J. Behcet's disease: Is there geographical variation? A review far from the Silk Road. Int J Rheumatol. 2015;**2015**:945262. DOI: 10.1155/2015/945262.

[7] Hatemi G, Yazici H. Behçet's syndrome and micro-organisms. Best Pract Res Clin Rheumatol. 2011;**25**:389–406. DOI:10.1016/j.berh.2011.05.002.

[8] Davatchi F. Diagnosis/classification criteria for Behcet's disease. Patholog Res Int. 2012;**2012**:607921. DOI: 10.1155/2012/607921.

[9] Uva L, Miguel D, Pinheiro C, Filipe P, Freitas JP. Mucocutaneous manifestations of Behçet's disease. Acta Reumatol Port. 2013;**38**:77–90.

[10] Mason RM, Barnes CG. Behçet's syndrome with arthritis. Ann Rheum Dis. 1969;**28**:95–103.

[11] O'Duffy J D. [Suggestion of diagnostic criterias in therapeutic management in Behcet Disease]. Rev Med Interne. 1974;**36**:2371–2379.

[12] Behçet's Disease Research Committee of Japan. Behçet's disease: guide to diagnosis. Japanese Journal of Ophthalmology. 1974;**18**:291–294

[13] International Study Group for Behcet's Disease. Criteria for diagnosis of Behcet's disease. Lancet. 1990;**335**:1078–1080.

[14] Davatchi F, Shahram F, Chams-Davatchi C, Shams H, Nadji A, Akhlaghi M, Faezi T, Ghodsi Z, Larimi R, Ashofteh F, Abdollahi BS. Behcet's disease in Iran: Analysis of 6500 cases. Int J Rheum Dis. 2010;**13**:367–373. DOI: 10.1111/j.1756-185X.2010.01549.x.

[15] Kokturk A. Clinical and pathological manifestations with differential diagnosis in Behçet's Disease. Patholog Res Int. 2012;**2012**:690390. DOI:10.1155/2012/690390.

[16] Hamdan A, Mansour W, Uthman I, Masri AF, Nasr F, Arayssi T. Behçet's disease in Lebanon: clinical profile, severity and two-decade comparison. Clin Rheumatol. 2006;**25**:364–367. DOI: 10.1007/s10067-005-0058-4.

[17] Houman MH, Neffati H, Braham A, Harzallah O, Khanfir M, Miled M, Hamzaoui K. Behçet's disease in Tunisia. Demographic, clinical and genetic aspects in 260 patients. Clin Exp Rheumatol. 2007;**25**:S58-64.

[18] Arida A, Vaiopoulos G, Markomichelakis N, Kaklamanis P, Sfikakis PP. Are clusters of patients with distinct clinical expression present in Behçet's disease? Clin Exp Rheumatol. 2009;27:S48-51.

[19] Vaiopoulos G, Konstantopoulou P, Evangelatos N, Kaklamanis PH. The spectrum of mucocutaneous manifestations in Adamantiades-Behçet's disease in Greece. J Eur Acad Dermatol Venereol. 2010;**24**:434–438. DOI: 10.1111/j.1468-3083.2009.03435.x.

[20] Oliveira AC, Buosi AL, Dutra LA, de Souza AW. Behçet disease: Clinical features and management in a Brazilian tertiary hospital. J Clin Rheumatol. 2011;**17**:416–420. DOI: 10.1097/RHU.0b013e31823a46ed.

[21] Hatemi G, Bahar H, Uysal S, Mat C, Gogus F, Masatlioglu S, Altas K, Yazici H. The pustular skin lesions in Behcet's syndrome are not sterile. Ann Rheum Dis. 2004;**63**:1450–1452. DOI: 10.1136/ard.2003.017467.

[22] Alpsoy E, Aktekin M, Er H, Durusoy C, Yilmaz E. A randomized, controlled and blinded study of papulopustular lesions in Turkish Behçet's patients. Int J Dermatol. 1998;**37**:839–842.

[23] Ergun T, Gürbüz O, Dogusoy G, Mat C, Yazici H. Histopathologic features of the spontaneous pustular lesions of Behçet's syndrome. Int J Dermatol. 1998;**37**:194–196.

[24] Boyvat A, Heper AO, Koçyiğit P, Erekul S, Gürgey E. Can specific vessel-based papulopustular lesions of Behçet's disease be differentiated from nonspecific follicular-based lesions clinically? Int J Dermatol. 2006;**45**:814–818.

[25] Ilknur T, Pabuççuoglu U, Akin C, Lebe B, Gunes AT. Histopathologic and direct immunofluorescence findings of the papulopustular lesions in Behçet's disease. Eur J Dermatol. 2006;**16**:146–150.

[26] Kalkan G, Karadag AS, Astarci HM, Akbay G, Ustun H, Eksioglu M. A histopathological approach: When papulopustular lesions should be in the diagnostic criteria of Behçet's disease? J Eur Acad Dermatol Venereol. 2009;**23**:1056–1060. DOI: 10.1111/j.1468-3083.2009.03256.x.

[27] Kutlubay Z, Mat CM, Aydin Ö, Demirkesen C, Calay Ö, Engın B, Tüzün Y, Yazici H. Histopathological and clinical evaluation of papulopustular lesions in Behçet's disease. Clin Exp Rheumatol. 2015;**33**:S101-106.

[28] Yamasaki O, Morizane S, Aochi S, Ogawa K, Oono T, Iwatsuki K. Granulysin-producing cytotoxic T cells in the mucocutaneous lesions of Behçet disease: A distinct inflammatory response from erythema nodosum. Clin Exp Dermatol. 2011;**36**:903–907. DOI: 10.1111/j.1365-2230.2011.04159.x.

[29] Park G, Kim HS, Choe JY, Kim SK. SUMO4 C438T polymorphism is associated with papulopustular skin lesion in Korean patients with Behçet's disease. Rheumatol Int. 2012;**32**:3031–3037.

[30] Demirseren DD, Ceylan GG, Akoglu G, Emre S, Erten S, Arman A, Metin A. HLA-B51 subtypes in Turkish patients with Behçet's disease and their correlation with clinical manifestations. Genet Mol Res. 2014;**13**:4788–4796. DOI: 10.4238/2014.July.2.8.

[31] Cho S, Kim J, Cho SB, Zheng Z, Choi MJ, Kim DY, Bang D. Immunopathogenic characterization of cutaneous inflammation in Behçet's disease. J Eur Acad Dermatol Venereol. 2014;**28**:51–57. DOI: 10.1111/jdv.12054.

[32] Zouboulis ChC, Kötter I, Djawari D, Krause L, Pleyer U, Stadler R, Kirch W, Wollina U, Kohl PK, Keitel W, Ochsendorf FR, Gollnick HP, Borgmann H, Turnbull JR, Keitzer R, Hölzle E, Proksch E, Söhnchen R, Blech H, Glosemeyer R, Gross GE, Hoch Y, Jung EG, Koch G, Pfeiff B, Reichrath J, Schaffartzik W, Weber H, Fritz K, Orfanos CE. Current epidemiological data from the German Registry of Adamantiades-Behçet's disease. Adv Exp Med Biol. 2003;**528**:43–48.

[33] Shahram F, Davatchi F, Nadji A, Jamshidi A, Chams H, Chams C, Shafaie N, Akbarian M, Gharibdoost F. Recent epidemiological data on Behçet's disease in Iran. The 2001 survey. Adv Exp Med Biol. 2003;**528**:31–36.

[34] Azizlerli G, Köse AA, Sarica R, Gül A, Tutkun IT, Kulac M, Tunç R, Urgancioglu M, Disci R. Prevalence of Behçet's disease in Istanbul, Turkey. Int J Dermatol. 2003;**42**:803–836.

[35] Tursen U, Gurler A, Boyvat A. Evaluation of clinical findings according to sex in 2313 Turkish patients with Behçet's disease. Int J Dermatol. 2003;**42**:346–351.

[36] Alpsoy E, Donmez L, Onder M, Gunasti S, Usta A, Karincaoglu Y, Kandi B, Buyukkara S, Keseroglu O, Uzun S,Tursen U, Seyhan M, Akman A. Clinical features and natural course of Behçet's disease in 661 cases: A multicentre study. Br J Dermatol. 2007;**157**:901–906. DOI: 10.1111/j.1365-2133.2007.08116.x.

[37] Alli N, Gur G, Yalcin B, Hayran M. Patient characteristics in Behçet disease: A retrospective analysis of 213 Turkish patients during 2001–2004. Am J Clin Dermatol. 2009;**10**:411–418. DOI: 10.2165/11310880-000000000-00000.

[38] Singal A, Chhabra N, Pandhi D, Rohatgi J. Behçet's disease in India: a dermatological perspective. Indian J Dermatol Venereol Leprol. 2013;**79**:199–204. DOI: 10.4103/0378-6323.107636.

[39] Hamzaoui A, Jaziri F, Ben Salem T, Said Imed Ben Ghorbel F, Lamloum M, Smiti Khanfir M, Houman Mohamed H. Comparison of clinical features of Behcet disease according to age in a Tunisian cohort. Acta Med Iran. 2014;**52**:748–751.

[40] Sula B, Batmaz I, Ucmak D, Yolbas I, Akdeniz S. Demographical and clinical characteristics of Behcet's Disease in southeastern Turkey. J Clin Med Res. 2014;**6**:476–481. DOI: 10.14740/jocmr1952w.

[41] Balta I, Akbay G, Kalkan G, Eksioglu M. Demographic and clinical features of 521 Turkish patients with Behçet's disease. Int J Dermatol. 2014;**53**:564–569. DOI: 10.1111/j.1365-4632.2012.05756.x.

[42] Ugurlu N, Bozkurt S, Bacanli A, Akman-Karakas A, Uzun S, Alpsoy E. The natural course and factors affecting severity of Behçet's disease: A single-center cohort of 368 patients. Rheumatol Int. 2015;**35**:2103–2107. DOI: 10.1007/s00296-015-3310-5. Epub 2015 Jun 18.

[43] Bonitsis NG, Luong Nguyen LB, LaValley MP, Papoutsis N, Altenburg A, Kötter I, Micheli C, Maldini C, Mahr A, Zouboulis CC. Gender-specific differences in Adamantiades-Behçet's disease manifestations: An analysis of the German registry and meta-analysis of data from the literature. Rheumatology (Oxford). 2015;**54**:121–133. DOI: 10.1093/rheumatology/keu247.

[44] Ndiaye M, Sow AS, Valiollah A, Diallo M, Diop A, Alaoui RA, Diatta BA, Ly F, Niang SO, Dieng MT, Kane A. Behçet's disease in black skin. A retrospective study of 50 cases in Dakar. J Dermatol Case Rep. 2015;**9**:98–102. DOI: 10.3315/jdcr.2015.1213.

[45] Fatemi A, Shahram F, Akhlaghi M, Smiley A, Nadji A, Davatchi F. Prospective study of articular manifestations in Behçet's disease: Five-year report. Int J Rheum Dis. 2014 May;**17**(4):355-7. doi: 10.1111/1756-185X.12378. Epub 2014 Apr 25

[46] Davatchi F, Chams-Davatchi C, Shams H, Nadji A, Faezi T, Akhlaghi M, Sadeghi Abdollahi B, Ashofteh F, Ghodsi Z, Mohtasham N, Shahram F. Adult Behcet's disease in Iran: Analysis of 6075 patients. Int J Rheum Dis. 2016;**19**:95–103.

[47] Davatchi F, Shahram F, Chams-Davatchi C, Shams H, Nadji A, Akhlaghi M, Faezi T, Ghodsi Z, Faridar A, Ashofteh F, Sadeghi Abdollahi B. Behcet's disease: From East to West. Clin Rheumatol. 2010;**29**:823–833. DOI: 10.1007/s10067-010-1430-6

[48] Durusoy C, Alpsoy E, Elpek O, Karpuzoglu G. Androgen receptor levels in the sebaceous glands of papulopustular lesions from patients with Behçet's disease and acne vulgaris: a controlled study. Adv Clin Path. 2002;**6**:87–93.

[49] Diri E, Mat C, Hamuryudan V, Yurdakul S, Hizli N, Yazici H. Papulopustular skin lesions are seen more frequently in patients with Behçet's syndrome who have arthritis: A controlled and masked study. Ann Rheum Dis. 2001;**60**:1074–1076.

[50] Karaca M, Hatemi G, Sut N, Yazici H. The papulopustular lesion/arthritis cluster of Behçet's syndrome also clusters in families. Rheumatology (Oxford). 2012;**51**:1053–1060. DOI: 10.1093/rheumatology/ker423.

[51] Calgüneri M, Kiraz S, Ertenli I, Benekli M, Karaarslan Y, Celik I. The effect of prophylactic penicillin treatment on the course of arthritis episodes in patients with Behçet's disease. A randomized clinical trial. Arthritis Rheum. 1996;**39**:2062–2065.

[52] Caravatti M, Wiesli P, Uebelhart D, Germann D, Welzl-Hinterkörner E, Schulthess G. Coincidence of Behçet's disease and SAPHO syndrome. Clin Rheumatol. 2002;**21**:324–327.

[53] Yabe H, Takano Y, Nomura E, Nakayama M, Kihara M, Miyakawa S, Horiuchi Y. Two cases of SAPHO syndrome accompanied by classic features of Behcet's disease and review of the literature. Clin Rheumatol. 2008;**27**:133–135. DOI: 10.1007/s10067-007-0697-8.

[54] Lolis MS, Bowe WP, Shalita AR. Acne and systemic disease. Med Clin North Am. 2009;**93**:1161–1181. DOI:10.1016/j.mcna.2009.08.008.

[55] Chun SI, Su WP, Lee S. Histopathologic study of cutaneous lesions in Behçet's syndrome. J Dermatol. 1990;**17**:333–341.

[56] Alpsoy E, Uzun S, Akman A, Acar MA, Memisoglu HR, Basaran E. Histological and immunofluorescence findings of non-follicular papulopustular lesions in patients with Behçet's disease. J Eur Acad Dermatol Venereol. 2003;**17**:521–524.

[57] Alpsoy E, Akman A. Behçet's disease: an algorithmic approach to its treatment. Arch Dermatol Res. 2009;**301**:693–702. DOI: 10.1007/s00403-009-0990-2

[58] Rotondo C, Lopalco G, Iannone F, Vitale A, Talarico R, Galeazzi M, Lapadula G, Cantarini L. Mucocutaneous involvement in Behçet's Disease: How systemic treatment has changed in the last decades and future perspectives. Mediators Inflamm. 2015;**2015**:451675. DOI: 10.1155/2015/451675.

[59] Alpsoy E. Behçet's disease: Treatment of mucocutaneous lesions. Clin Exp Rheumatol. 2005;**23**:532–539.

[60] Dessinioti C, Antoniou C, Katsambas A. Acneiform eruptions. Clin Dermatol. 2014;**32**:24–34. DOI: 10.1016/j.clindermatol.2013.05.023.

Chapter 8

The Use of Topical Retinoids in Acne

Dilek Bayramgurler, Selda Pelin Kartal and Cemile Altunel

Additional information is available at the end of the chapter

http://dx.doi.org/10.5772/108205

Abstract

Acne vulgaris is the most common skin disease in adolescents and young adults and has serious influence on quality of life of the patients. Acne vulgaris is the most common skin disease in adolescents and young adults and has serious influence on quality of life of the patients. The initial lesions of acne are the microcomedones that can be observed histologically in normal-appearing skin. The first step in the treatment of acne is to understand the pathophysiology of disease and to act on the factors involved in the development of acne. Increased sebum secretion from sebaceous glands, secretion of inflammatory mediators, altered keratinization and follicular plugging, and follicular colonization of *Propionibacterium acnes* are major four steps of acne pathogenesis. Topical retinoids have multiple effects in the treatment of acne and act on more than one factor implicated in the etiology of acne. They prevent the formation of microcomedones and reduce their number, reduce macrocomedones, promote the normal desquamation of follicular epithelium, exert anti-inflammatory effects, enhance the penetration of other topical acne drugs, and prolong the remission periods of acne by inhibiting the formation of microcomedone formation and preventing the development of new lesions and bacterial resistance. Therefore, topical retinoids have been the first-line treatment for most forms of acne vulgaris either alone or together with other agents.

Keywords: acne, retinoids, topical treatment

1. Acne

1.1. Introduction

Acne vulgaris is the most common skin disease in adolescents and young adults with 70–95% prevalence rate. Adult or postadolescent acne occurs in 12–14% of this population and is seen as the continuation of acne from adolescence into adulthood or starts in the adult life [1, 2].

Acne has a serious influence on quality of life of the patients. The negative impact of acne on behavioral and social functions has found to be greater than medical conditions such as asthma and epilepsy. Additionally, compared to unemployment, acne has been shown to be more highly associated with anxiety and depression [2, 3]. Fortunately, it is possible to improve the quality of life of patients with successful treatment. Over the past few decades, a large spectrum of local and systemic drugs has been introduced and a lot of efforts have been devoted to reach a consensus on the treatment approach of acne. As new drugs are constantly being added to the list, it is critical to update the current recommendations.

1.2. The global alliance to improve outcomes in acne

The Global Alliance to Improve Outcomes in Acne Group ("Global Alliance") is an international group of dermatologists with clinical and research expertise in acne vulgaris. The first consensus guidelines were published in 2003 in JAAD and were very well received as an evidence-based and thoughtful document [1]. In the 2009 and 2016 guidelines updated information on pathogenesis, mechanism of action of therapies, and clinical results are presented [2, 4].

For this purpose, Global Alliance to Improve Outcomes in Acne Group ("Global Alliance") was formed and the recommendations of the group have been published in 2003 as a supplement in the Journal of the Academy of Dermatology [2]. In the light of novel evidence-based studies, these recommendations have been updated recently [4]. On the other hand, racial and regional differences may affect the therapeutic approach to acne. Accordingly, in this ongoing process regional treatment guidelines are also being published [1, 2, 5–10].

1.3. Clinical features of acne vulgaris

Acne vulgaris is characterized by the presence of comedones and suggested to be a chronic disease. It has been traditionally thought that comedones are the noninflammatory lesions which present as either open or closed form. Inflammatory lesions of acne are papules, pustules, and nodules. In the previous guidelines, acne was graded into four levels as follows "Comedonal acne, mild to moderate papulopustular acne, severe papulopustular/moderate nodular acne, severe nodular acne/acne conglobata" [1, 7].

In the last guideline [4], acne has been divided simply as "Mild, moderate, and severe".

1.4. Pathophysiology of acne

The first step in the treatment of acne is to understand the pathophysiology of disease and to act on all factors involved in the development of acne. The initial lesions of acne are the microcomedones that already exist in normal-appearing skin. These microcomedones can only be observed histologically [1–3, 8]. Additionally, the role of inflammatory cytokine such as interleukin-1 (IL-1), relative deficiency of linoleic acid, and hormonal and genetic factors has been reported [7].

Four major steps that have been hypothesized in the pathogenesis of acne are outlined in **Table 1**. Although the inflammatory step was previously believed to occur at the end of these stages, now it is thought to occur after the increased sebum secretion from sebaceous glands

Increased sebum secretion from sebaceous glands
Secretion of inflammatory mediators
Altered keratinization and follicular plugging
Follicular colonization of *P. acnes**
*P. acnes: Propionibacterium acnes

Table 1. Four major steps in the pathogenesis of acne.

because of the proinflammatory properties of lipids of hyperseborrhea as well as some other factors including excess androgen and smoking [1–4, 11].

1.5. Topical treatment of acne

Reviewing the guidelines on the treatment of acne, a recommended common approach is outlined in **Table 2** [1–4].

Start with topical treatment, if appropriate
Give systemic treatment when necessary
Limit the use of local and systemic antibiotic concomitantly OR add topical BPO*
*BPO: Benzoyl peroxide

Table 2. Recommended general approach for the treatment of acne.

There is a large spectrum of topical agents for the treatment of acne (**Table 3**).

1.6. The importance of topical retinoids in the treatment of acne

Topical retinoids have multiple effects in the treatment of acne and act on more than one factor implicated in the etiology of acne (**Table 4**) [1–4, 12–14].

Topical retinoids have been the first-line treatment for most forms of acne vulgaris. They are used either alone or together with other agents as a first-line treatment in the treatment of acne forms other than severe nodular acne and acne conglobata. Alternative retinoids are included in alternative treatment options as well. In maintenance treatment, topical retinoids are used alone or in combination with BPO [1–4].

1. Antimicrobials: Azelaic acid (20%), BPO, clindamycin, dapsone (5%), erythromycin, sodium sulfacetamide, sulfur
2. Topical retinoids: Isotretinoin, tretinoin, adapalene, tazarotene
3. Combination drugs: Adapalene-benzoyl peroxide, BPO-clindamycin, BPO-erythromycin, sodium sulfacetamide-sulfur, tretinoin-clindamycin
4. Keratolytic agents: Salicylic acid

Table 3. Topical agents for the treatment of acne.

1.	Prevent the formation of microcomedones and reduce their number
2.	Reduce macrocomedones
3.	Promote the normal desquamation of follicular epithelium
4.	Exert anti-inflammatory effects
5.	Enhance the penetration of other drugs
6.	Prolong the remission periods of acne by inhibiting the of microcomedone formation and preventing the development of new lesions
7.	Prevents bacterial resistance

Table 4. Multiple effects of topical retinoids in the treatment of acne.

2. Topical retinoids

2.1. Introduction

Retinoids are vitamin A (retinol) or functional analogs with vitamin A activity. The abnormal keratinization in animals with vitamin A deficiency has exposed the importance of vitamin A in antikeratinization. As the systemic retinols given in effective dose have resulted in severe side effects, synthetic retinoids and their topical forms have been developed with similar clinical effect and fewer side effects. The first retinoid synthesized is all-trans-retinoic acid (ATRA, tretinoin) but as it has no significant advantages over retinol, it is used generally in topical form. ATRA is the natural metabolite of retinol. Isotretinoin has both systemic and topical forms. Today various topical retinoids are available for different purposes [14–16]. Human skin has retinoid receptors, belonging to thyroid receptor family, which have the capacity to store and metabolize retinoids [17]. The biologic effects of topical retinoids are mediated through nuclear hormone receptors and cytosolic binding proteins because human skin expresses RAR (RAR-γ > RAR-α) and RXR (RXR-α > RXR-β) [14–16]. **Table 5** outlines retinoid receptors and their main endogenous ligands.

2.2. Topical retinoids used in the treatment of acne

Tretinoin and isotretinoin are the first-generation retinoids whereas adapalene and tazarotene are the third-generation retinoids. Retinaldehyde and retinol are found in cosmetic formulations [5]. Commercially available topical retinoids for acne treatment are presented in **Table 6**.

The receptors of retinoids	Main endogenous ligand
RAR α, β, γ	Retinoic acid, 9-cis retinoic acid
RXR α, β, γ	9-cis retinoic acid
RAR, retinoic acid receptor; RXR, retinoid X receptor.	

Table 5. Retinoid receptors and their endogenous ligands.

Tretinoin
13-cis retinoic acid (isotretinoin)
Adapalene
Tazarotene

Table 6. Topical retinoids used in the treatment of acne.

2.2.1. *Tretinoin*

Tretinoin is the first retinoid studied and has been used more than 30 years in the treatment of acne. It induces the breakage of bonds between keratinized cells and enables the disintegration and the removal of the keratin plug. Besides comedolytic effect, it exerts anti-inflammatory effect; however, it does not have an effect on sebaceous gland activity. It binds to RARs on cytosol and regulates the expression of genes after moving to nucleus. It can bind all three types of RARs, namely, α, β, and γ [13–15]. Tretinoin can be used alone or in combination with other agents. As it enhances the penetration of other drugs, it creates a synergistic effect in combined use. Different formulations of tretinoin molecule have been introduced including 0.025, 0.05, and 0.1% cream, 0.025 and 0.1 gel, 0.05% solution, microsphere gel, and polymer cream [13–16].

2.2.2. *Adapalene*

Adapalene is a third-generation retinoid. It is available in 0.1 and 0.3 % gel and 0.1% cream form [1–4, 13–15, 18].

2.2.3. *Isotretinoin*

13-cis retinoic acid is produced from the isomerization of retinoic acid. The effects and efficacy are similar to retinoic acids. Other than oral form, it is available in 0.05% gel, and 0.05 and 0.1% cream form [1–4, 13–15].

2.2.4. *Tazarotene*

Tazarotene is a third-generation retinoid and its active metabolite is tazarotenic acid and it can bind all three types of RARs. It has not only anti-inflammatory effect like other retinoids, but also antiproliferative properties and normalizes the Filaggrin expression. Therefore, it is used also in the treatment of psoriasis. It is available in 0.05 and 0.1% cream form [1–4, 13–15].

2.2.5. *Others*

Retinaldehyde has a pivotal role in the natural vitamin A metabolism of keratinocytes. It is converted into all-trans retinoic acid and acts as topical retinoic acid in lower concentrations and generally found in cosmetic formulations. It has a mild comedolytic effect and has an antibacterial activity against Gram-positive bacteria including *P. acnes* due to its aldehyde group [19]. It is generally used in cosmetic formulations. Retinol and retinoic acid are metabolized into retinoyl beta-glucuronide. Motretinid is a second-generation monoaromatic retinoid. The clinical and side effects of motretinid are less than tretinoin [1–4].

2.2.6. *Combination formulations*

After the superiority of combining erythromycin 2% solution with 0.05% tretinoin to the monotherapy of each had been shown, fixed combination formulations of topical retinoids have been in production since 1978. Then, 0.025% tretinoid-4% erythromycin and 0.005% isotretinoin-2% erythromycin fixed combination formulations have been introduced [5]. It was reported that the usage of combination products were associated with better patient compliance. Recently, adapalene 0.1% and BPO 2.5% combination has been introduced. Theoretically, retinoid and BPO combination has been suggested to be advantageous due to the lack of bacterial resistance [1, 4, 13, 14].

2.2.7. *The evaluation of comparative studies*

Nast et al. conducted an evidence-based guideline for the treatment of acne in 2012 [7]. In this study, previous treatments were compared; superior efficacy was defined as a difference of more than 10% reduction of lesions in head-to-head comparisons.

2.2.7.1. *Comedonal acne*

Topical retinoids were found to show comparable-to-superior efficacy on noninflammatory lesions when compared to benzoyl peroxide [7].

Adapalene has shown comparable efficacy against noninflammatory lesions compared with tretinoin. Isotretinoin was effective as adapalene in the treatment of noninflammatory lesions, whereas it was found to be superior to tretinoin. Combination of adapalene and BPO shows a comparable-to-superior efficacy compared with BPO or adapalene alone. There was no trial comparing fixed-dose combinations of erythromycin and isotretinoin; however, using both erythromycin and isotretinoin was found to show comparable efficacy compared to erythromycin or isotretinoin alone [7].

Fixed-dose combination of adapalene-BPO has shown comparable-to-superior efficacy compared to adapalene or BPO alone, however, it was associated with lower patient tolerance [7].

2.2.7.2. *Papulopustular acne*

The efficacy of adapalene against inflammatory lesions was comparable to azelaic acid, BPO, tretinoin, and isotretinoin. Tretinoin was found to show comparable efficacy compared to isotretinoin. Fixed-dose combination of adapalene-BPO was superior to adapalene alone and was effective as BPO or clindamycin-BPO combination [7].

Combination of erythromycin and isotretinoin was superior to isotretinoin alone and was effective as erythromycin alone [7].

2.2.8. *Patient tolerability and safety*

Adapalene was found to display the best tolerability and safety among the topical retinoids followed by isotretinoin and tretinoin [7]. The tolerability and safety profile of fixed-dose adapalene-BPO preparation was lower than adapalene or BPO alone. The tolerability and safety of erythromycin-isotretinoin combination was comparable to erythromycin or isotretinoin alone [7].

2.2.8.1. *Factors affecting therapeutic compliance of patients*

Treatment with less irritant topical retinoids was associated with better patient tolerance. To increase tolerance, it is advised to increase the dose gradually [5]. The carrier is also important as the active ingredient in topical formulation. Drugs with same active ingredient but different carriers were reported to show different tolerability profile [6, 13]. As these factors affect patient compliance they even influence the efficacy of the drug. Therefore, preparations with less irritant properties are more effective due to increased patient adherence. The other factors involved in treatment compliance are cosmetic products and skin cleaning habits. Application of drying agents was associated with the increased side effects of topical products. Also, racial differences were reported to affect the tolerance to topical retinoids. Asians are more prone to the irritation effect of topical retinoids compared to Caucasians [1, 3, 6].

2.2.9. *The safety profile of topical retinoids*

The major side effects of topical retinoids are local skin reactions such as erythema, scaling, dryness, burning, and stinging; rarely, they can cause pustular eruption. In comparative studies, adapalene with lower irritation rates has showed better tolerability profile compared to tretinoin or isotretinoin. Patient preferred adapalene over tretinoin [1, 7, 13].

2.2.9.1. *Safety in pregnancy and systemic absorption*

Even in long-term usage local retinoids were absorbed percutaneously only 1–2% and found in the range of natural endogenous levels in plasma [13]. However, congenital anomalies have been reported after the usage of local retinoids in the first trimester [20]. On the other hand, according to two retrospective cohort study topical retinoic acids were found not to associate with minor malformations in first trimester [21, 22]. According to many studies, systemic absorption of 0.05 and 1% isotretinoin gel is negligible even in 12 times greater than the normal dose. Adapalene is a derivative of naphthoic acid. It contains methoxyphenyl adamantyl chain and is stable against oxygen and light. Its cutaneous absorption is low due to its chemical structure. It could not be found in plasma after the application of 0.1% gel form [13]. In animal experiments, only systemic and high dose adapalene was reported to induce teratogenicity. However, as no studies have been carried out in pregnant subjects, potential risk cannot be excluded. In the literature, anophthalmia and abortion on 22nd week have been reported in a pregnant woman who used adapalene in 13th week of pregnancy [23]. Percutaneous absorption of tazarotene is less than 6%. No teratogenicity has been reported so far. Pregnancy category of tretinoin and adapalene is C, so they should be prescribed during pregnancy only if the potential benefit justifies potential risk to the fetus. On the other hand, erythromycin, azelaic acid, and BPO can be used during pregnancy, and retinoids are not recommended during pregnancy [13, 14, 24]. As no studies have been conducted on breastfeeding women, they should be avoided during lactation period. The pregnancy category of oral isotretinoin and tazarotene is X and their topical formulations are contraindicatory [21, 22].

2.2.10. Practical applications

According to an investigation, dermatologists prescribe topical retinoids as second-line treatment after clindamycin, oral minocycline, and topical BPO [25]. Since topical retinoids inhibit microcomedones that are the precursor lesions of acne, they are recommended in most forms of acne. In acne patients, microcomedones are observed histopathologically even in normal-appearing skin. This underlines the fact that topical acne drugs can also be applied to normal-appearing skin [26].

Mild, noninflammatory acne can be treated by topical retinoids alone. If the comedonal lesions present together with inflammatory lesions topical retinoids should be combined with antimicrobial agents. As the combination treatment targets multiple pathophysiological factors, it is possible to get faster and permanent results. In the first-line treatment of moderate inflammatory acne, topical retinoids are recommended in combination with antimicrobial agents. Topical retinoids are the essential part of the maintenance treatment of acne [1–4, 13, 14].

Author details

Dilek Bayramgurler[1]*, Selda Pelin Kartal[2] and Cemile Altunel[3]

*Address all correspondence to: dbayramgurler@yahoo.com

1 Department of Dermatology, Kocaeli University, Izmit-Kocaeli, Turkey

2 Dermatology Department, Ministry of Health Ankara Diskapi Yildirim Beyazit Education and Research Hospital, Ankara, Turkey

3 Department of Dermatology, Ankara Nato Hospital, Ankara, Turkey

References

[1] Thiboutot D, Gollnick H, Bettoli V, et al. New insights into the management of acne: an update from the Global Alliance to Improve Outcomes in Acne Group. J Am Acad Dermatol. 2009;**60**:1–50.

[2] Gollnick H, Cunliffe W, BersonD, et al. Management of acne: a report from Global Alliance to Improve Outcomes in Acne. J Am Acad Dermatol. 2003;**49**:1–37.

[3] Eskioglu F, Kartal Durmazlar SP. Akne vulgaris: algoritmik yaklasım. Turkiye Klinikleri Dermatoloji Dergisi. 2004;**14**:96–9.

[4] Zaenglein AL, Pathy AL, Schlosser BJ, Alikhan A, Baldwin HE, Berson DS, et al. Guidelines of care for the management of acne vulgaris. J Am Acad Dermatol. 2016;**74**:945–73.

[5] Eichenfield LF, Fowler JF, Fried RG et al. Perspectives on therapeutic options for acne: an update. Semin Cutan Med Surg. 2010;**29**:13–6.

[6] Abad-Casintahan F, Chow SKW, Goh CL, et al. Toward evidence-based practice in acne: consensus of an Asian acne group. J Dermatol. 2011;**38**:1041–8.

[7] Nast A, Dreno B, Bettoli V, et al. European evidence-based (S3) guidelines for the treatment of acne. J Eur Acad Dermatol Venereol 2012;**26**:1–29.

[8] Yan AC, Baldwin HE, Eichenfield LF, et al. Approach to pediatric acne treatment: an update. Semin Cutan Med Surg. 2011;**30**:16–21.

[9] Friedlander SF, Baldwin HE, Mancini AJ, et al. The acne continuum: an age-based approach to therapy. Semin Cutan Med Surg. 2011;**30**:6–11.

[10] Preneau S, Dreno B. Female acne – a different subtype of teenager acne? J Eur Acad Dermatol Venereol. 2011;**26**:277–82.

[11] Zouboulis CC. Acne and sebaceous gland function. Clin Dermatol. 2004;**22**:360–6.

[12] Gollnick H, Finlay AY, Shear N. Global alliance to improve outcomes in acne. Can we describe acne as a chronic disease? If so, how and when? Am J Clin Dermatol. 2008;**9**:279–84.

[13] Thielitz A, Abdel-Naser MB, Fluhr JW, et al. Topical retinoids in acne-an evidence-based overview. J Dtsch Dermatol Ges. 2008;**6**:1023–31.

[14] Tzellos T, Toulis KA, Dessinioti C, et al. Topical retinoids for the treatment of acne vulgaris. Cochrane Database of Systematic Reviews 2011; Issue 12. No: CD009470. DOI: 10.1002/14651858. CD009470.

[15] Bikowski JB. Mechanism of the comedolytic and anti-inflammatory properties of topical retinoids. J Drugs Dermatol. 2005;**4**:41–7.

[16] Kong S. The mechanism of action of topical retinoids. Cutis. 2005;**75**:10–3.

[17] Slominsky A, Wortsman J. Neuroendocrinology of the skin. Endocr Rev. 2000:**21**:457–87.

[18] Thielitz A, Helmdach M, Rapke EM, Gollnick H. Control of microcomedone formation throughout a maintenance treatment with adapalene gel 0.1%. J Eur Acad Dermatol Venereol. 2007;**21**:747–53.

[19] Pechere M, Pechere JC, Siegentholer G, Germanier L, Saurat JH. Antibacterial activity of retinaldehyde against Propionibacterium acnes. Dermatology. 1999;**1**:29–31.

[20] Lipson AH, Collins F, Webster WS. Multiple congenital defects associated with maternal use of topical tretinoin. Lancet. 1993;**341**:1352–3.

[21] Jick SS, Terris BZ, Jick H. First trimester topical tretinoin and congenital disorders. Lancet. 1993;**341**:1181–2.

[22] Loureiro KD, Kao KK, Jones KL, et al. Minor malformations characteristic of the retinoic acid embryopathy and other birth outcomes in children of women exposed to topical tretinoin during early pregnancy. Am J Med Genet A. 2005;**136**:117–21.

[23] Autret E, Berjot M, Jonville-Bera Ap, Aubry MC, Moraine C. Anophthalmia and agenesis of optic chiasma associated with adapalene gel in early pregnancy. Lancet. 1997;**350**:339.

[24] Kartal Durmazlar SP, Eskioglu F. Cosmetic procedures in pregnancy: review. Turkiye Klinikleri J Med Sci. 2008;**28**:942–6.

[25] Yentzer BA, Irby CE, Fleischer AB Jr, Feldman SR. Differences in acne treatment prescribing patterns of pediatricians and dermatologists: An analysis of nationally representative data. Pediatr Dermatol. 2008;**25**:635–9.

[26] Cunliffe WJ, Holland DB, Clark SM, Stables GI. Comedogenesis: some new aetiological, clinical and therapeutic strategies. Br J Dermatol. 2000;**142**:1084–91.

Chapter 9

Treatment of Acneiform Eruptions, Acne and Acne Scars with Surgery, Lasers and Light-Based Devices

Erol Koc and Asli Gunaydin Tatliparmak

Additional information is available at the end of the chapter

http://dx.doi.org/10.5772/66923

Abstract

Acne is a common skin disease that affects pilosebaceous unit, and it is characterized as comedones, inflammatory papules, pustules and occasionally nodulocystic lesions. Acne scar lesions have adverse effects on psychosocial life despite the latest treatment options.

Keywords: acne, eruption, laser, scar treatment

1. Treatment of acne with surgery.

Although acne surgery term is used for acne scar treatment methods, it could also be used in active acne lesions to support medical therapy. Surgical therapy is used to minimize inflammation and scar risk and to fasten the healing. Below are four categories of active acne lesions for surgical therapy guidelines [1]:

- Grade 1 (comedonal acne)
  - Comedone extraction
- Grade 2 (inflammatory papules)
  - Cryotherapy
  - Laser and light therapy

- Grade 3 (inflammatory pustules)
  - Cryotherapy
  - Nonablative lasers
  - Light therapy
- Grade 4 (nodulocystic acne)
  - Incision/drainage
  - Intralesional corticosteroids
  - Cryotherapy

1.1. Comedone extraction

Comedone extraction is a method where the clogged content in pilosebaceous unit is mechanically drained using a comedone extractor.

After wiping the surface with alcohol, comedone extractor is centered over the comedone and pressure is applied to the direction of hair follicle to drain the contest. If closed comedones present a small hole on the surface of the lesion, they should be opened by 21 gauge needles to make the extraction less traumatic.

The important considerations in the extraction process to minimize the risk of scarring and inflammation are to avoid applying undue pressure and pay attention to antisepsis rules [1, 2].

1.2. Cryotherapy

Cryotherapy can be applied with cryoslush or cryopeel methods in nodulocystic acne. In cryoslush method, crushed carbon dioxide and a few drops of acetone are added to make a paste. This paste is spooned on the lesions for 2–10 s with a gauze ball. It consists of superficial peeling effect due to epidermal necrosis, which causes desquamation of comedones and resolution of inflammatory lesions. The degree of peeling effect is determined by the amount of time the slush contacted with the lesions [3].

In the cryopeel method, liquid nitrogen spray is applied to lesions for 2–3 s. However, the risk of postinflammatory pigmentation (hypo or hyper), persistent erythema and scarring should be noted with this method. In particular, the patients with Fitzpatrick skin type 4–5 have greater risk of pigmentation and scar formation [1].

1.3. Incision/drainage/aspiration

Incision/drainage/aspiration of the cystic lesions can be applied with or without phenolization. After surgical cleaning of the area, a small incision is made with a no.15 surgical blade and cysts are drained. After draining, cyst wall is chemically cauterized with 88% phenol applied swab stick and neutralized with povidone-iodine to prevent from recurrence. Intralesional and perilesional triamcinolone acetonide 5–10 mg/ml is injected to reduce the risk of fibrous scarring in some cases [1, 2].

http://dx.doi.org/10.5772/66923

1.4. Intralesional corticosteroids

Intralesional corticosteroids are used in nodular and cystic acne patients to reduce the inflammation and minimize scarring. Triamcinolone acetonide is diluted with lidocaine 1% or sterile water to obtain 2.5 mg/ml concentration.

If the lesion is tensed, it should be drained before the injection. Injection is repeated after 3 weeks if there is an incomplete resolution. Hematoma, infection, atrophy and hypopigmentation are the complications that can be seen after the treatment [1, 4, 5].

2. Treatment of acne with lasers

2.1. Infrared lasers

Near-infrared (IR) light (700–1000 nm) penetrates deeper dermis than the red light. And during this penetration, it makes a minimal effect on the epidermis. This wavelength targets the tissue water in sebaceous glands and reduces the sebum secretion by thermal damage.

Infrared lasers (1064, 1320, 1450, 1540 nm) are generally used in facial skin rejuvenation, but there are also literatures showing reduction in the inflammatory acne lesions [6].

2.2. Pulse dye laser

Pulse dye lasers are nonablative, 585–595 nm wavelength systems that target the oxyhemoglobin in microvessels. They are generally used in the treatment of vascular lesions. The mechanism of action in acne treatment is still unknown, and the respond rates range between 40 and 49% [6–8]. Pain and postinflammatory hyperpigmentation are the most common adverse effects. The risk of discoloration is higher in patients with Fitzpatrick type IV and V skin. The treatment parameters are 4–7.5 J/cm^2 fluence, 350 μs to 6 ms pulse duration, and 585 or 595 nm wavelength [6, 7].

2.3. Potassium titanyl phosphate laser

Potassium titanyl phosphate lasers (KTP) are the laser devices with 535 nm wavelength and often used in the treatment of rosacea and telangiectasia. Response rates ranging from 32 to 20% have been reported with 1 or 2 time sessions per week.

The mechanism of action may be related to the destruction of blood vessels or laser-stimulated photodynamic reaction. Before the treatment, the use of aminolevulinic acid (ALA) as a photosensitizer response rate rises to 52% [6, 9].

3. Treatment of acne with light-based devices

Use of light-based devices for acne is based on the effect of photoabsorption of porphyrin produced by *Propionibacterium acnes*. This basic pathogenic Gram-positive bacterium in acne produces porphyrin, and when this substance absorbs the light, it reveals highly reactive oxygen radicals and leads to death of bacteria.

Porphyrin has two photo absorption peaks. The highest absorption is seen in the middle of blue light wavelengths in other words at Soret band, 415 nm. The second major absorption peak occurs at 630 nm, red light [10]. Red light has less effect on the activation of porphyrin; however, it reaches deeper into the skin, and by this means, it may lead to direct effect on inflammatory mediators [11].

3.1. Intense pulsed light (IPL)

IPL is an intense pulsed light system used in a number of dermatological cases such as vascular lesions, acneiform eruptions, pigmentary diseases, premalignant lesions and adnexal diseases. In the single pulse mode, the fluence will be delivered in single mode, and in burst mode, the fluence will be divided into series of pulses. It works in single pulse mostly, and pulse duration identifies energy output. However, in one of the study reports, 56% of reduction was achieved in acne scores in burst mode, and this rate was reported as 40% in the single pulse mode [9, 10].

It is considered that IPL has an impact by means of photoactivation of porphyrin secreted by *P. acnes*. Free oxygen radicals as a result of this photoactivation reduce production of sebum from sebaceous glands.

At the same time, it was shown that suppression of IL-8 and TNF-alpha production has a significant role in inflammatory acne pathogenesis and increased expression of IL10 has an anti-inflammatory effect [12]. In the studies conducted, it was reported that IPL was especially effective for inflammatory acne lesions. Safe use for skin type 3–4 patients is one of the advantages of IPL.

Recently, application of vacuum IPL to target pilosebaceous unit better has came into question. It was indicated that vacuum apparatus would reduce the debris in pilosebaceous unit and offer the opportunity of easier application in curled regions such as nose and forehead sides. However, risk of transient mild erythema is higher in vacuum IPL [6].

3.2. Narrowband blue light

Ultraviolet (UV) radiation has a therapeutic effect in inflammatory acne. This effect is considered as related to follicular Langerhans cell suppression and destruction of *P. acnes*.

Blue light is in 400–500 nm wavelength and can penetrate into upper epidermis. Light with such wavelength inhibits keratinocyte inflammation and also results in mitochondrial damage in nonpigmented epithelial cells and creates toxic effect. It slows down proliferation of keratinocyte in pilosebaceous unit. Anti-inflammatory effect on keratinocyte occurs by reducing IL-1 and ICAM markers. As stated before, when porphyrin produced by *P. acnes* absorbs light, it produces free oxygen radicals being toxic for the bacteria [13, 14].

Rate of response to the treatment was reported up to 77% in moderate inflammatory acne. Administration dose in the studies varies between 2 and 29 J/cm^2 for the inhibition of occurrence of new lesion or to prevent inflammation in the active lesion [6, 9].

http://dx.doi.org/10.5772/66923

3.3. Narrowband red light

Red light can penetrate into sebaceous glands in dermis (620–660 nm). Its basic effect is the activation of protoporphyrin IX and reducing release of inflammatory cytokine. Although it penetrates deeper than blue light, higher concentration light is necessary for *P. acnes* eradication.

It reduces inflammation in inflammatory and noninflammatory acne; however, it cannot achieve resolution completely. For this reason, it should be used in combination with ALA, not alone [6, 15].

3.4. Blue-red light-emitting diode

Blue-red light is more effective for the treatment of inflammatory acne alone than blue (415 nm) or red light (630 nm). Reported rates of response to treatment vary between 77 and 90%. Blue-red light achieves 34–54% reduction in noninflammatory acne lesions. Synergic effect of combined treatment was observed as decrease in cell proliferation in in vitro cultured sebaceous cells and lipogenesis [6, 16].

Phototherapy is administered to the patients 1 or 2 times a week for 15–20 min totally for 4 weeks, and it is reported that efficiency of the treatment lasts for average 8 weeks more [16].

3.5. Photodynamic therapy

When photosensitizing agents are applied to acne lesions, protoporphyrin IX production by *P. acnes* increases and free oxygen radicals appear. These free oxygen radicals damage mitochondria, nucleus and cell membrane and create cytotoxic effect on *P. acnes*.

A number of light sources were used in photodynamic therapy (PDT) with varying success rates. All light sources may lead to erythema, stinging, peeling, oozing, pruritus and pustule formation [6, 9].

Aminolevulinic acid (ALA) is a photosensitizer used in PDT frequently and is transformed into protoporphyrin IX by *P. acnes* if applied to inflammatory lesions. The biggest advantages of ALA are the short duration of photosensitizing effect within 24 h and low risk of side effects due to topical usage [17, 18].

There are a number of variations related to ALA-PDT combination. Some of them include the concentration of medicine used, incubation time and type of light source used (LED, IPL, red light, blue light or combined light). For this reason, an optimal therapy regime is not applicable for PDT in acne treatment.

Before starting ALA-PDT treatment, it should be proven that basic bacterium in the lesions is *P. acnes* because the response to the treatment depends on the presence of *P. acnes*. For this reason, lesional skin should be examined with wood lamp before the treatment and it should be examined whether spontaneous fluorescence is positive or not [17].

One of the most significant parameters determining the treatment response is which light source will be used. While depth of sebaceous glands in the skin is ≤2 mm, it is deeper than 2 mm in elevated acne papule or pustule. For this reason, wavelengths affecting deeper should be used [8, 17].

Success rate was reported as 68–95% in PDT with red light. Success rate of PDT with blue light is 7–21% better than blue light alone. However, ALA-PDT with blue light has relatively shorter effectiveness and longer side effect profile [6, 8].

4. Treatment of acne scars with surgery

Acne scars vary from superficial rolling scars to deep ice pick and boxcar scars due to their morphology and depth. Most of the patients have more than one type of scars. Atrophic scars are grouped as ice pick, boxcar and rolling scars and those characterized with collagen overproduction are grouped as hypertrophic and keloid scars [17]. While selecting the treatment, acne scar type and duration of the disease should be considered. Previous treatments, keloid history, past or active herpes simplex infection, habit of smoking and sun exposure should be questioned certainly.

If the patient has HSV infection history, acyclovir or famciclovir treatment should be started 2 days prior to the procedure and carried on 7–10 days after the procedure. Informed consent form should be obtained from every case, and if possible, pre- and posttreatment photographs should be taken.

Surgical treatment options for acne scars are subcision, punch excision, dermabrasion, filling, intralesional steroid injection, silicone gel coating and scar revision [4].

4.1. Subcision

The purpose of this treatment is to break down the fibrotic bands connecting the scar to the subcutaneous tissue. It is mostly preferred for rolling scars.

Firstly, scar area is marked with a pen. Then, local anesthesia is applied, and 18 or 20 gauge needle is proceeded to deep dermis parallel to the border of the scar marked.

It is continued along the border marked, side-to-side needle motion called 'fanning motion' is applied, and fibrous bands are made free. There are publications in the literature, indicating that better response (50% cure rate) is achieved with 18 and 21 gauge cannula [19]. The doctor should be more careful in preauricular, temporal and mandibular regions because of the placement of facial nerve branches and major arterioles.

'Blunt blade subcision' is also another technique for the treatment of atrophic acne scars. The authors hypothesized that using a blunt blade reduces the risk of trauma of neurovascular structures.

After local anesthesia, 18 gauge needle is used to puncture the entrance of the blade. Up to three-fourths of the blade could enter into the skin, and the blade should be moved back and forth subdermally to release the fibrotic tissue [20, 21].

4.2. Punch excision techniques

These techniques are used for depressed scars such as ice pick and boxcar. There are punch excision types varying in the diameter and surface of the scar:

http://dx.doi.org/10.5772/66923

I: Punch excision and closure: If the scar is bigger than 3–5 mm, it is excised to subcutaneous fat layer firstly and sutured after undermining. The doctor should be careful to avoid new scar formation.

II: Punch incision and elevation: If the depressed scar has a normal surface structure, it is incised to subcutaneous tissue (incised up) and elevated to the level of peripheral tissue.

III: Punch excision and grafting: Depressed pitted ice pick scars with the diameter of 4 mm are excised and then placed into autologous, full layer punch grafts. Donor sites are mostly post-auricular site or hip [2, 4, 5].

4.3. Dermabrasion

Dermabrasion is the peeling of skin from epidermis to dermal layers to the level desired by use of electrical dermabrader. Manual dermabrader is used only for spot dermabrasion.

Re-epithelialization starts from the border of scar and sebaceous gland, sweat gland and hair follicle residuals. Since facial area is rich of these glands, recovery is faster than other regions.

Spot dermabrasion is applied under local anesthesia and at outpatient clinic; however, full-face dermabrasion should be performed in the hospital where we have the opportunity of immediate intervention. After the consent of the patient is obtained, the treatment area is cleaned, local anesthesia is done, and scars are marked. Dermabrasion is applied to the marked regions. Dermabrasion should be applied to maximum upper and midreticular dermis joining region to prevent postprocedure formation.

Wider bleeding focus, firmer surface and parallel line and break in grooves are observed in this joining region. According to the depth of dermabrasion, crusting starts within 7–10 days. Infection, persistent dyschromia, hypo-/hyperpigmentation, erythema and scarring are the complications.

Even if dermabrasion remains in the background after ablative lasers started to be used, it is still an efficient option for properly selected patients [1, 2, 5].

4.4. Filling (soft tissue augmentation)

A number of fillers are used for depressed scars, and these are mainly hyaluronic acid, hydroxyapatite, collagen, tricalcium phosphate, autologous fibroblasts and silicone gel. Fillers are chosen for minimal downtime and fast response.

Dermal filler is placed under the scar and injected till the scar level becomes the same as the surrounding tissue. It can be used alone and also can be applied after subcision or ablative laser treatment [2, 5].

Hyaluronic acid is a hydrophilic polysaccharide that occurs in the connective tissue naturally. Injection of hyaluronic acid stimulates the collagen synthesis and activation of dermal fibroblasts [4].

Calcium hydroxyapatite is a semipermanent dermal filler that stimulates fibroblast production of collagen. This filler can improve the appearance of atrophic acne scars but not deeper ice pick scars [1].

4.5. Intralesional steroids

In 10–20 mg/ml dilution, intralesional triamcinolone for hypertrophic scars and keloids can be applied with or without cytotoxic agents (like 5-fluoroauracil). The procedure is repeated for 3- to 4-week period till the lesion is regressed, but risk of atrophy should be considered [1, 2].

The proposed mechanisms of action are decreased fibroblast proliferation and collagen synthesis [4].

4.6. Silicone gel sheeting

It is considered that silicon sheets are effective to correct surfaces of hypertrophic scars and keloids and reduce the discoloration [1].

Silicone provides the therapeutic effect by pressure and hydration. Silicone sheets are cut to the size of scar and should be worn for 12 h per day for 2 months [4].

4.7. Scar revision

In the selected cases, surgical techniques such as Z, M and Y plasty can be used if the scar is linear or extensive. However, the procedure should be performed by an experienced dermatosurgeon [1].

5. Treatment of acne scars with lasers

This issue will be mentioned under the headlines of ablative, nonablative and fractional lasers.

5.1. Ablative lasers

Er:YAG (2940 nm) and infrared CO_2 (10,600 nm) lasers are the treatment choices for ablative nonfractional skin resurfacing. The depth of efficacy depends on the number of passes. The energy is absorbed by the intercellular tissue water, and with this photodermal effect, neocollagenesis and collagen remodeling are stimulated. Thermal skin injury with Er:YAG laser is less than CO_2 laser. Because of this limitation of short-pulsed Er:YAG lasers, long pulses were developed.

But Er:YAG laser has still some advantages like rapid healing time and less complications compared to CO_2laser [22].

Absolute contraindications for the ablative laser treatment are as follows:

- Active cutaneous infection (bacterial, viral or fungal)
- Inflammatory skin condition (psoriasis, eczema, etc) on the treatment area
- History of keloid
- Isotretinoin use in last 6 months

After laser ablation, topical antibacterials should not be used due to risk of contact dermatitis [4, 9].

Postinflammatory hyper- or hypopigmentation, acne flare up and erythema are the most common side effects that can be seen after ablative nonfractional laser treatments [23]. Most of the authors suggest the use of topical retinoic acid and/or hydroquinone cream to reduce the risk of hyperpigmentation [4, 22].

5.2. Nonablative lasers

The most popular nonablative lasers are Nd:YAG 1320 nm, diode 1450 nm and Nd:YAG 1064 nm lasers. These lasers deliver the energy through dermis without epidermal damage and target the tissue water. Dermal fibroblasts in the papillary and midreticular dermis are thermally stimulated leading to collagen remodeling. They have minimal postrecovery time, and this makes them safe but less effective on the atrophic acne scars than ablative lasers [23, 24].

Pulsed dye laser (PDL) has been used especially for hypertrophic, erythematous acne scars. The mechanism of effect depends on reducing transforming growth factor beta expression, fibroblast proliferation and collagen type III deposition.

The most common adverse effect of PDL treatment is purpura, which persists for several days. Edema is another side effect that can be seen but usually regresses in 48 h [9].

5.3. Fractional lasers

These lasers are classified into two categories: nonablative fractional lasers (NAFL) and ablative fractional lasers (AFL).

Fractional lasers have started to be used in 2004 firstly. These devices create vertical, cylindrical and multiple thermal damage areas called microthermal zone (MTZ) in dermis. MTZ is the zone being 1.5 mm in depth, 100–400 μm in width and having 6400 particles per square centimeter [25]. Fractional lasers are the most preferred treatment method, especially for atrophic acne scars [2]. Rolling scars are caused by subcuticular fat destruction, and they are treated with the lasers that penetrate up to the papillary dermis. Ice pick scars are narrow, deep and sharply marginated lesions.

They extend vertically to the deep dermis and do not respond well to fractional lasers. Shallow boxcar scars and most of the deep boxcar scars are amenable to fractional lasers [26].

Ablation is described as fast cellular heating and tissue vaporization during laser application. Nonablative fractional lasers have 1320–1927 nm wavelength, while ablative fractional lasers have 2940–10,600 nm wavelength.

While fractional ablative lasers are more efficient in treatment, they have longer recovery period compared to fractional nonablative lasers and higher risk of posttreatment, postinflammatory hyperpigmentation [2, 25]. Points to be considered for better response during treatment with fractional lasers are the number of passes per session and the number of sessions. While average 3–4 passes per session over four monthly sessions are preferred for fractional Er:YAG lasers, for fractional CO_2 lasers, fewer passes and sessions and longer time must be left between the treatments [2, 27, 28].

By means of intact tissue surrounding MTZ in fractional ablative lasers compared to classical ablative lasers, re-epithelialization and therefore postprocedure recovery are faster [29].

In this study, varying rates for efficiency of fractional lasers in acne scars are reported. In a review, it was reported that success rate for acne scar treatment with ablative fractional laser is varied between 26 and 83% and varied between 26 and 50% in nonablative fractional lasers [8, 30, 31].

6. Treatment of acne scars with light-based devices

Fractional radiofrequency is a new and noninvasive treatment method used for all atrophic acne scar types. When radiowave energy is transmitted to subcutaneous tissue, it will result in heating of water in skin cells, stimulation of heat-shock protein production and therefore wound healing.

Possible side effects include transient erythema, dryness, bruising, crusting and postinflammatory hyperpigmentation [2].

IPL treatment was tried for hypertrophic acne scars and keloid. Possible mechanism of action is to suppress vascular proliferation, which has a role in artificial pigmentation and collagen overgrowth. Sufficient literature about hypertrophic and keloid acne scars is not present, but in a study with 109 patients, it was reported that IPL achieved 59.7% good/excellent recovery in hypertrophic scars and keloid.

For this reason, it was claimed that IPL treatment to be started in early period after cutaneous surgical procedures prevented hypertrophic scars [32].

Author details

Erol Koc* and Asli Gunaydin Tatliparmak

*Address all correspondence to: drerolkoc@yahoo.com

Department of Dermatology, Bahcesehir University, Istanbul, Turkey

References

[1] Khunger N. Standard guidelines of care for acne surgery. Indian J Dermatol Venerol Leprol 2008;74:28–36.

[2] Viera MS. Management of acne scars: fulfilling our duty of care for patients. Br J Dermatol 2015;172:47–51.

[3] Kaminsky A. Less common methods to treat acne. Dermatology 2003;206:68–73.

[4] Levy LL, Zeichner JA. Management of acne scarring, Part II. Am J Clin Dermatol 2012;13:331–340.

[5] Goodman GJ. Treatment of acne scarring. Int J Dermatol 2011;50:1179–1194.

[6] Handler MZ, Bloom BS, Goldberg DJ. Energy based devices in the treatment of acne vulgaris. Dermatol Surg 2016;42:573–585.

[7] Voravutinon N, Rojanamatin J, Sadhwani D, Iyengar S, Alam M. A comparative split-face study using different mild purpuric and subpurpuric fluence level of 595-nm pulsed dye laser for treatment of moderate to severe acne vulgaris. Dermatol Surg 2016;42:403–409.

[8] Hadersal M, Bo TK, Wulf HC. Evidence based review of lasers, light sources and photodynamic therapy in the treatment of acne vulgaris. J Eur Acad Dermatol Venerol 2008;22:267–278.

[9] Sobanko JF, Alster TS. Management of acne scarring, Part I. Am J Clin Dermatol 2012;13:319–330.

[10] Kumerasan M, Srinivas CR. Efficacy of IPL in treatment of acne vulgaris: comparison of single and burst pulse mode in IPL. Indian J Dermatol 2010;55:370–372.

[11] Hamilton FL, Car J, Lyons C, Car M, Layton A, Majeed A. Laser and other light therapies for the treatment of acne vulgaris: systematic review. Br J Dermatol 2009;160:1273–1285.

[12] Taylor M, Porter R, Gonzalez M. Intense pulsed light may improve inflammatory acne through TNF α down regulation. J Cosmet Laser Ther 2014;16:96–103.

[13] Ash C, Harrison A, Drew S, Whittall R. A randomized controlled study for the treatment of acne vulgaris using high intensity 414 nm solid state diode arrays. J Cosmet Laser Ther 2015;17:170–176.

[14] Tremblay JF, Sire DJ, Lowe NJ, Moy RL. Light emitting diode 415 nm in the treatment of inflammatory acne: an open label, multisentric, pilot investigation. J Cosmet Laser Ther 2006;8:31–33.

[15] Choi MS, Yun SJ, Beom HJ, Park HR, Lee JB. Comparative study of the bactericidal effects of 5-aminolevulinic acid with blue and red light on *Propionibacterium acnes*. J Dermatol 2011;38:661–666.

[16] Goldberg DJ, Russell BA. Combination blue (415 nm) and red (633 nm) LED phototherapy in the treatment of mild to severe acne vulgaris. J Cosmet Laser Ther 2006;8:71–75.

[17] Dong Y, Zhou G, Jihan C, et al. A new LED device used for photodynamic therapy in treatment of moderate to severe acne vulgaris. Photodiagnosis Photodyn Ther 2016;13:188–195.

[18] Ma Y, Liu Y, Wang Q, Ren J, Xiang L. Prospective study of 5-aminolevulinic acid photodynamic therapy for the treatment of severe adolescent acne in Chinese patients. J Dermatol 2015;42:504–507.

[19] Nilforoushzadeh M, Lofti E, Nickkholgh E, Salehi B, Shokrani M. Can subcision with the cannula be an acceptable alternative method in treatment of acne scars? Med Arh 2015;69:384–386.

[20] Engin B, Kutlubay Z, Karakus O, et al. Evaluation of effectiveness of erbium-yttrium-aluminium-garnet laser on atrophic facial acne scars with 22 MHz digital ultrasonography in a Turkish population. J Dermatol 2012;39:982–988.

[21] Barikbin B, Akbari Z, Yousefi M, Dowlati Y. Blunt Blade Subcision: An Evolution in the Treatment of Atrophic Acne Scars. Dermatol Surg. 2017 Jan;43 Suppl 1: 57–63.

[22] Lee SJ, Kang JM, Chung WS, Kim YK, Kim HS. Ablative non fractional lasers for atrophic acne scars: a new modality of erbium YAG laser resurfacing in Asians. Lasers Med Sci 2014;29:615–619.

[23] Rogachefsky AS, Hussain M, Goldberg DJ. Atrophic and a mixed pattern of acne scars improved with a 1320 nm Nd:YAG laser. Dermatol Surg 2003;29:904–908.

[24] Asilian A, Salimi E, Faghihi G, et al. Comparison of Q switched 1064 nm Nd YAG laser and fractional CO2 laser efficacies on improvement of atrophic facial acne scar. J Res Med Sci 2011;16:1189–1195.

[25] Stewart N, Lim AC, Lowe PM, Goodman G. Lasers and laser-like devices: part one. Aust J Dermatol 2015;54:173–183.

[26] Sardana K, Garg VK, Arora P, Khurana N. Histological validity and clinical evidence for use of fractional lasers for acne scars. J CutanAesthetSurg 2012;5:75–90.

[27] Ong MWS, Bashir SJ. Fractional laser resurfacing for acne scars: a review. Br J Dermatol 2012;166:1160–1169.

[28] Nimal B, Pai SB, Sripathi H, et al. Efficacy and safety of erbium doped yttrium aluminium garnet fractional resurfacing laser for treatment of facial acne scars. Indian J Dermatol Venerol Leprol 2013;79:193–198.

[29] Qıan H, Lu Z, Dıng H, Yan S, Xıang L, Gold MH. Treatment of acne scarring with fractional laser. J Cosmet Laser Ther 2012;14:162–163.

[30] Cachafeiro T, Escobar G, Maldonado G, Cestari T, Corleta O. Comparison of nonablative fractional erbium laser 1,340 nm and microneedling for the treatment of atrophic acne scars. A randomized clinical trial. Dermatol Surg 2016;42:232–241.

[31] Cho SB, Lee SJ, Cho S, et al. Non ablative 1550 nm erbium glass and ablative 10.600 nm carbon dioxide fractional lasers for acne scars: a randomized split face study with blinded response evaluation. J Eur Acad Dermatol Venerol 2010;24:921–925.

[32] Erol OO, Gurlek A, Agaoglu G, Topcuoglu E, Oz H. Treatment of hypertrophic scars and keloids using intense pulsed light (IPL). Aesth Plast Surg 2008;32:902–909.

Chapter 10

Histopathologic Evaluation of Acneiform Eruptions: Practical Algorithmic Proposal for Acne Lesions

Murat Alper and Fatma Aksoy Khurami

Additional information is available at the end of the chapter

http://dx.doi.org/10.5772/65494

Abstract

Acneiform lesions are encountered in different chapters in various dermatology and dermatopathology textbooks. The most common titles used for these disorders are diseases of the hair, diseases of cutaneous appendages, folliculitis, acne, and inflammatory lesions of dermis and epidermis. In this chapter, first of all we will discuss folliculitis, and then acne vulgaris that is a kind of folliculitis will be described. After acne vulgaris, other acneiform eruptions and demodicosis will be studied. At the end, simple algorithmic schemes by assembling clinical, pathological, and microbiological data will be shared.

Keywords: acneiform lesions, algorithm, histopathologic evaluation

1. Introduction

1.1. Histology of pilar unit

Pilar unit is a structure generally made up of three subunits which are hair follicle, sebaceous gland, and arrector pili muscle. Hair follicle is divided in to three parts: infundibulum, isthmus, and inferior part. Infundibulum extends between entrance of sebaceous gland duct to the follicular orifice in epidermis. Isthmus: extends between entrance of sebaceous duct to hair follicle and insertion of arrector pili muscle. The basal part of hair follicle is called the inferior segment or inferior part. Histologic structure and function of hair follicle is very intriguing. *Demodex folliculorum* mites, *Staphylococcus epidermis*, and yeast of *pityrosporum* can be seen and can be a normal component of pilosebaceous unit.

The life cycle of hair follicle is divided into three phases: anagen (growth phase), catagen (regressing phase), and telogen (resting phase). The sebaceous gland attached to hair follicle produces holocrine-type secretions. They excrete the sebum through excretory ducts into hair follicle [1]. Sebum that inhibits the reproduction of bacteria and fungi is rich in triglyceride. When the increased number of *Propionibacterium acnes* is present, triglyceride is hydrolyzed and the biochemical conditions are altered [2].

1.2. Routine clinical and pathological conditions

There are bazillion hair and pilosebaceous units on the body surface. As a matter of course, hair follicle-related pathologies (especially inflammatory diseases) comprise one of the most popular topics in dermatology clinics.

In a big pathology center where daily around 40 cases of skin materials and annually a total of 35,000–40,000 different biopsy materials are examined, we rarely do histopathologic examination of disorders in inflammatory pilosebaceous units. It is mainly because the clinicians diagnose clinically and do not need much tissue correlation with their differential diagnosis in these disorders.

We retrospectively searched the information system of our hospital for the last 3 years and found 154 reports in which the term "acne" was aforementioned (132 cases were categorized as acne rosacea). For the last 3 years, approximately 23,000 skin samples have been sent by dermatology or plastic and reconstructive surgery departments (punch biopsies, shave biopsies, incisional biopsies, excisional biopsies included). Although general approach do not persuade for biopsy, sometimes in our clinic there is a little tendency to biopsying central face lesions for differential diagnosis.

2. Histopathology of acneiform lesions

2.1. Folliculitis, subtypes, differential diagnosis

In follicular eruptions adnexocentric inflammation, microabscesses and pustules on epidermis can be seen [3]. Peri- and intrafollicular inflammatory cells consist: lymphocytes, plasmocytes, histiocytes, polymorphonuclear, leukocytes, and multinuclear giant cells. Most folliculitis emerges as a result of follicular orifice occlusion by normal flora of the skin.

Although different categorization can be found in various textbooks, folliculitis can be divided into two groups: infectious and noninfectious (sterile). Furthermore noninfectious folliculitis can be grouped as neutrophilic, eosinophilic, etc. according to the predominant cell component present in the lesion. Infectious folliculitis can be grouped as bacterial (Gram-negative, Gram-positive), fungal, viral, and symbiotic (demodex) folliculitis [4].

The most common cause of Gram-positive folliculitis is *Staphylococcus aureus*. Similarly, *Enterobacter, Klebsiella, Escherichia, Serratia, Proteus*, etc., can cause Gram-negative folliculitis. Gram-negative folliculitis is generally caused in consequence of long-term antibiotic treatment. Hot tub folliculitis is a special form of bacterial folliculitis, which arises 24–48 hours after hot water contact and is caused by *Pseudomonas aeruginosa*. The most common cause of viral folliculitis is herpes simplex virus, varicella zoster virus, and the most common cause of fungal folliculitis is pityrosporum.

According to some other studies, folliculitis can be classified as superficial and both superficial and deep [5].

Independent of etiology, the primer lesion of folliculitis is generally an erythematous papule or pustule. Histologically in all types of folliculitis, inflammation is seen either in follicular epithelia and/or perifollicular area (**Figure 1**).

Whenever the cause is a bacterium, a neutrophilic infiltrate is dominantly seen in the follicular epithelia and dermis (**Figure 2**). Granuloma formation can be seen in consequence of follicular epithelial rupture and passing of pilosebaceous unit components into the dermis.

In viral folliculitis, cytopathic effects such as acantolysis, dyskeratosis, multinucleation, inclusions, chromatin marginalization, nuclear molding, etc., can be seen in infundibulum. In early lesions, cytopathic effects cannot be seen [5]. In a viral folliculitis, a lower concentration of inflammation is noticeable. In some cases, hyperplasia of epidermis, necrosis of follicular epithelia or sebaceous gland can be visible.

Fungal folliculitis is commonly seen in adult women living in warm and humid climates. Immunosuppression, diabetes and antibiotic use can be predisposing factors. The cause is

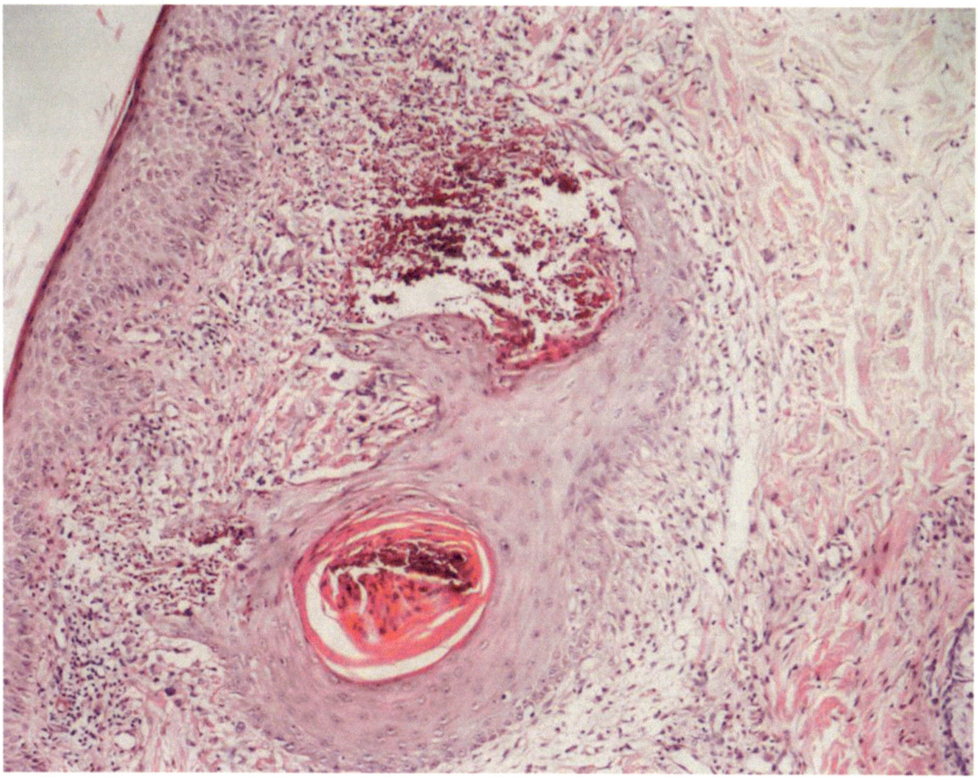

Figure 1. Mixed type inflammation that surrounded the follicle, attacked the follicular epithelia, and destroyed the hair follicle (HE ×100).

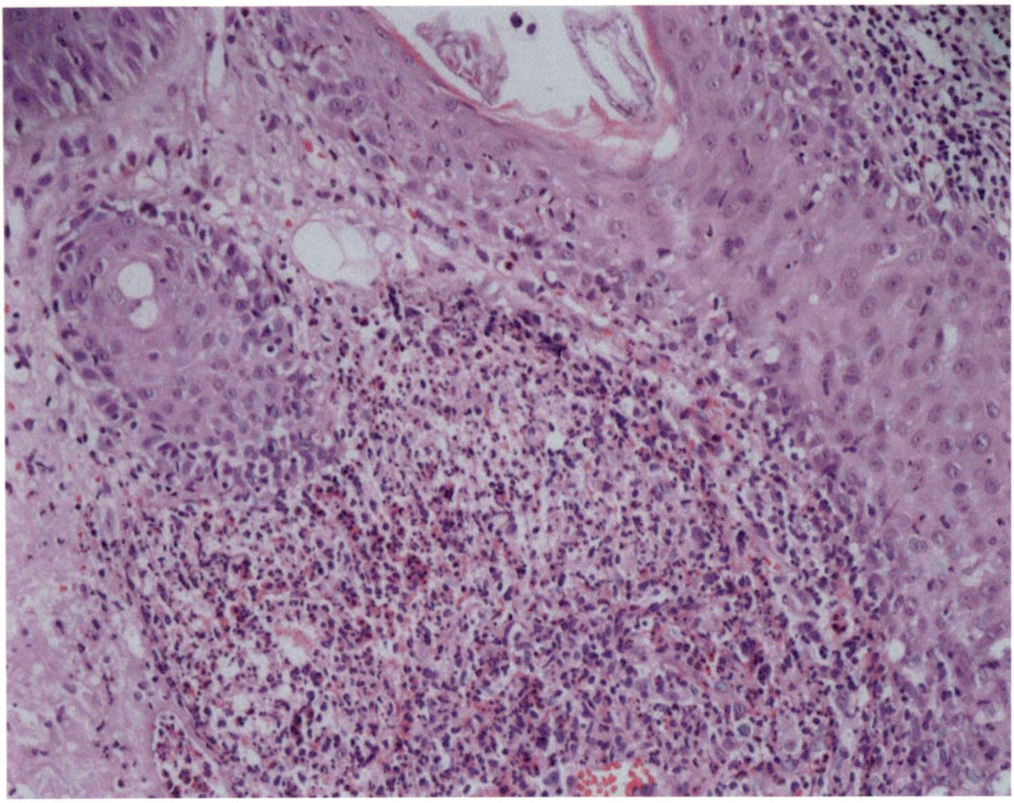

Figure 2. In a bacterial folliculitis case, predominantly neutrophilic infiltrate is present in the upper dermis and invades the follicular epithelia (HE ×100).

mostly *Malassezia globosa* (*Malassezia furfur*). Inside the dilated hair follicle due to keratin plug, numerous yeasts are visible (**Figure 3**). Around hair follicle mild chronic inflammation (including eosinophils) can be seen. The rupture of follicle transforms chronic inflammation to acute inflammation consequently abscess formation and granulation tissue can be seen [4].

In the syphilitic folliculitis, plasma cells are dominant [6].

There are some possible and practical methods for finding the cause of folliculitis such as: Gram staining (for bacteria), PAS or silver stain (for fungi) and immunohistochemistry (for viral causes). However, the sensitivity of these methods can be low. The more sensitive and specific methods such as fresh tissue culture, PCR, etc., can be used for microorganism typology [6].

Folliculitis can also be classified according to microanatomic structure of the skin which is involved. Most of bacterial folliculitis involves the superficial part of hair follicle that is why they are called superficial bacterial folliculitis. The superficial folliculitis caused by *S. aureus* is also called impetigo of Bockhart. In deep folliculitis tenderness, warmth, and erythema are visible in a wide area. Nodules are formed. They are most commonly seen in buttocks, axilla,

http://dx.doi.org/10.5772/65494

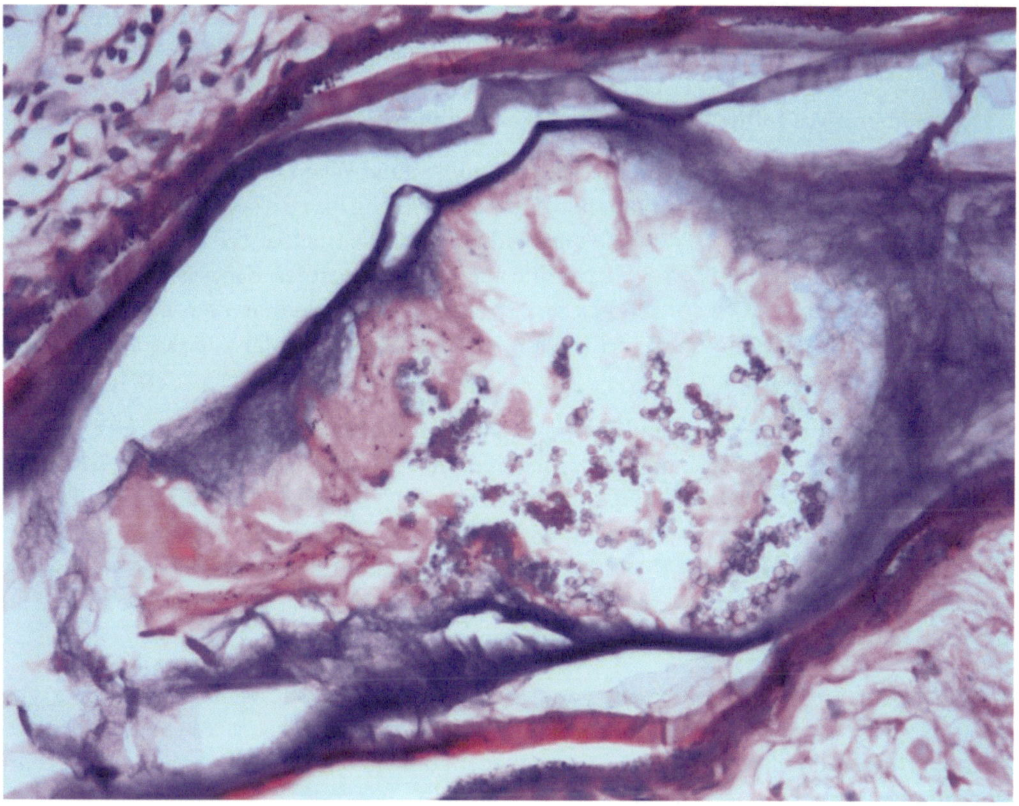

Figure 3. Keratin plug of hair follicle contains numerous yeast forms of fungi (HE ×400).

and legs. Furuncle: deep folliculitis includes only one hair follicle. More than one furuncle combines to form carbuncle [5].

In some textbooks the term "acneiform folliculitis" can be seen. This term means that there is an acneiform dilatation in the hair follicle (e.g., pityrosporum folliculitis).

In demodex folliculitis, besides the mites located inside the hair follicle, follicular spongiosis, perifollicular lymphohistiocytic inflammation also draws attention. An isolated folliculitis is generally self-limited. In old and advanced lesions of all folliculitis perifollicular fibrosis can be visible.

When clinically folliculitis is among the differential diagnosis but histopathologically the lesion is not seen in biopsy sections, deeper and serial sections must be taken. When histopathologically folliculitis diagnosis is made but no microorganism is detected, additional histochemical and immunohistochemical stains can be implemented. Acneiform lesions should be thought primarily when no microorganisms detected microscopically and by applying additional methods (culture, etc.). On the other hand, for diagnosis of acneiform lesions a hundred percent clinical correlation is required.

During investigation if a microorganism is detected, cure rate is very high with appropriate treatment (topical antibiotic, topical antifungal, and systemic antiviral drugs).

2.2. Special types of folliculitis and acneiform eruptions

Eosinophils are predominant in some kinds of folliculitis. When eosinophils are predominantly seen in folliculitis, the first step should not be searching for microorganisms. *Eosinophilic folliculitis* is mostly seen in HIV-positive patient whose CD4 T helper cell count <200–300/μl. *E. folliculitis* is characterized by severe pruritic papules and pustules. Bacteria and yeast fungi can accompany this clinic course. *Ofuji disease* (eosinophilic pustular dermatosis) is a rare disease generally detected in Japan, characterized by pruritic follicular papules and pustules located on the face and scalp [5].

Histopathologically follicle infundibulum is surrounded by inflammation which is predominantly composed of eosinophils and few lymphocytes. The follicle can be ruptured but granuloma formation is not expected. In the past few years, studies have recommended exclusion of fungal folliculitis with PAS-D and/or GMS (Gomori methenamine silver) staining. Eosinophilia in peripheral blood and increased serum IgE levels can be detected in eosinophilic folliculitis. There is also a self-limiting variant of eosinophilic folliculitis presenting on the scalp of children with numerous papules and pustules.

Folliculitis decalvans (perifolliculitis capitis abscedens et suffodiens/dissecting cellulitis of scalp): is a type of deep folliculitis, generally affects the scalp and commonly seen in black race. In the year 1952, Brunstig described folliculitis decalvans a component of the *follicular occlusion triad*. Other components of the triad include: acne conglobata (a kind of nodulocystic acne) and hidradenitis suppurativa (acne inversa or apocrine acne). The histology of these disorders is similar. In all three disorders, abscess formation, suppurative granulomas, and finally sinus tracts are formed as a result of follicular hyperkeratinization [3]. Generally, culture is negative in these three disorders.

Acne conglobata: giant comedones, cysts, and nodules are located on the neck and chest. These lesions leave large irregular scars and can end up with epidermal cysts.

Hidradenitis suppurativa is actually a wrong nomenclature because apocrine and eccrine sweat glands are generally affected secondarily. It favors axilla and groins. Histopathologically, the hair follicle is dilated and the apocrine gland duct is plugged with keratin.

Some authors accept *pilonidal sinus* as a component of *follicular occlusion triad*. In pilonidal sinus disease, hair shafts are embedded in fibrosis they continue growing and elongating inside fibrosis (**Figure 4**). Histopathologically dense suppurative inflammation, fragmented hairs, abscess formation, and necrosis are seen one within the other.

Acne keloidalis nuchae and acne conglobata (component of follicular occlusion triad) are frequently seen together and generally seen in the black race. Acne keloidalis nuchae favors posterior part of scalp and neck. Lesions end up with scars. In the beginning, discrete papules and pustules are detected [5]. This condition is also called *folliculitis keloidalis nuchae*. This is among the causes of scarring alopecia [4]. In curly hairs, the hair infundibulum is believed to grow backwards

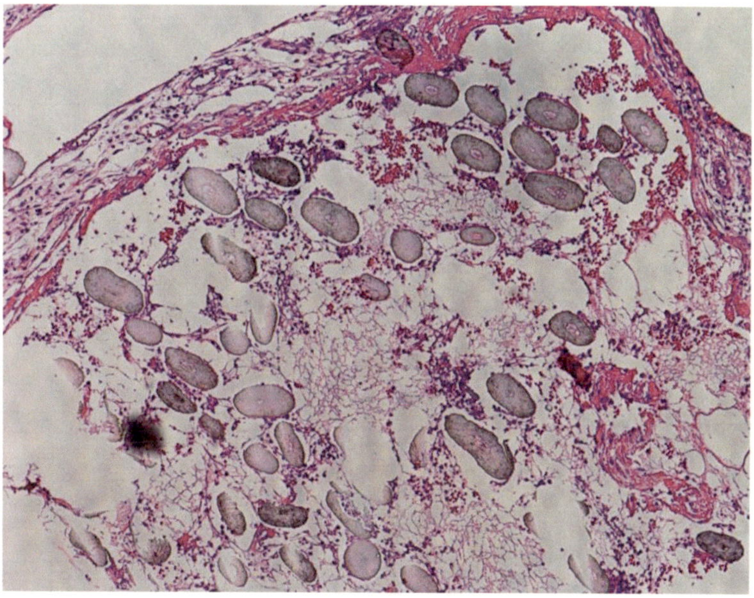

Figure 4. Chronic abscess which is formed by hair shafts and chronic inflammatory cells (HE ×100).

and cause a reaction in dermis which in turn triggers scarring. Follicle is surrounded by lymphocytes and plasma cells. Inflammation is observed in the upper part of the follicle. Ruptured follicles cause secondary granuloma formation. Abscess formation and sinus tracts can also be formed. Dense hypertrophic scar and collagenosis is noticeable (**Figure 5**). Exactly a true keloid formation is not seen [6]. Dystrophic calcification can be seen in scarring acne lesions.

Pseudofolliculitis barbae is another entity which has similarities with acne/folliculitis keloidalis nuchae [5]. *P. barbae* is seen in people who have thick and curly hair in beard area. The lesions are formed due to the transition of hair from infundibulum to the surrounding epidermis. Histopathologically mixed type inflammatory cells and foreign-body-type giant cells are seen in the intrafollicular and perifollicular area.

Acne/folliculitis necrotica (acne varioliformis): It is a folliculitis that ends up with scarring and alopecia. The lesions present as umbilicated erythematous papules and pustules. The lesions are located in the follicle. Comedones are not expected [2]. The term acne is misnomer. Histopathologically perifollicular lymphocytic infiltrate is seen. This infiltrate makes exocytosis into follicular epithelia and causes dense necrosis in keratinocytes. In advanced lesions, necrosis of the follicles can be confluent and clinically ends up with formation of depressed scars [6].

There are some acne forms that are induced or developed by drugs, sunlight exposure, impulsive skin picking, or different materials.

Acne cosmetica (pomade acne): this clinical entity is a temporary follicular occlusion that ends up with acneiform eruption. Acne cosmetica is caused by dense cosmetic usage. The follicle infundibulum is dilated and thin.

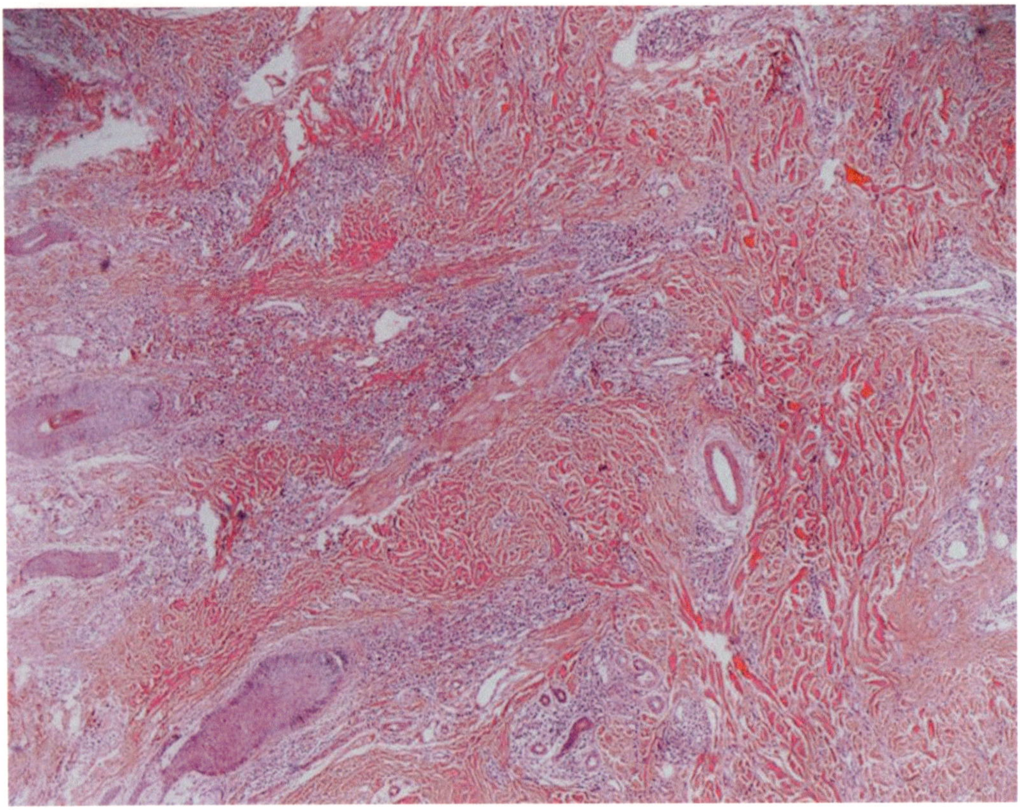

Figure 5. Fibrosis in the dermis which can turn into a hypertrophic scar (clinically an acne keloidalis nuchae case) (HE ×100).

Overuse of bromides triggers severe acneiform lesions which is called *halogenoderma/iododerma/bromoderma/fluoroderma*. Histopathologically in addition to classical acne findings, pseudoepitheliomatous hyperplasia, intraepithelial small abscess and granulomatous inflammation can be seen [3].

Chemical exposure to mineral oils and dioxin can cause acneiform eruptions predominantly comedones, this is called *chloracne*. The comedones are shaped as a bottle or column. Follicular keratin stasis and increased melanocytic activity is detected in epidermis and hair infundibulum [7]. *Steroid-induced acne* is caused as a result of high dose corticosteroid treatment. In contrast to chloracne comedones are not expected. Generally monomorphic pustules are observed [8]. EGFR inhibitors can cause acneiform drug reaction [3].

Acne aestivalis (Mallorcan acne): presents with papules and pustules, favors head and neck, sun exposure triggers the lesions. Histopathologically folliculitis and necrosis of follicular epithelia is noticeable [9, 10].

Acneiform lesions can be seen both in Behcet's and Wegener's diseases.

http://dx.doi.org/10.5772/65494

Morbus Morbihan (Morbihan disease): is a clinical form of severe acne which presents with solid facial edema and favors primarily the central face area.

Acne fulminans: characterized by abrupt onset of tender nodules, plaques, and ulcers. Clinically fever, lymphadenopathy, hepatosplenomegaly, weight loss, etc., can accompany.

Acne Excoriee: scratched acneiform lesions seen in young women due to impulsive picking emotion.

Acne mechanica: acneiform lesions are observed secondary to hair friction caused by hat, helmet, etc. [3].

Nevus comedonicus (acne nevus): is a term used when multiple open comedones are gathered together on a plaque lesion [3]. This lesion can also be evaluated as a hamartoma made up of small infundibular cysts [6].

In conclusion, a comprehensive dermatological examination and detailed history taking is indispensable in all clinical entities mentioned above.

Flowchart 1 summarizes all the above-mentioned clinical entities.

2.3. Acne vulgaris/pimples

Acne vulgaris is the prototype of acneiform lesions and is the inflammatory disease of sweat glands and pilosebaceous units, mostly observed in teenagers and young adults. In contrast to age predilection, race and sex predilection do not exist. The clinical course is severe in male

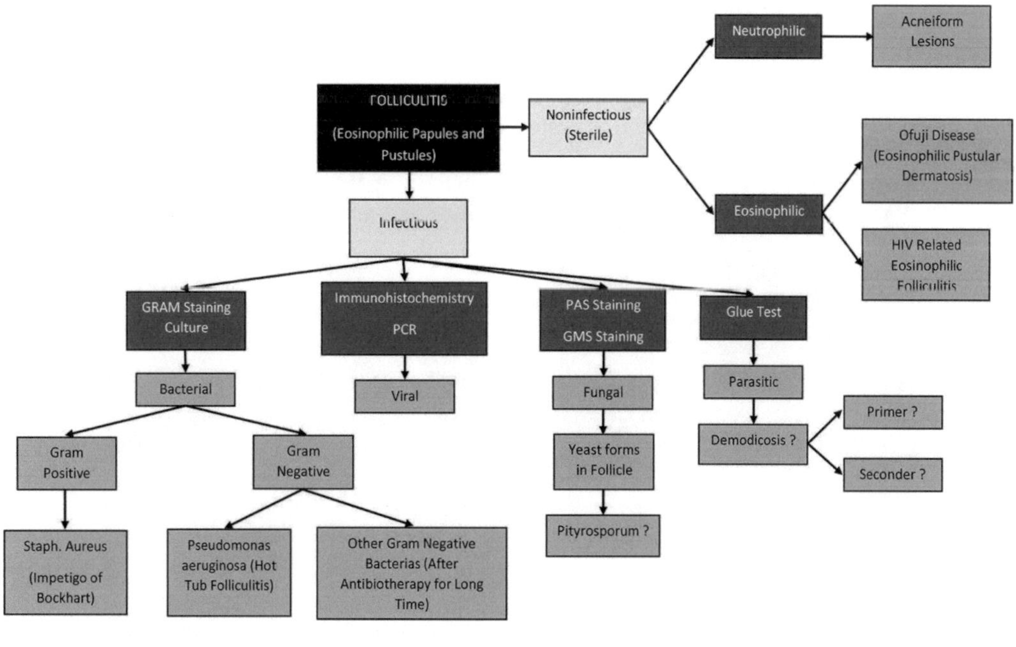

Flowchart 1. A simple, practical approach to basic kinds of folliculitis.

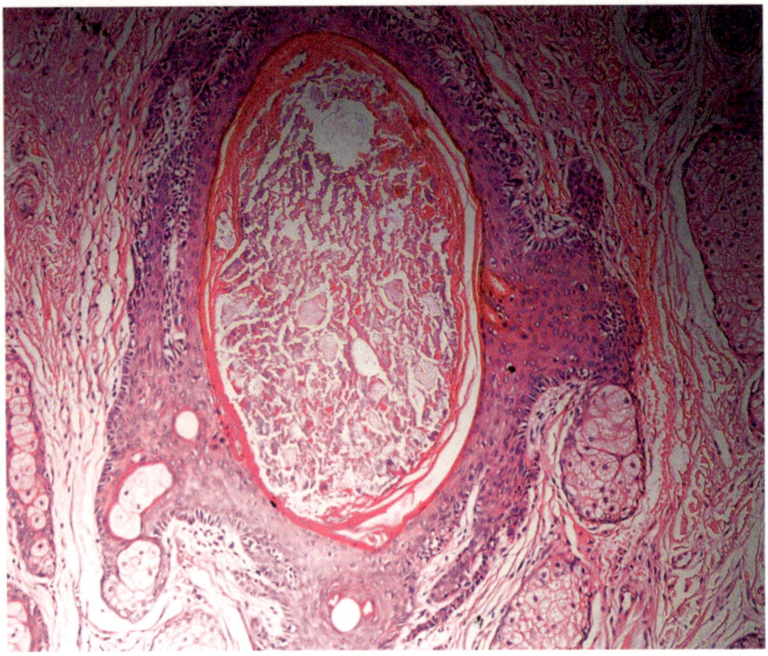

Figure 6. Pilosebaceous unit has started to be dilated with keratin plugging, also a mild perifollicular inflammation can be seen (HE ×100).

patients [2]. Acne lesions favor forehead, chin, cheek, chest, shoulder, and back. Family history may be present. In most patients, the lesions regress in a few years period.

The lesions are generally presented as erythematous papules, pustules, blackheads, and whiteheads. In severe cases, tender and painful nodules and cysts can be apparent. Because hair follicle is plugged with keratin, excreted sebum is accumulated in addition to *P. acnes*

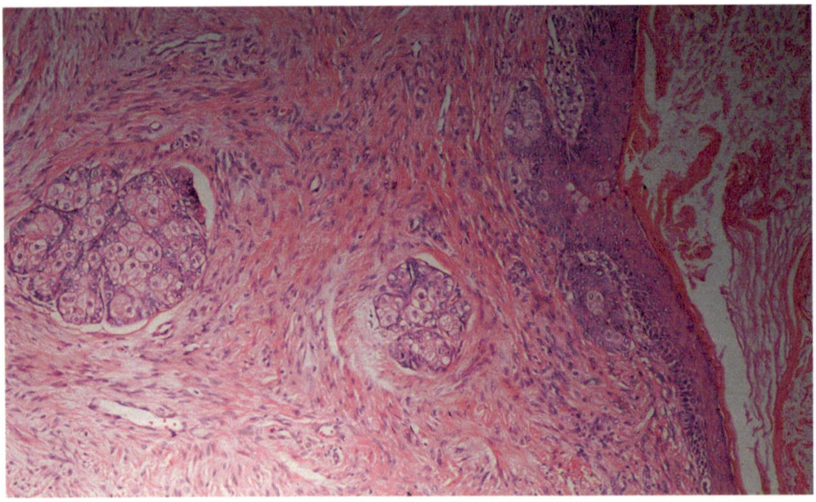

Figure 7. A kind of fibrotic process at the neighborhood of dilated follicle can be noticed (HE ×100) (Same case with **Figure 6**).

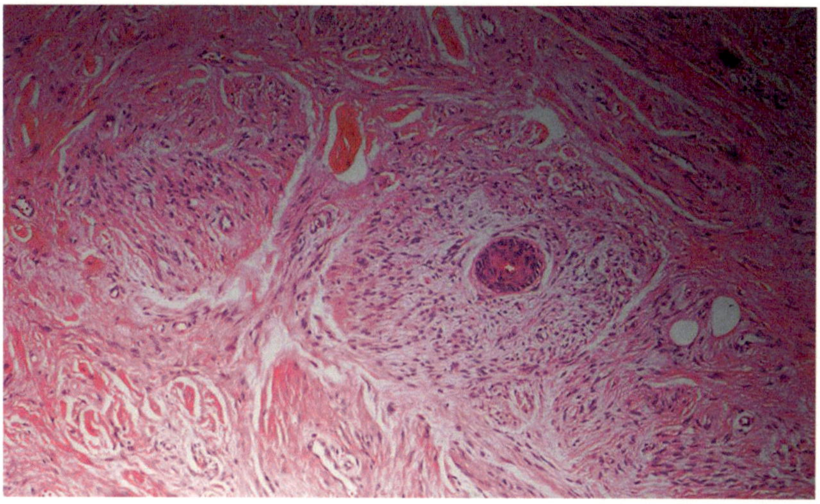

Figure 8. Deeper part of the same lesion in Figures 6 and 7. Scar formation and an entrapped tiny hair follicle can be defined (HE ×100).

colonization and all these steps lead the follicle to folliculitis. Severe desquamation of follicle epithelia and sebaceous gland epithelia also plays a role in pathogenesis.

Acne vulgaris lesions are studied in two groups: noninflammatory (blackheads and whiteheads or comedones) and inflammatory (folliculitis, etc.). Acne lesions can end up with postinflammatory hyperpigmentation and scars (**Figures 6–8**). Keloid formation is quite rare.

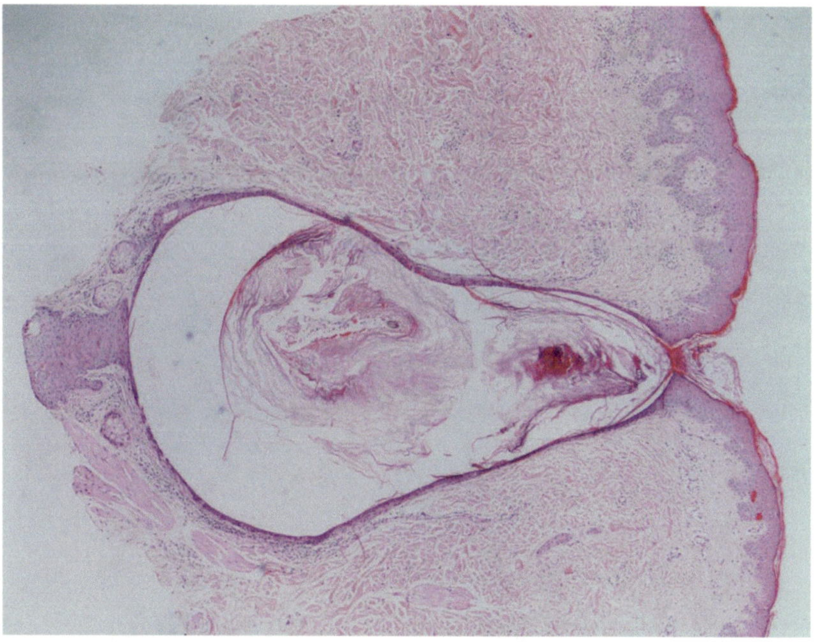

Figure 9. A closed comedone that has a narrow orifice on epidermal side (HE ×40).

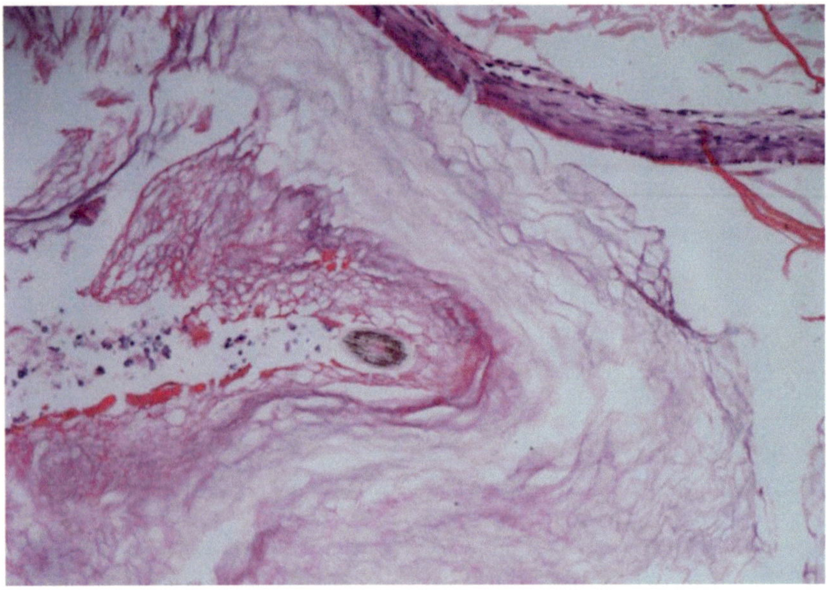

Figure 10. Comedone consists of lamellar keratin, hair shaft, and some bacteria (HE ×200).

Acne is diagnosed clinically, and biopsy confirmation is generally not required. Histopathologically noninflammatory lesions (comedones) are a kind of follicular retention cysts. These tiny cysts may consist of cornified cells, hair shafts, sebum, *P. acnes*, and other bacteria. Closed comedones' orifices on epidermis can be normal in size, mild wider, or narrower (**Figures 9–11**). However, open comedones' orifices on epidermis are definitely dilated (**Figure 12**) [6]. The precursors of inflammatory lesions are generally closed comedones or subclinical microcomedones. Open

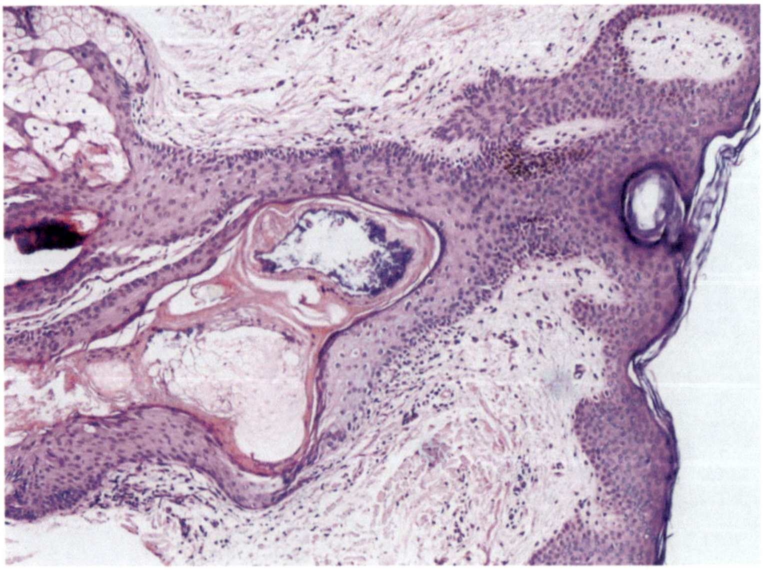

Figure 11. Microcomedone that has a smaller dilatation of follicle opening and a few mononuclear inflammatory cells basically around the follicular epithelia (HE ×100).

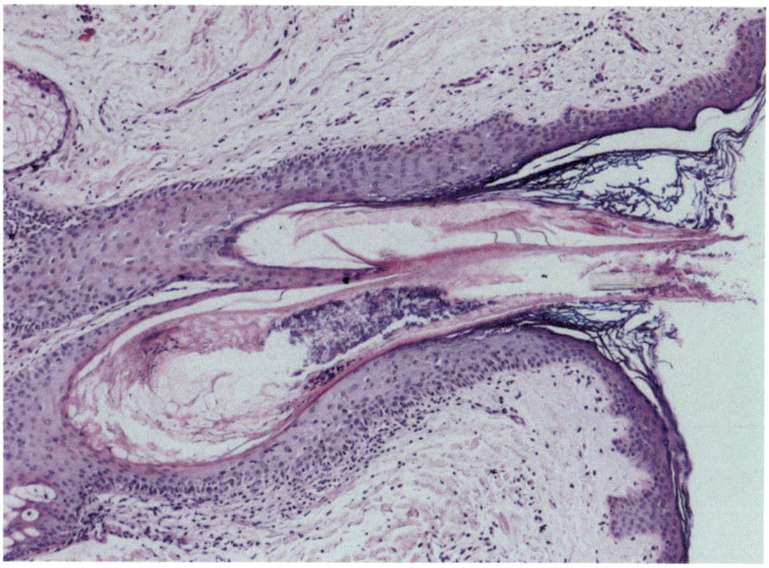

Figure 12. An opened comedone with keratin plugging, wider orifice on epidermis, and mild perifollicular inflammation (HE ×100).

comedones do not trigger the inflammatory process. In comedonal lesions around the affected hair follicle, few inflammatory cells may be present.

Inflammatory lesions may progress in the following pattern: papule→pustule→nodule→cyst.

Comedonal lesions due to retention the follicular wall is quite thin and the follicular content oozes into adjacent dermis which in turn causes accumulation of inflammatory cells in dermis. This process plays the major role in the formation of inflammatory lesions. When the follicle wall becomes much thinner, the follicle may rupture and lead to pustule (**Figure 13**) and by the time, nodule formation is in deep dermis. Depending on follicular damage and severity of inflammatory response scar formation, dermal necrosis, and confluent abscesses formation can be observed. Perifollicular elastolysis can be noticed in acne vulgaris scars [8].

In a noninflammatory lesion if the follicular opening does not expand the follicular wall becomes thinner thus follicular rupture becomes inevitable [8]. Spongiosis is noticeable in follicular epithelia of both inflammatory and noninflammatory lesions. In inflammatory lesions the inflammatory cells attacking follicular epithelia or perifollicular inflammatory cells are composed of mixed type cells (polymorphonuclear leucocytes, lymphocytes, histiocytes). Foreign-body-type multinuclear giant cells and/or granulomatous reactions can be observed as a result of follicular rupture (**Figure 14**).

2.4. Acne rosacea (adult onset acne)

Rosacea is a disease characterized by macular erythema and flushing of central face generally affecting adult population. Some authors classify acne rosacea as a vascular and follicular disease. In a true rosacea, typical acneiform lesions such as papules and pustules are observed. However, comedones are not an important component of acne rosacea. In contrast to acne vulgaris, increased sebum is not the subject in acne rosacea. Sometimes acne rosacea can lead

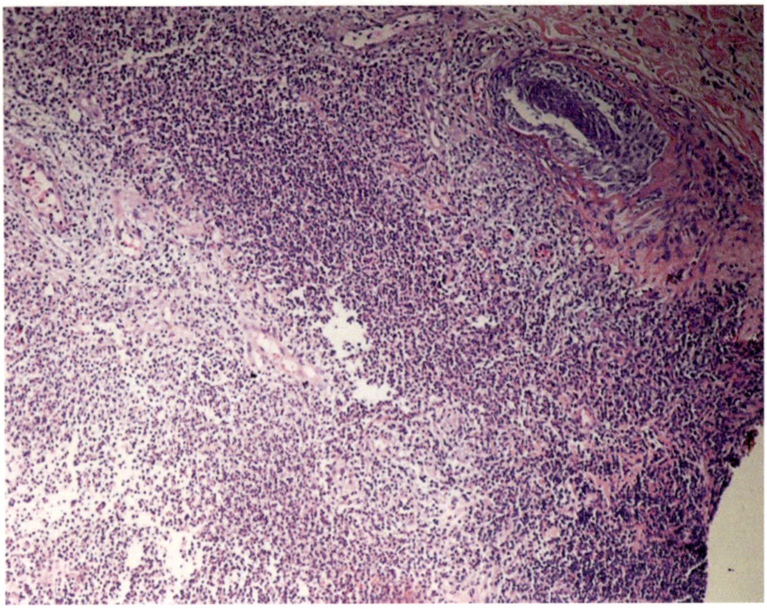

Figure 13. A deep ruptured folliculitis, severe mixed type inflammation and a destroyed hair follicle (HE ×100).

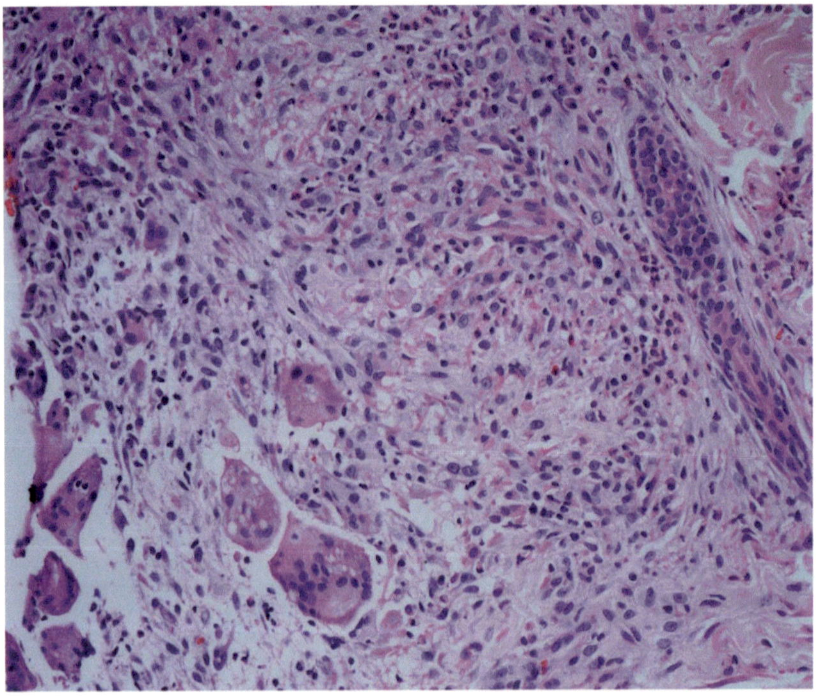

Figure 14. After the rupture of hair follicle, foreign body type inflammatory reaction can be seen (HE × 200).

to blepharitis and phyma formation. In acne rosacea, flushing can be triggered by warmth, cold, alcohol intake, and spicy foods. Granulomatous lesions can be confronted within acne rosacea which present as yellow-brown nodular lesions [5].

Histopathological findings differ according to the stage of disorder.

In early nonpustular lesions, telangiectasia is in the foreground also perifollicular and perivascular mixed type inflammation (lymphocytes, plasmocytes, macrophages, eosinophils, and polymorphonuclear leucocytes) draw attention (**Figures 15** and **16**). Abnormal dermal vessel regulation hypothesis is postulated but there is no objective method for evaluating telangiectasia [11, 12]

Acne rosacea can rarely be extrafascial and/or generalized [2]. Acne rosacea more commonly affects women who have type 1 celtic descent skin phenotype. Some methods are present for clinical staging and severity scoring of acne rosacea [2, 13].

In pustular lesions, an increased amount of polymorphonuclear leucocytes are observed. In severe rosacea (rosacea fulminans, pyoderma faciale), polymorphonuclear leucocytes are predominant cells. In the epithelia of hair follicle, spongiosis can be seen in infundibulum part (**Figure 17**). Follicular rupture can cause granulomatous reactions. Sometimes caseification necrosis can be observed in the center of granulomatous reaction. Solar elastosis can be generally present in rosacea lesions. However, solar elastosis can be a coincidence rather than a specific finding of acne rosacea because solar elastosis is generally present in patients above 40 years of age, in addition to central face is under dense exposure of sunlight throughout life [2].

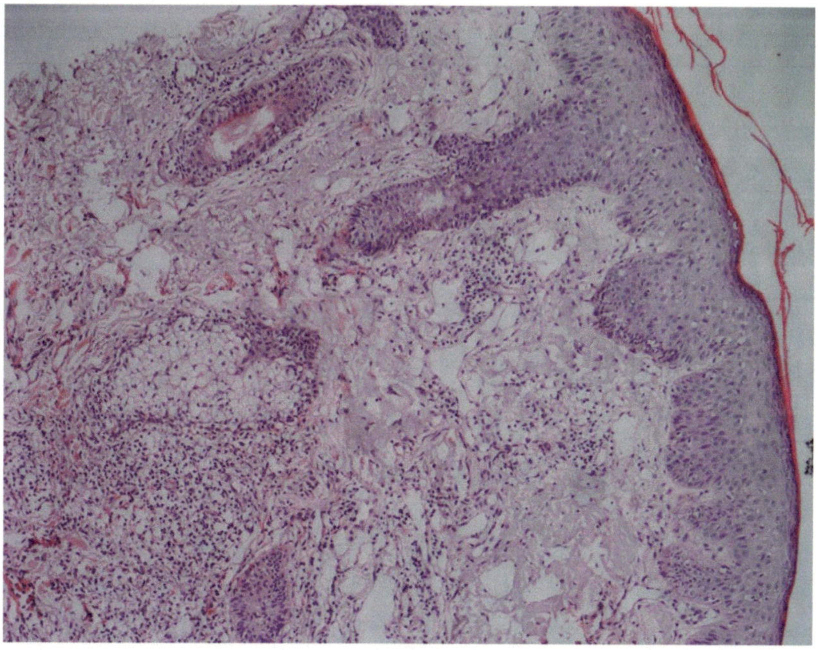

Figure 15. There is a mild-moderate inflammation in dermis and also telangiectatic vascular structures with solar elastosis in the upper dermis (HE ×100).

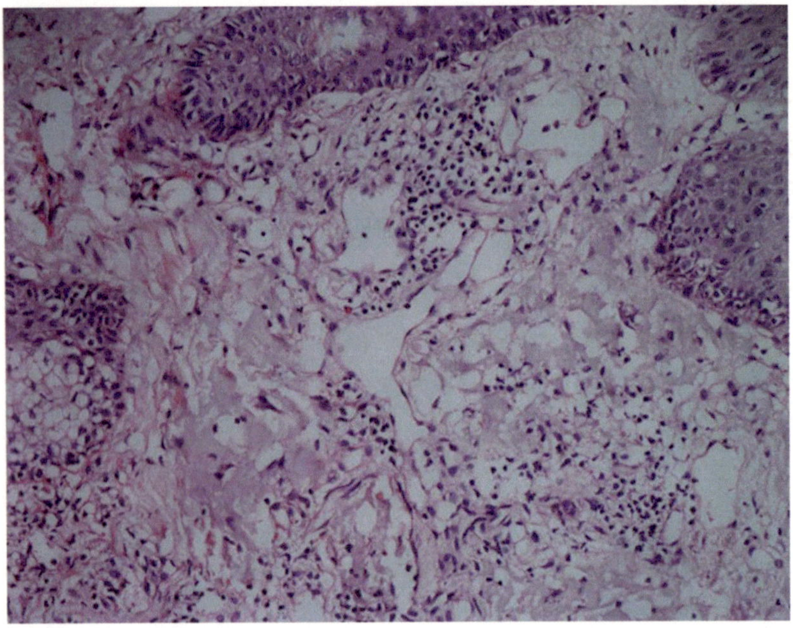

Figure 16. Lymphocyte predominant inflammation in the upper dermis, around the telangiectatic vessels (HE ×200).

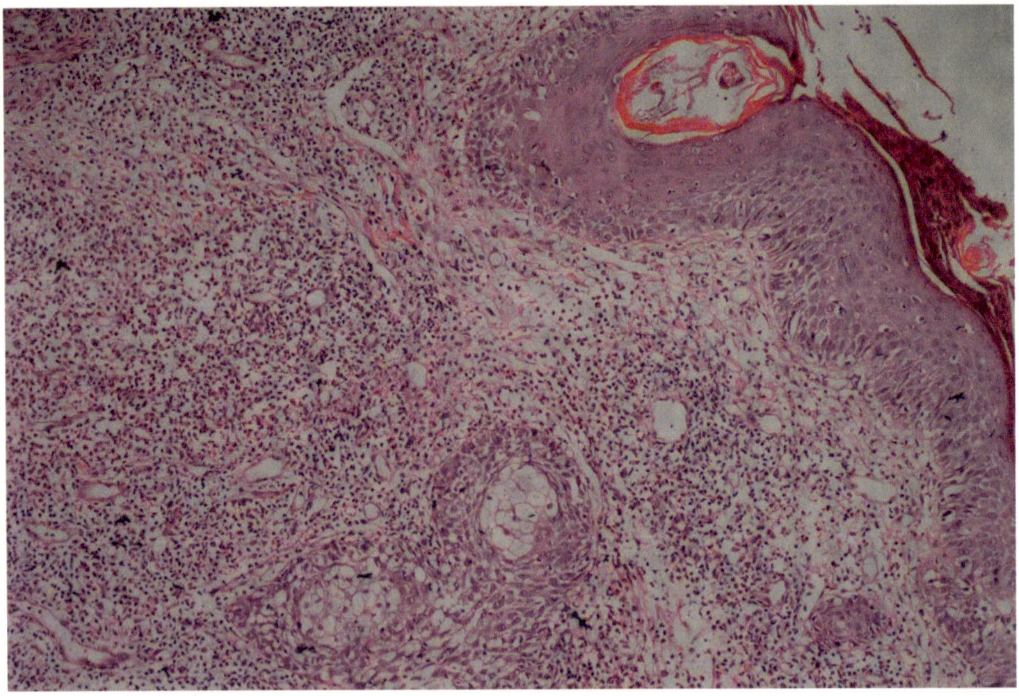

Figure 17. A severe rosacea case that has intensive inflammatory infiltrate (polymorphonuclear leucocytes are dominant) (HE ×100).

http://dx.doi.org/10.5772/65494

Most of resources use the clinical classification method [14, 15] that has four types of acne rosacea:

1. Erythematotelangiectatic
2. Papulopustular
3. Phymatous
4. Ocular

Rhinophyma or phyma formation (*nose*, chin, auricle, and forehead) can be seen in the most advanced stages of acne rosacea.

In order to reach this stage, episodic flushing → persistent flushing → papulopustular stages must be passed.

In the histopathologically evaluation of rhinophyma, different amounts of lymphocytic inflammation, sebaceous hypertrophy, nodular ectatic vessels, hyperkeratosis [4], fibrosis, solar elastosis [6], and mucin accumulation can be observed [8]. Rhinophyma is generally irreversible and surgical intervention is required.

Telangiectatic vascular structures surrounding the rhinophymatous papules may evoke the suspicion of basal cell carcinoma for a clinician [16]. In this case, a biopsy can be done for the exclusion of basal cell carcinoma.

In granulomatous rosacea where long-term phymatous lesions are present in the face, *acne agminata (lupus miliaris disseminatus faciei, acnitis)* [5] *or* FIGURE *(facial idiopathic granuloma with regressive evolution)* [2] can also be observed. In this disease, caseification necrosis is seen in the

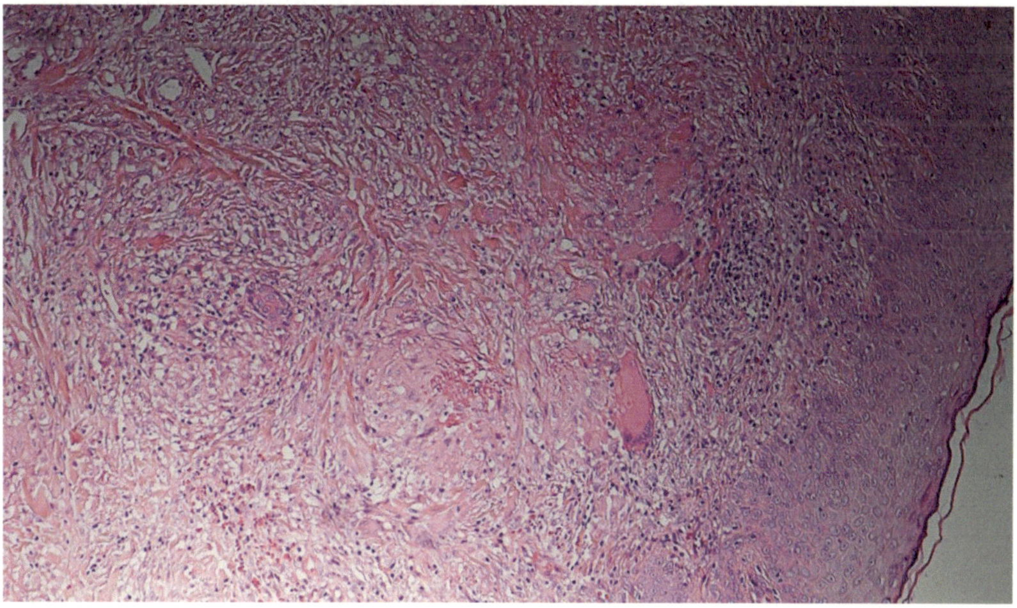

Figure 18. There are granulomas that have caseification necrosis in their center and multinuclear histiocytic giant cells in dermis (HE ×100).

center of pealike granulomas (**Figure 18**). The granulomas are ARB (acid resistant bacteria) negative; no microorganisms are found in PCR. Because of the caseific and amorphic eosinophilic material, the morphology of the granuloma is similar to that of rheumatoid nodule [17]. Acne agminata is the best identified form of granulomatous rosacea. Acne agminata do not involve extrafascial areas, within years the lesions undergo resolution.

Perioral-periocular dermatitis: is very similar to acne rosacea, some authors acknowledge this as the same entity with acne rosacea [5]. Symmetrically distributed erythematous papules and pustules are observed around mouth and eyes. Steroid abuse can induce perioral-periocular dermatitis. Telangiectasia is not expected in perioral dermatitis. Histopathologically mild acanthosis in epidermis, parakeratosis (especially in the ostium of hair follicle) with perivascular and perifollicular lymphocytic inflammation is present. The presence of a relation between demodex mite and acne rosacea or other acne forms has been observed.

3. Demodex and demodicosis

Demodex can be found in the normal fauna of the pilosebaceous unit. For this reason, generally it is not mentioned in the pathology reports. However, changing degrees of inflammatory reactions (from accumulation of lymphocytes up to suppurative and granulomatous reactions) are related to demodex mites [3]. Demodex favors sebaceous areas. Density of demodex mites increases with age.

Two species of demodex inhabit in human: *Demodex folliculorum* and *Demodex brevis*.

Life cycle of demodex mite is as follows: ova→larvae→protonymph→nymph→adult [16].

The aid of its mouth, *D. folliculorum* moves inside the follicle. The tail is in the caudal part (**Figure 19**). *D. folliculorum* has eight ova, and each ovum has an arrowhead-like structure and is big in size. *Demodex folliculorum* is the most frequent demodex living on human beings. In each hair follicle so many *D. folliculorum* can live.

D. brevis is smaller than *D. folliculorum*, and the ovum is oval shaped. This type is not as frequent as *D. folliculorum*. In each follicle, one or two *D. brevis* can inhabit. *D. folliculorum* and *D. brevis* can live together in the same host. Mites are nourished from epithelial and glandular cells.

In 1993 Bonnar et al. [18], removed the stratum corneum of the skin by the help of cyanoacrylate glue and investigated the follicular contents. The mite count was significantly increased in patients who had acne rosacea compared to normal people. This study showed the relation between acne rosacea and demodex mites. This study is one of the studies that conclude the relationship between acne rosacea and demodex mites [17].

The pathogenetic mechanisms of Demodex in rosacea can be:

- foreign body reaction against the parasite
- immune reaction of the host toward the parasite
- the parasite serving as a vector for bacteria [18].

http://dx.doi.org/10.5772/65494

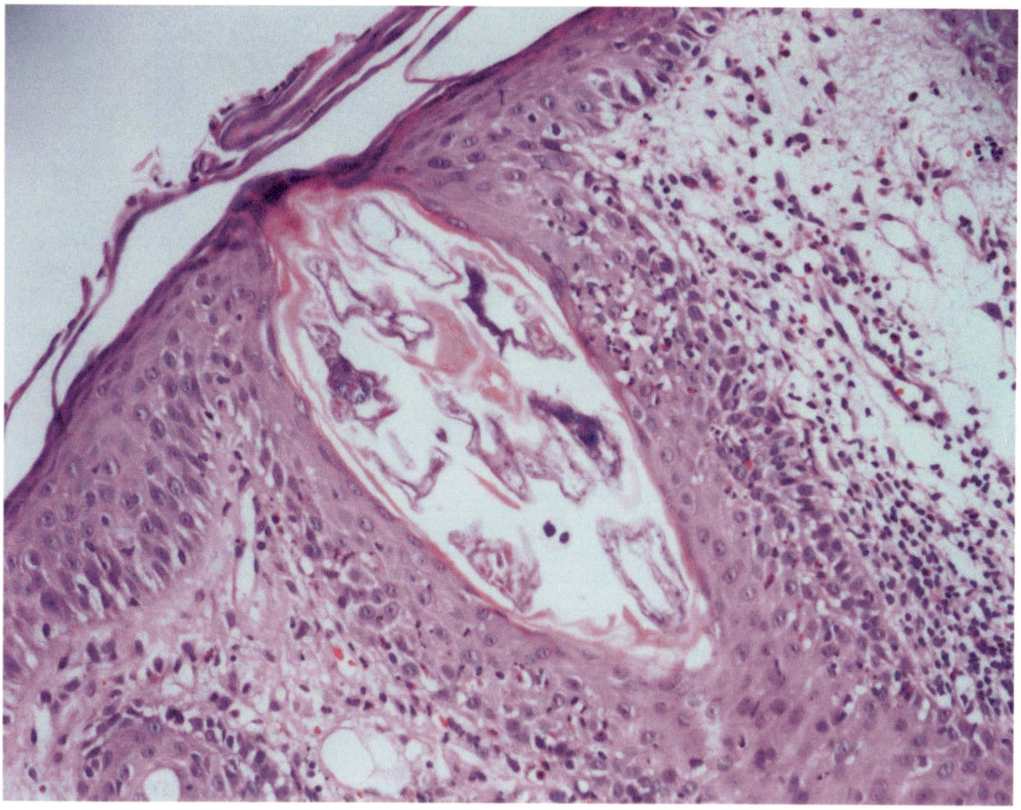

Figure 19. Demodex mites inside the hair follicle, perifollicular inflammatory cells and exocytosis of these inflammatory cells (HE ×200).

Clinically demodicosis also can be divided into primary and secondary demodicosis.

Primary demodicosis: *D. folliculorum* is found in the disease-free T region of the face (there is no sign and symptom).

Secondary demodicosis: more than 30% of the face is affected. Signs and symptoms of the disease are present (erythema, pruritus, etc.), this clinic course is thought to be induced by *D. brevis* [19].

Furthermore, there are three forms of traditionally identified demodicosis:

- pityriasis folliculorum,
- rosacea like demodicosis,
- demodicosis gravis [2].

In **Flowcharts 2** and **3**, we tried to establish a simple algorithm for making diagnosis easier.

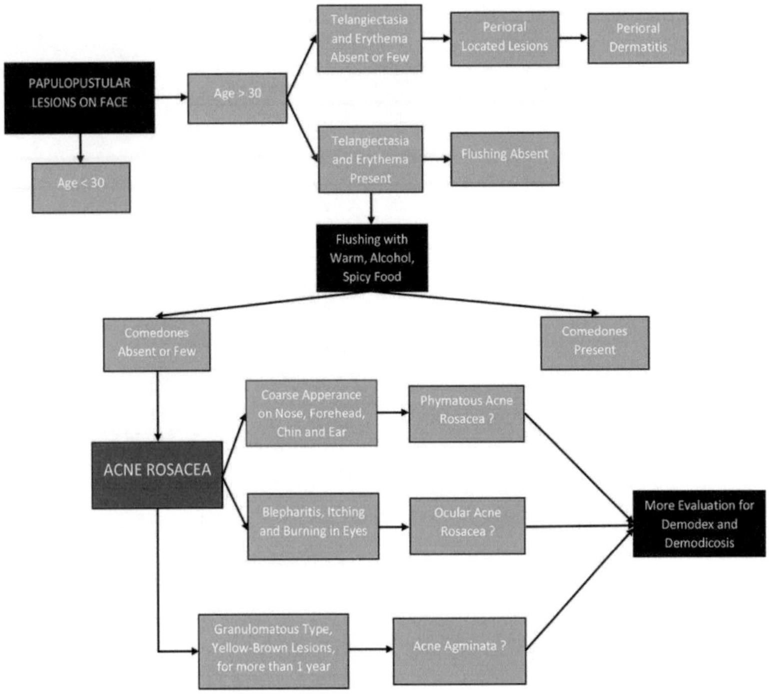

Flowchart 2. A simple clinicopathological approach to central facial lesions.

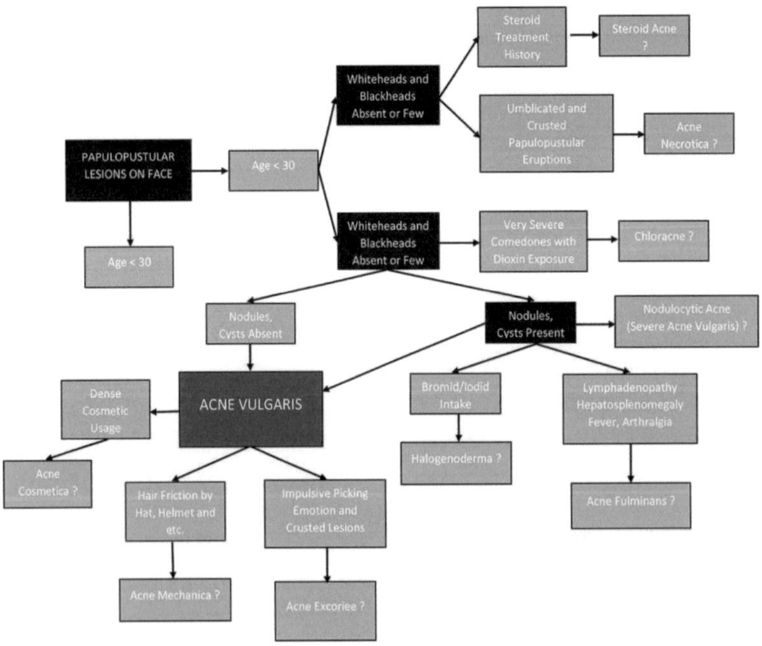

Flowchart 3. Acne vulgaris and related diseases.

Author details

Murat Alper* and Fatma Aksoy Khurami

*Address all correspondence to: muratalper70@gmail.com

Diskapi Yildirim Beyazit Research and Training Hospital, Altindag, Ankara, Turkey

References

[1] Mills ES. Histology for Pathologists, 4th edition. Philadelphia: Wolters Kluwer Health/ Lippincott Williams & Wilkins, 2012; pp. 10–2.

[2] Calonje E, Brenn T, Lazar A. McKee P.H. McKee's Pathology of the Skin, 4th edition. Elsevier/Saunders, 2012.

[3] Rapini RP. Practical Dermatopathology, 2nd edition. Edinburgh: Elsevier/Saunders, 2012.

[4] Brinster NK, Liu V, Diwan AH, McKee PH. Dermatopathology, 1st edition. Philadelphia: Elsevier/Saunders, 2011.

[5] Barnhill RL, Crowson AL, Magro CM, Piepkorn MW. Dermatopathology, 3rd edition. New York: McGraw Hill, 2010.

[6] Busam KJ. Dermatopathology, 1st edition. Philadelphia: Elsevier/Saunders, 2010.

[7] Mooi WJ, Krausz T. Pathology of Melanocytic Disorders, 2nd edition. London: Hodder Arnold, 2007.

[8] Elder ED, Elenitsas R, Johnson BL, Murphy GF, Xu X. Lever's Histopathology of Skin, 11th edition. Philadelphia: Lippincott Williams & Wilkins, 2014.

[9] Hjorth N, Sjolin KE, Sylvest B, Thomsen K. Acne Aestivalis, Mallorca Acne. Acta Derm Venereol. 1972;52(1):61–3.

[10] Veysey EC, George S. Actinic folliculitis. Clin Exp Dermatol. 2005;30(6):659–61. DOI: 10.1111/j.1365-2230.2005.01899.x

[11] Marks R. Concepts in the pathogenesis of rosacea. Br J Dermatol. 1968;80:170. DOI: 10.1111/j.1365-2133.1968.tb12288.x

[12] Qureshi AA, Lerner LH, Lerner EA. Nitric oxide and the cutis. Arch Dermatol. 1996;132:889. DOI: 10.1001/archderm.1996.03890320037005

[13] Wilkin J, Dahl M, Detmar M et al. National Rosacea Society Expert Committee. Standard grading system for rosacea: report of the National Rosacea Society Expert Committee on the Classification and Staging of Rosacea. J Am Acad Dermatol. 2004;50:907–912. DOI: 10.1016/j.jaad.2004.01.048

[14] Wilkin J, Dahl M, Detmar M, et al. Standard classification of rosacea: report of the National Rosacea Society Expert Committee on the Classification and Staging of Rosacea. J Am Acad Dermatol. 2002;46:584. DOI: 10.1067/mjd.2002.120625

[15] Crawford GH, Pelle MT, James WD et al. Rosacea: I. Etiology, pathogenesis, and subtype classification. J Am Acad Dermatol. 2004;51:327. DOI: 10.1016/j.jaad.2004.03.030

[16] Brehmer-Andersson E. Dermatopathology, A Resident's Guide, 1st edition. New York: Springer, 2006.

[17] Elston DM, Ferringer T, Peckham S, High WA, DiCaudo DJ, Ko C. Dermatopathology, 2nd edition. Philadelphia: Elsevier/Saunders, 2014.

[18] Bonnar E, Eustace P, Powell FC. The Demodex mite population in Rosacea. J Am Acad Dermatol. 1993;28:443. DOI: 10.1016/0190-9622(93)70065-2

[19] Akilov OE, Butov YS, Mumcuoglu KY et al. A clinico-pathological approach to the classification of human demodicosis. J Dtsch Dermatol Ges 2005;3:607. DOI: 10.1111/j.1610-0387.2005.05725.x

Chapter 11

Acne-Associated Syndromes

Nazan Emiroglu

Additional information is available at the end of the chapter

http://dx.doi.org/10.5772/65635

Abstract

Introduction: Acne, a chronic inflammatory disorder of pilosebaceous unit, is characterized by comedones, pustules, papules, nodules, cysts, and scars. It affects nearly 85% of adolescents. High sebaceous gland secretion, follicular hyperproliferation, high androgen effects, propionibacterium acnes colonization, and inflammation are major pathogenic factors. Systemic disease or syndromes that are associated with acne are less commonly defined. Therefore, these syndromes may not be usually recognized easily.

Research methods: Acne-associated syndromes prove the nature of these diseases and are indicative of pathogenesis of acne. Polycystic ovary (PCOS), synovitis-acne-pustulosis-hyperostosis-osteitis (SAPHO), hyperandrogenism-insulin resistance-acanthosis nigricans (HAIR-AN), pyogenic arthritis-pyoderma gangrenosum-acne (PAPA), pyoderma gangrenosum-acne vulgaris-hidradenitis suppurativa-ankylosing spondylitis (PASS), pyoderma gangrenosum-acne conglobate-hidradenitis suppurativa (PASH), seborrhea-acne-hirsutism-androgenic alopecia (SAHA), and Apert syndromes are well-known acne-associated syndromes. Endocrine disorders (insulin resistance, obesity, hyperandrogenism, etc.) can be commonly seen in these syndromes, and there are too many unknown factors that must be investigated in the formation of these syndromes.

Conclusion—key results: If we are aware of the component of these syndromes, we will recognize those easily during dermatological examination. Knowledge of clinical manifestations and molecular mechanisms of these syndromes will help us to understand acne pathogenesis. When acne pathogenesis is explained clearly, new treatment modalities will be developed.

Keywords: acne, syndrome, PCOS, HAIRAN, PAPA, PASH, Apert, SAPHO, SAHA, acne-associated syndromes

1. Introduction

Acne vulgaris is a common chronic inflammatory disease of the pilosebaceous unit. Acne is typically thought as an adolescent disease but it is also seen in adulthood anymore [1].

Although there are lots of studies about the pathogenesis of acne, all pathogenetic factors are not known very well. Four main pathways are described in acne pathogenesis: increased sebum production, abnormal keratinization, *Propionibacterium acnes* colonization, and inflammation [2]. Acne is a multifactorial disease and sometimes associated with systemic disorders. Acne may be a potential skin marker of internal disease or a component of syndromes such as PCOS, HAIR-AN, PAPA, PASH, SAPHO, SAHA, and Apert. To know about the pathogenesis of those will help us to understand the acne pathogenesis [3, 4].

Herein, we aim to mention about acne-associated syndromes and their clinical and pathogenetic features.

2. Polycystic ovary syndrome (PCOS)

Polycystic ovary syndrome (PCOS) is an ovarian disease characterized by hyperandrogenism, chronic anovulation, and polycystic ovaries. It is one of the most common endocrinopathy that affects 4–12% of women of reproductive age [5].

Its etiology is unknown, but it was first described by Drs Irving Stein and Michael Leventhal in 1935. They discovered polycystic ovaries in seven patients who had anovulation during surgery and described this disorder as the name of Stein-Leventhal syndrome [6]. Later diagnostic criteria were developed.

The National Institutes of Health (NIH), the Rotterdam, and the Androgen Excess Society Criteria are used for the diagnosis of PCOS [7, 8]. Nowadays, NIH criteria are the preferred diagnostic criteria in adolescents [9].

NIH criteria are the presence of oligoovulation or anovulation and biochemical or clinical signs of hyperandrogenism [9]. Before the diagnosis with using these criteria, some conditions must be excluded that result in anovulation and hyperandrogenism, such as congenital adrenal hyperplasia, Cushing's syndrome, and androgen secreting tumors [9]. Thyroid disease, hyperprolactinemia must also be excluded.

Although pathogenesis of PCOS is not understood very well, it is thought that hormonal pathways contribute to this process. The pulse frequency of gonadotropin-releasing hormone (GnRH) increases in PCOS and stimulates to the anterior pituitary gland to secrete luteinizing hormone (LH) more than follicle-stimulating hormone (FSH), resulting in an increased ratio of LH to FSH. The increase in LH relative to FSH stimulates the ovarian theca cells to synthesize androstenedione. Consequently, the net ovarian androgen production increases [10]. Insulin has also a role in the pathogenesis of PCOS by stimulating the ovarian theca cell to secrete androgens as LH and also inhibits hepatic production of sex hormone binding globulin (SHBG). As a result, free and total androgen level increases.

Obesity is another component of this syndrome and contributes pathogenesis via insulin resistance [10].

Insulin resistance and hyperandrogenism are responsible for the cutaneous involvement of PCOS. Insulin resistance causes acanthosis nigricans (AN), and hyperandrogenism leads

http://dx.doi.org/10.5772/65635

to hirsutism, acne, oily skin, seborrhea, and hair loss (androgenic alopecia). It is estimated that 72–82% of women with PCOS have cutaneous signs [11]. PCOS has also multisystemic effects and is associated with lots of diseases including infertility, endometrial cancer, obesity, depression, sleep-disordered breathing/obstructive sleep apnea (OSA), nonalcoholic fatty liver disease (NAFLD), and nonalcoholic steatohepatitis (NASH), type 2 diabetes mellitus (T2DM), and cardiovascular diseases [9]. Patients with PCOS are usually first seen by a dermatologist. Because of the above comorbidities, dermatologists should know the diagnosis and clinical findings of PCOS very well.

Cutaneous findings in women with PCOS are related to abnormalities of the pilosebaceous unit. Increased androgen levels activate abnormal development of the pilosebaceous unit, and hirsutism, acne or androgenic alopecia. Androgenic alopecia is luckily rare among women with PCOS because of its complex etiology. Acanthosis nigricans (AN) and skin tags are the other skin disorders in PCOS [12].

Although acne, hirsutism, and AN were the most common skin manifestations, hirsutism and AN were the most sensitive for PCOS diagnosis [13]. In previous reports, the range of acne prevalence in PCOS is 15–95%. While hirsutism affects 5–15% of women in the general population, previous reports showed hirsutism prevalence between 8.1 and 77.5% in women with PCOS. In patients with PCOS, hirsutism is also a sign of metabolic abnormalities [13].

AN is also associated with substantial metabolic dysfunction (increased insulin resistance, glucose intolerance, body mass index, and dyslipidemia).

Therefore, the presence of AN and hirsutism should warn us regarding a patient's potential metabolic risk factors. A broad range in the prevalence of AN among women with PCOS (2.5% in the United Kingdom, 39 5.2% in Turkey, 16 and 17.2% in China) were observed [13].

Although patients with PCOS frequently refer to dermatologists with cutaneous concerns, it is important to educate them about the metabolic and fertility-related implications of PCOS.

Hormonal therapy (combination estrogen and progesterone oral contraceptives, antiandrogens: spironolactone, cyproterone acetate, drospirenone, flutamide, and inhibition of peripheral androgen conversion: finasteride), insulin-sensitizing agents (metformin, thiazolidinediones), and nonhormonal therapy (standard acne, hirsutism, androgenetic alopecia therapy) are treatment options [14].

Pharmacologic treatment is not every time necessary for all patients with PCOS. Mild forms of hirsutism, acne, and androgenetic alopecia may be controlled with standard nonhormonal agents and life style changes (weight loss, diet, exercise, glucose control) [14].

3. Hyperandrogenism-insulin resistance-acanthosis nigricans syndrome (HAIR-AN syndrome)

Hyperandrogenism-insulin resistance-acanthosis nigricans syndrome (HAIR-AN syndrome) is a subphenotype of polycystic ovary syndrome. It is clinically characterized by acne, obesity, hirsutism, and acanthosis nigricans. It usually manifests in early adolescence. Although etiology is not known very well, genetic, environmental factors, and obesity are estimated to cause HAIR-AN syndrome. The primary abnormality in patients with HAIR-AN syndrome is thought to be severe insulin resistance. In those patients, insulin levels increase and stimulate the overproduction of androgens in the ovaries [15].

Patients may also present with amenorrhea and signs of virilization. Although adrenal function is normal, the levels of insulin, testosterone, and androstenedione may be high. Adolescents with HAIR-AN syndrome usually have normal levels of luteinizing hormone (LH) and follicle-stimulating hormone (FSH) but the ratio of LH to FHS is usually more than one [16].

Clinical findings are related to insulin resistance and hyperandrogenism so patients first refer to dermatologist, endocrinologist, or gynecologist with hyperandrogenism signs (hirsutism, androgenic alopecia, male body habitus acne, menstrual dysfunction, increased libido, clitorimegaly) or insulin resistance signs (polydipsia, polyuria (often subclinical), acanthosis nigricans, skin tags, and obesity [17] (**Figure 1**).

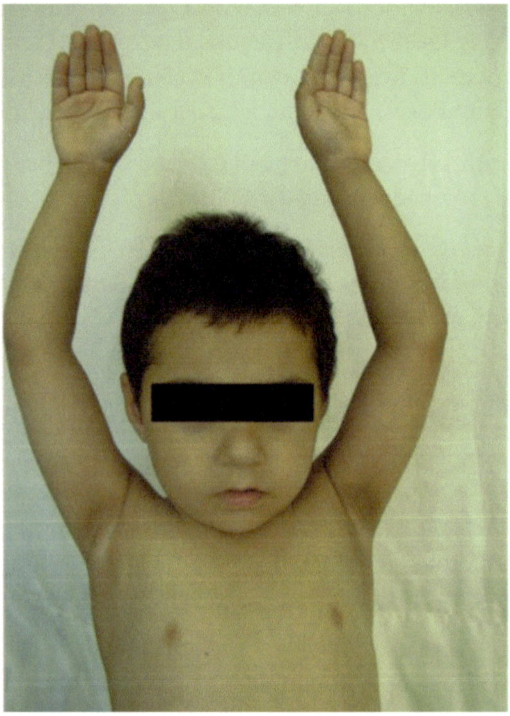

Figure 1. Acanthosis nigricans, *from Nahide Onsun's photos.*

Polycystic ovary syndrome (71–86%), congenital hyperplasia of the adrenal (3–10%), adrenal and ovarian tumors (0.3%), and idiopathic hirsutism (10%) are, respectively, the most common reasons of hyperandrogenism. Except those, HAIR-AN syndrome should also keep in mind as a reason of hyperandrogenism that is seen in almost 5% of females with hyperandrogenism [18].

http://dx.doi.org/10.5772/65635

For HAIR-AN syndrome diagnosis and follow-up, in addition to history and physical examination, a complete blood cell count, thyroid screen, serum prolactin, glucose and insulin measurements, serum electrolyte, and lipid panel should be evaluated [17] because Cushing's syndrome, Hashimoto's thyroiditis, Grave's disease, and congenital adrenal hyperplasia may accompanied with HAIR-AN syndrome [4]. To investigate the origin of hyperandrogenism, total testosterone, levels of 17-hydroxyprogesterone, dehydroepiandrosterone sulfate (DHEAS), levels of luteinizing and follicle-stimulating hormones, and morning cortisol after a low dose of dexamethasone should be analyzed [17].

High level of DHEAS should warn us about the possibility of an androgen-producing tumor of the adrenal gland. Increased 17-hydroxyprogesterone is usually seen in congenital adrenal hyperplasia. Patients with Cushing's syndrome have elevated levels of circulating androgen, and abnormal secretion of cortisol. In those, increased basal levels of cortisol and failure of suppression after stimulation with dexamethasone are observed. In polycystic ovarian syndrome, LH/FSH ratio is usually >2.5 (may see in normal patients as well). Although there is not an underlying virilizing tumor (ovarian or adrenal) in HAIR-AN syndrome, plasma testosterone level is high [19].

In the treatment, lifestyle changes like exercise, lower-calorie diet rich in fiber and protein are advised to patients. Metformin can also be prescribed. Other choices are estroprogestatif pills and antiandrogens [20].

4. SAHA syndrome

SAHA syndrome was first described in 1982, characterized by seborrhea, acne, hirsutism, and androgenetic alopecia [21]. The SAHA syndrome is classified into four types: idiopathic, ovarian, adrenal, and hyperprolactinemic [21], and it can be associated with polycystic ovaries, cystic mastitis, obesity, insulin resistance, and infertility [4, 21].

In the pathogenesis of SAHA, increased androgen synthesis in adrenals and ovaries, disturbed peripheral metabolism of androgens, or induction of metabolism and activation of androgens in the skin may play important role [4].

Approximately 20% of the patients have all four major signs of SAHA syndrome. Seborrhoea is observed in all of patients, androgenetic alopecia is seen in 21% of the patients, and acne in 10% and hirsutism in 6% of the patients [4].

The management of disorder resembles HAIR-AN and PCOS [22].

5. APERT syndrome

Apert syndrome is a rare congenital type I acrocephalosyndactyly syndrome (acrocephalosyndactyly type I). It was first described in 1906 by the French physician Eugène Apert, characterized by the premature fusion of the craniofacial sutures and syndactyly of the hands and feet [23].

The syndrome is inherited in an autosomal dominant fashion, a rare congenital disease. It is caused by a genetic mutation in the FGFR2 gene, and approximately 98% of all patients have specific missense mutations of FGFR2 [24].

FGFR2 is responsible for the development of embryonic skeleton, epithelial structures, and connective tissue [25]. Craniofacial deformities, hypertelorism, dental and palatal abnormalities, proptosis of the eyes, different skeletal deformities, hydrocephalus, abnormal brain development, mental retardation, blindness, cardiovascular, urogenital, gastrointestinal, respiratory, and skin abnormalities can be seen in patients with Apert syndrome [25].

Dermatologic associations of Apert syndrome was not known when first described in 1906 [26]. In 1970, Solomon first reported the dermatologic manifestation of this disorder, which is severe acneiform lesions [27]. The other skin manifestations are hyperhidrosis, hypopigmentation, and hyperkeratosis of plantar surfaces [27].

In this syndrome, the pathogenesis of acne is not understood very well but increased fibroblast growth factor receptor-2 (FGFR2)-signaling is suspected to be of pathophysiological importance in acne vulgaris because it was reported that in skin cultures, keratinocyte-derived interleukin-1α stimulated fibroblasts to secrete FGF7 which stimulated FGFR2b-mediated keratinocyte proliferation [28]. In acne pathogenesis, increased levels of interleukin-1α (IL-1α) are seen in comedones, and an important pro-inflammatory cytokine stimulates keratinocyte proliferation, hyperkeratinization, and decreased desquamation of comedo formation [28]. Patients with Apert syndrome usually have oily skin. Moderate to severe acne, occurring in childhood or early adolescence, affecting the forearms, which is an unusual site for conventional acne, is often observed [23, 28]. Comedones, papules, pustules, furunculoid cysts, and scars as seen in conglobate acne can be seen. It is very difficult to treat, and often unresponsive to therapy but good response to oral isotretinoin [23, 26, 28].

Although isotretinoin therapy has good treatment option, it has serious adverse effects such as teratogenicity, hepatic dysfunction, elevation of cholesterol and triglyceride levels, visual changes, pseudotumor cerebri, musculoskeletal pain, hyperostosis, mucocutaneous dryness, and dryness of the eyes. Therefore, the risk/benefit ratio in treatment of acne lesions with isotretinoin in children with Apert syndrome should be evaluated well [26].

6. Synovitis, acne, pustulosis, hyperostosis, and osteitis (SAPHO) syndrome

SAPHO syndrome was first defined in 1987 by Chamot et al. and its characteristic clinical findings are synovitis, acne, pustulosis, hyperostosis, and osteitis [29]. The etiology is controversial [30]. Although infections (Propionibacterium acnes, Corynebacterium sp.), seronegative spondyloarthropathies (psoriasis, sacroiliitis, enthesitis, inflammatory bowel disease, axial involvement), genetic factors, and stress were responsible for the pathogenesis, those are only hypothesis [30].

Propionibacterium acnes is estimated to play a pathogenic role in SAPHO syndrome. Productions of microbial determinants of P. acnes stimulate innate immune response through TLR-2. TLR-2 induces inflammatory cytokines via NF-jB and mitogen-activated protein kinase pathway [31]. Recent reports also showed that SAPHO syndrome had similar features with other autoinflammatory disease. IL-1β, TNF-α, and IL-8 were suggested to be important in the pathogenesis of SAPHO [32].

Two cohort studies investigated genes PSTPIP2, LPIN2, NOD2, PSTPIP1, and PTPN22, but did not show causal mutations. Therefore, SAPHO syndrome is thought as a polygenic disease [33].

SAPHO syndrome is a rare disease so usually misdiagnosed because this syndrome have similar clinical features with infectious discitis, seronegative SpA, and psoriatic arthritis (PsA), and skin and bone lesions may appear at different times [34].

Standard diagnostic criteria are also controversial such as etiology. The commonly used diagnostic criteria of SAPHO syndrome: (i) local bone pain with gradual onset; (ii) multifocal lesions, especially in the long, tubular bones and spine; (iii) failure to culture an infectious microorganism; (iv) a protracted course for several years with exacerbations and improvement with anti-inflammatory drugs; and (v) neutrophilic skin eruptions, mostly palmoplantar pustulosis (PPP), nonpalmoplantar pustulosis, psoriasis vulgaris, or severe acne [30] (**Figure 2**).

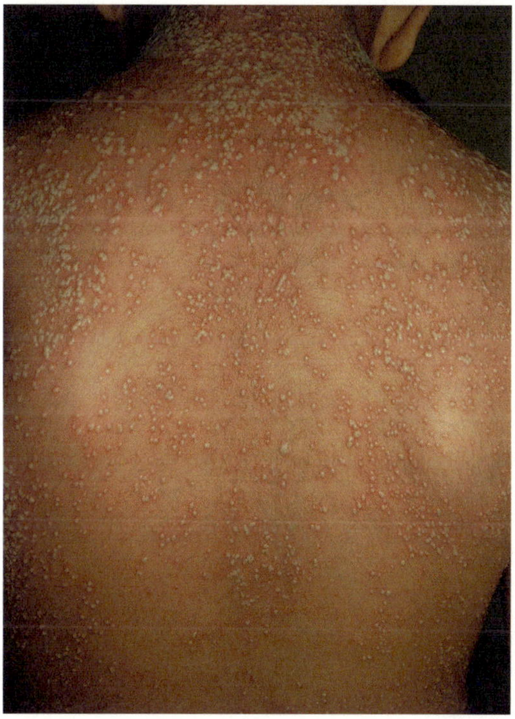

Figure 2. Pustular psoriasis, *from Nahide Onsun's photos.*

The skin manifestations are those of different neutrophilic dermatoses. PPP is the most common skin involvement, including pustular psoriasis, representing 50–75% of all dermatologic manifestations, psoriasis vulgaris may also be seen among the dermatologic manifestations of SAPHO. One fourth of patients have acne conglobata and fulminans with men clearly predominating [34]. Hidradenitis suppurativa may also be seen.

PG, Sweet's syndrome, and Sneddon-Wilkinson disease are the other rare cutaneous manifestations. IBD especially Crohn's disease may also be accompanied with SAPHO syndrome [34].

The most of author agree about that SAPHO could be classified within the spectrum of autoinflammatory diseases. Therefore, intra-articular or systemic corticosteroids, disease-modifying antirheumatic drugs (DMARDs) such as methotrexate, sulfasalazine, cyclosporine, and leflunomide are the treatment options but there are no randomized controlled clinical trials for the treatment. Doxycycline can also be thought as a treatment option for P. acnes eradication [33] Infliximab (INFX), an anti-TNF-α monoclonal antibody, has been showed effective for the treatment SAPHO patients especially unresponsive or refractory to conventional drugs. In recent case series, remarkable improvement of bone, joints, and skin inflammatory manifestations was observed with Infliximab (INFX) therapy. In resistant SAPHO cases, the IL-1 antagonist anakinra can be also tried [35, 36].

7. PAPA syndrome

PAPA syndrome (pyogenic arthritis, pyoderma gangrenosum, and acne) is an autosomal dominant, autoinflammatory disorder. PAPA syndrome was first described as a hereditary disease in 1997 [37]. There is a PSTPIP1/CD2BP1 mutation on chromosome 15q that causes an increased binding affinity to pyrin and induces the assembly of inflammasomes [37]. The caspase, a protease, is activated and converts inactive prointerleukin (IL)-1 beta to its active isoform IL-1 beta. Overproduction of IL-1 beta induces to release pro-inflammatory cytokines and chemokines. Those are responsible for the recruitment and activation of neutrophils, leading to a neutrophil-mediated inflammation [38].

PAPA syndrome is usually presents with severe self-limiting pyogenic arthritis in early childhood. Pyoderma gangrenosum (**Figure 3**) and nodular-cystic acne may be seen around puberty and adulthood [37]. Pathergy test is positive in PAPA syndrome and clinically appears as pustule formation followed by ulceration [34]. There is not a diagnostic test but acute phase reactants and white blood cell count may be elevated because of systemic inflammation [34].

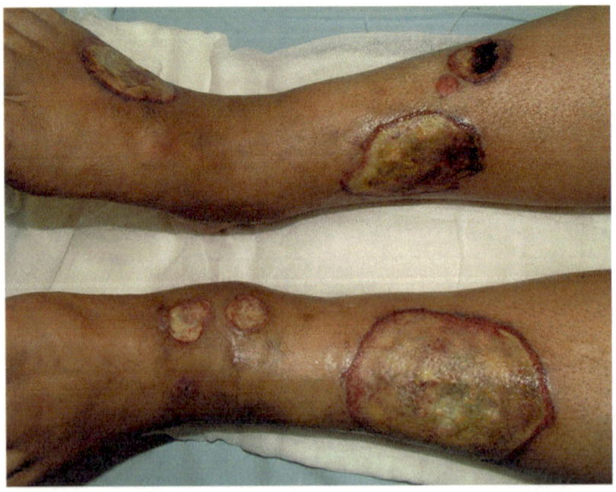

Figure 3. Pyoderma gangrenosum, *from Nahide Onsun's photos.*

Arthritis usually gives good response to therapy with corticosteroids. Pyoderma gangrenosum is treated with topical or systemic immunosuppressant drugs. In addition, a few reports showed that anti-TNF-α and anti-IL-1 agents are effective in the treatment [39].

8. PASH syndrome

The clinical trial of pyoderma gangrenosum, acne conglobata, and hidradenitis suppurativa was described as PASH syndrome by Braun-Falco et al. in 2012. PASH syndrome clinically resembles pyoderma gangrenosum, acne conglobata, and pyogenic arthritis (PAPA) syndrome, but arthritis is not observed [40].

The molecular basis of PASH syndrome is not known very well. It is accepted as autoinflammatory disease. PAPA (pyogenic arthritis, pyoderma gangrenosum, and acne), PAPASH (pyogenic arthritis and PASH), and PASH (pyoderma gangrenosum, acne conglobata and hidradenitis suppurativa) syndromes clinically have similar components. The absence of pathogenic mutations in the PSTPIP1 gene may be used for distinguishing this syndrome from other AIDs [41, 42]. Although a genetic mutation was not discovered clearly in PASH syndrome, in some case series, NCSTN gene, NOD (nucleotide-binding oligomerization domain) genes, the immunoproteasome, and MEFV mutations were reported in PASH syndrome [41, 42].

Systemic corticosteroids, traditional antineutrophilic agents (dapsone and colchicine), and metformin may be tried at first but standard therapy options for autoinflammatory diseases are not usually enough to treat patients with PAPA and PASH syndrome whereas anti-TNF therapies and anti-IL-1 therapy are promising new treatment options for drug resistant cases [43].

Author details

Nazan Emiroglu

Address all correspondence to: dr.nazanyilmaz@hotmail.com

Department of Dermatology, Bezmialem Vakif University, Istanbul, Turkey

References

[1] Cerman AA, Aktaş E, Altunay İK, Arıcı JE, Tulunay A, Ozturk FY. Dietary glycemic factors, insulin resistance, and adiponectin levels in acne vulgaris. J Am Acad Dermatol. 2016; 75(1):155–62. Doi: 10.1016/j.jaad.2016.02.1220.

[2] Araviiskaia E, Dréno B. The role of topical dermocosmetics in acne vulgaris. J Eur Acad Dermatol Venereol. 2016; 30(6):926–35. Doi: 10.1111/jdv.13579

[3] Pace JL. Acne—a potential skin marker of internal disease. Clin Dermatol. 2015; 33(5):572–8. Doi: 10.1016/j.clindermatol.2015.05.010.

[4] Chen W, Obermayer-Pietsch B, Hong JB, Melnik BC, Yamasaki O, Dessinioti C et al. Acne-associated syndromes: models for better understanding of acne pathogenesis. J Eur Acad Dermatol Venereol. 2011; 25(6):637–46. Doi: 10.1111/j.1468-3083.2010.03937.x.

[5] Norman RJ, Dewailly D, Legro RS, Hickey TE. Polycystic ovary syndrome. Lancet. 2007; 370(9588):685–97. Doi: 10.1016/S0140-6736(07)61345-2.

[6] Dastur Adi E, Tank P D. Irving Stein, Michael Leventhal and a slice of endocrine history. J Obstet Gynecol India. 2010; 60(2):121–122. Doi: 10.1007/s13224-010-0016-1.

[7] Rotterdam ESHRE/ASRM-Sponsored PCOS Consensus Workshop Group. Revised 2003 consensus on diagnostic criteria and long-term health risks related to polycystic ovary syndrome. Fertil Steril. 2004; 81(1):19–25. Doi:10.1016/j.fertnstert.2003.10.004

[8] Azziz R, Carmina E, Dewailly D, Diamanti-Kandarakis E, Escobar-Morreale HF, Futterweit W, et al. The androgen excess and PCOS society criteria for the polycystic ovary syndrome: the complete task force report. Fertil Steril. 2009; 91(2):456–88. Doi: 10.1016/j.fertnstert.2008.06.035.

[9] Legro RS, Arslanian SA, Ehrmann DA, Hoeger KM, Murad MH, Pasquali R. Diagnosis and treatment of polycystic ovary syndrome: an endocrine society clinical practice guideline. J Clin Endocrinol Metab. 2013; 98(12):4565–92. Doi: 10.1210/jc.2013-2350.

[10] Housman E, Reynolds RV. Polycystic ovary syndrome: a review for dermatologists: Part I. Diagnosis and manifestations. J Am Acad Dermatol. 2014; 71(5):847. Doi: 10.1016/j.jaad.2014.05.007.

[11] Schmidt TH, Shinkai K. Evidence-based approach to cutaneous hyperandrogenism in women. J Am Acad Dermatol. 2015; 73(4):672–90. Doi: 10.1016/j.jaad.2015.05.026.

[12] Lee AT, Zane LT. Dermatologic manifestations of polycystic ovary syndrome. Am J Clin Dermatol. 2007; 8(4):201–219. Doi: 10.2165/00128071-200708040-00003.

[13] Schmidt TH, Khanijow K, Cedars MI, Huddleston H, Pasch L, Wang ET, et al. Findings and systemic associations in women with polycystic ovary syndrome. JAMA Dermatol. 2016; 152(4):391–8. Doi: 10.1001/jamadermatol.2015.4498.

[14] Buzney E, Sheu J, Buzney C, Reynolds RV. Polycystic ovary syndrome: a review for dermatologists: Part II. Treatment. J Am Acad Dermatol. 2014; 71(5):859. Doi: 10.1016/j.jaad.2014.05.009

[15] Dédjan AH, Chadli A, El Aziz S, Farouqi A. Hyperandrogenism-Insulin resistance-acanthosis nigricans syndrome. Case Rep Endocrinol. 2015; 193097. Doi: 10.1155/2015/193097.

[16] Omar HA, Logsdon S, Richards J. Clinical profiles, occurrence, and management of adolescent patients with HAIR-AN syndrome. Sci World J. 2004 Jul 8; 4:507–11. Doi: 10.1100/tsw.2004.106

[17] Elmer KB, George RM. HAIR-AN syndrome: a multisystem challenge. Am Fam Physician. 2001 Jun 15; 63(12):2385–90.

[18] Escobar-Morreale HF, Carmina E, Dewailly D, Gambineri A, Kelestimur F, Moghetti P, et al. Epidemiology, diagnosis and management of hirsutism: a consensus statement by the androgen excess and polycystic ovary syndrome society. Hum Reprod Update. 2012; 18(2):146–70. Doi: 10.1093/humupd/dmr042.

[19] Chang RJ, Katz SE. Diagnosis of polycystic ovary syndrome. Endocrinol Metab Clin North Am. 1999; 28(2):397–408, vii.

[20] Zemtsov A, Wilson L. Successful treatment of hirsutism in HAIR-AN syndrome using flutamide, spironolactone, and birth control therapy. Arch Dermatol. 1997; 133(4):431–3. Doi:10.1001/archderm.1997.03890400023003.

[21] Dalamaga M, Papadavid E, Basios G, Vaggopoulos V, Rigopoulos D, Kassanos D, et al. Ovarian SAHA syndrome is associated with a more insulin-resistant profile and represents an independent risk factor for glucose abnormalities in women with polycystic ovary syndrome: a prospective controlled study. J Am Acad Dermatol. 2013; 69(6):922–30. Doi: 10.1016/j.jaad.2013.09.014.

[22] Lowenstein EJ. Diagnosis and management of the dermatologic manifestations of the polycystic ovary syndrome. Dermatol Ther. 2006; 19(4):210–23. Doi:10.1111/j.1529-8019.2006.00077.x.

[23] DeGiovanni CV, Jong C, Woollons A. What syndrome is this? Apert syndrome. Pediatr Dermatol. 2007; 24(2):186–8. Doi:10.1111/j.1525-1470.2007.00372.x.

[24] Ko JM. Genetic syndromes associated with craniosynostosis. J Korean Neurosurg Soc. 2016; 59(3):187–91. Doi:10.3340/jkns.2016.59.3.187.

[25] Dolenc-Voljc M, Finzgar-Perme M. Successful isotretinoin treatment of acne in a patient with Apert syndrome. Acta Derm Venereol. 2008; 88(5):534–5. Doi: 10.2340/00015555-0501.

[26] Benjamin LT, Trowers AB, Schachner LA. Successful acne management in Apert syndrome twins. Pediatr Dermatol. 2005; 22(6):561–5. Doi: 10.1111/j.1525-1470.2005.00141.x.

[27] Cohen MM Jr., Kreiborg S. Cutaneous manifestations of Apert syndrome. Am J Med Genet. 1995; 31; 58(1):94–6. Doi: 10.1002/ajmg.1320580119.

[28] Melnik BC. Role of FGFR2-signaling in the pathogenesis of acne. Dermatoendocrinol. 2009; 1(3):141–56.

[29] Chamot AM, Benhamou CL, Kahn MF, Beraneck L, Kaplan G, Prost A. Acne-pustulosis-hyperostosis-osteitis syndrome. Results of a national survey. 85 cases. Rev Rhum Mal Osteoartic. 1987; 54(3):187–96.

[30] Zhao Z, Li Y, Li Y, Zhao H, Li H. Synovitis, acne, pustulosis, hyperostosis and osteitis (SAPHO) syndrome with review of the relevant published work. J Dermatol. 2011 Feb; 38(2):155–9. Doi: 10.1111/j.1346-8138.2010.00931.x.

[31] Yamamoto T. Pustulotic arthro-osteitis associated with palmoplantar pustulosis. J Dermatol. 2013; 40(11):857–63. Doi: 10.1111/1346-8138.12272.

[32] Hurtado-Nedelec M, Chollet-Martin S, Nicaise-Roland P, Grootenboer-Mignot S, Ruimy R, Meyer O, et al. Characterization of the immune response in the synovitis, acne, pustulosis, hyperostosis, osteitis (SAPHO) syndrome. Rheumatology (Oxford). 2008; 47(8):1160–7. Doi: 10.1093/rheumatology/ken185.

[33] Firinu D, Garcia-Larsen V, Manconi PE, Del Giacco SR. SAPHO syndrome: current developments and approaches to clinical treatment. Curr Rheumatol Rep. 2016; 18(6):35. Doi: 10.1007/s11926-016-0583-y.

[34] Marzano AV, Borghi A, Meroni PL, Cugno M. Pyoderma gangrenosum and its syndromic forms: evidence for a link with autoinflammation. Br J Dermatol. 2016; 23. Doi: 10.1111/bjd.14691.

[35] Firinu D, Murgia G, Lorrai MM, Barca MP, Peralta MM, Manconi PE, et al. Biological treatments for SAPHO syndrome: an update. inflamm allergy drug targets. 2014; 13(3):199–205. Doi: 10.2174/1871528113666140520100402

[36] Wendling D, Prati C, Aubin F. Anakinra treatment of SAPHO syndrome: short-term results of an open study. Ann Rheum Dis. 2012; 71(6):1098–100. Doi: 10.1136/annrheumdis-2011-200743

[37] Lindor NM, Arsenault TM, Solomon H, Seidman CE, McEvoy MT. A new autosomal dominant disorder of pyogenic sterile arthritis, pyoderma gangrenosum, and acne: PAPA syndrome. Mayo Clin Proc. 1997;72(7):611–5. Doi: 10.1016/S0025-6196(11)63565-9

[38] Smith EJ, Allantaz F, Bennett L, Zhang D, Gao X, Wood G, et al. Clinical, molecular, and genetic characteristics of PAPA syndrome: a review. Curr Genomics. 2010;11(7):519–27. Doi: 10.2174/138920210793175921.

[39] Geusau A1, Mothes-Luksch N, Nahavandi H, Pickl WF, Wise CA, Pourpak Z, et al. Identification of a homozygous PSTPIP1 mutation in a patient with a PAPA-like syndrome responding to canakinumab treatment. JAMA Dermatol. 2013; 149(2):209–15. Doi: 10.1001/2013.jamadermatol.717.

[40] Braun-Falco M, Kovnerystyy O, Lohse P, Ruzicka T. Pyoderma gangrenosum, acne, and suppurative hidradenitis (PASH)—a new autoinflammatory syndrome distinct from PAPA syndrome. J Am Acad Dermatol. 2012;66(3):409–15. Doi: 10.1016/j.jaad.2010.12.025.

[41] Marzano AV, Trevisan V, Gattorno M, Ceccherini I, De Simone C, Crosti C. Pyogenic arthritis, pyoderma gangrenosum, acne, and hidradenitis suppurativa (PAPASH): a new autoinflammatory syndrome associated with a novel mutation of the PSTPIP1 gene. JAMA Dermatol. 2013;149(6):762–4. Doi: 10.1001/jamadermatol.2013.2907.

[42] Calderón-Castrat X, Bancalari-Diaz D, Román-Curto C, Romo-Melgar A, Amorós-Cerdán D2, A Alcaraz-Mas L2, et al. PSTPIP1 Gene mutation in a pyoderma gangrenosum, acne and suppurative hidradenitis (PASH) Syndrome. Br J Dermatol. 2016; 175(1):194–8. Doi: 10.1111/bjd.14383.

[43] Staub J, Pfannschmidt N, Strohal R, Braun-Falco M, Lohse P, Goerdt S, et al. Successful treatment of PASH syndrome with infliximab, cyclosporine and dapsone. J Eur Acad Dermatol Venereol. 2015; 29(11):2243–7. Doi: 10.1111/jdv.12765

Chapter 12

Acne Conglobata

Fatma Pelin Cengiz and Funda Kemeriz

Additional information is available at the end of the chapter

http://dx.doi.org/10.5772/67044

Abstract

Acne conglobata is the severe form of acne, located on the face, back, and chest with large, painful, pus-filled cysts deep in the skin. The abscesses and sinuses result in pain, inflammation, and hypertrophic and atrophic scars. In this chapter, we aimed to clarify the pathways of acne conglobata and review the treatment options based on the literature.

Keywords: acne, nodule, severe, scar, treatment

1. Introduction

Acne conglobata (AC) is a severe chronic inflammatory disorder characterized by the presence of comedones, cysts, and scars on the face, back, and chest. It affects deep skin tissue and can result in swelling, bleeding, pain, and scarring. The clinical effects of treatment options for acne conglobata are often unsatisfactory because of a long course of therapy, side effects, the high rate of recurrence, and failure to prevent scar formation. Therefore, we aim to discuss the treatment options based on the literature in this chapter.

2. Clinical presentation

Acne conglobata (AC) is the uncommon and severe form of acne, characterized by large, tender nodules; draining sinuses; and interconnecting abscesses with seropurulent discharge. These lesions are generally located on the back, chest, and face. Healing of the nodules, abscesses usually causes hypertrophic and atrophic scars. Besides, chronic scars of AC may result in squamous cell carcinoma [1]. This disease is common in males more than females. The disease affects young adults and adolescents more frequently than elder people.

Acne conglobata may develop owing to acute flare of existing acne, or it may occur as the rebound of acne that has been latent for a long time.

Synovitis, pustulosis, acne conglobata, hyperostosis, and osteitis are clinically specific inflammatory disorders that may be seen barely in the same patient in a syndrome known as SAPHO syndrome [2].

Acne conglobata may also be associated with the PAPA syndrome, which consists of pyogenic arthritis, acne conglobata, and pyoderma gangrenosum [3].

The primary causes of acne conglobata are still unknown. The HLA-A and HLA-B phenotypes were evaluated in six patients with acne conglobata and hidradenitis suppurativa, in four of whom had HLA-B7 cross-reacting antigens and all had HLA-DRw4 [4]. Other causes include using anabolic steroids, withdrawal of testosterone therapy, nutrition or medications that contain bromine or iodine, aromatic hydrocarbons, and adrenal gland tumors which release large amount of androgens [5].

Acne conglobata can be malodorous, and patients may eliminate themselves from community. Severe scarring can lead to psychological problems, such as anxiety, depression, and low self-esteem in many patients.

3. Treatment

Isotretinoin (13-cis retinoic acid) is an oral pharmaceutical drug primarily preferred in the treatment of severe nodular acne. The adverse effects are the flare of acne, cheilitis, xerosis, an increased susceptibility to sunburn, muscle aches, myalgias, and headaches. The patients need to be monitored for blood lipids and liver enzymes especially closely. It has an X category for pregnancy.

Isotretinoin, generally combined with prednisone, is the approved therapy for severe acne conglobata. The recommended dosage of isotretinoin is 0.5–1.0 mg/kg/day for at least 4–5 months [6].

Gollnick et al. compared the effectiveness and safety profile of combined azelaic acid cream plus oral minocycline with oral isotretinoin in severe acne. Their study involved 85 patients with nodular papulopustular acne or acne conglobata who were treated for 6 months. AA cream was applied twice daily, and minocycline was taken twice daily in a dose of 50 mg (daily 100 mg). The doses of isotretinoin were 0.8 mg/kg for the first month, 0.7 mg/kg for the second month, 0.5–0.7 mg/kg for the third month, and 0.5 mg/kg for the fourth to sixth months per day [7].

In the 6-month course, 50 patients in the combined therapy group achieved median reduction of facial comedones, 70%; of papules and pustules, 88%; and of deep inflammatory acne lesions, 100%, while 35 patients in the oral isotretinoin group achieved reduction of comedones, 83%; of papules and pustules, 97%; and of deep inflammatory acne lesions, 100%. Overall, oral isotretinoin was more effective than the combined treatment. The local side effects observed under the combination of AA and minocycline were significantly lower than that seen with

http://dx.doi.org/10.5772/67044

isotretinoin (36.5% versus 65.7%). The incidence of systemic side effects was lower under the combined therapy than under isotretinoin (8% versus 14.3%). They suggested that the combination of topical 20% AA cream and oral minocycline is a highly effective treatment in severe forms of acne, and it is better tolerated and associated with fewer risks than oral isotretinoin [7].

TNF-α is one of the important cytokines involved in the pathogenesis of acne conglobata. Graham et al. found that *Propionibacterium acnes* stimulated keratinocytes to produce interleukin (IL)-1α, IL-8, and TNF-α [8]. Caillon et al. showed that levels of TNF-α and IL-8 secretion in peripheral blood mononuclear cells were significantly higher than in patients with acne vulgaris than controls [9].

As a result of the role of the TNF-α in proliferation of the immune response with the inflammatory infiltrate including neutrophils, lymphocytes, and histiocytes, it was hypothesized that acne conglobata might benefit from anti-inflammatory therapy. Notable results with adalimumab have been reported for the treatment of dissecting cellulitis of the scalp and hidradenitis suppurativa [10, 11].

On the other hand, anti-TNF therapy can stimulate paradoxical inflammatory skin conditions, of which the most frequent is a psoriasiform eruption. There have been three patients with Crohn's disease, psoriasis vulgaris, and rheumatoid arthritis who were treated with adalimumab in the literature. As a result of adalimumab therapy, acneiform eruptions were occurred in these cases [12]. It was suggested that genetic predisposition and overlap with the primary inflammatory disease and autoimmune sensitivity induced interferon-α and cytokine imbalance [13].

Given the previous success reported with hidradenitis suppurativa, Shirakawa et al. considered infliximab therapy in a patient with acne conglobata and rheumatoid arthritis. The patient had experienced flares of the acne conglobata and side effects of oral isotretinoin. The patient was started on the 300 mg (3 mg/kg) of infliximab for the treatment of rheumatoid arthritis. The same dose was repeated at weeks 2 and 6. They observed a significant improvement in the size and number of his cystic lesions after the third dose. Subsequently, the same doses were repeated every 8 weeks and continued for at least 6 months. The patient had achieved a decrease in the number of lesions and pain symptoms [14].

Yiu et al. reported a patient with recalcitrant acne conglobata, who was commenced on subcutaneous adalimumab at 80 mg loading dose, followed by 40 mg every other week, in combination with 15 mg prednisolone. Most of the inflammatory nodules resolved within 4 weeks of commencing treatment with adalimumab, and this response was maintained at the 12-week follow-up [15].

Sand et al. reported another unresponsive patient to doxycycline, oral isotretinoin, combination of prednisolone and isotretinoin, and combination of isotretinoin and dapsone. They initiated monotherapy with adalimumab using an initial loading dose of 80 mg, followed by 40 mg monthly twice. They observed a significant decrease in the size and degree of inflammation of the nodular lesions 4 weeks after initial treatment and disappearance of all nodular lesions after 12 weeks of therapy. The patient had received continuous monotherapy with adalimumab, 40 mg, twice monthly for a total of 12 months, and no recurrence of acne lesions had appeared [16].

Vega et al. reported a 14-year-old adolescent with recalcitrant acne conglobata on the face, neck, and upper chest. That patient had experienced acne fulminans and flares of severe acne while on the isotretinoin and prednisone therapies. Then, twice weekly injections of etanercept 50 mg combined with oral isotretinoin 40 mg/d were started. They observed a clear improvement after 2 months of treatment. The patient had completed the isotretinoin cycle of 9600 mg over 8 months. They continued etanercept (50 mg/wk) 3 months more, and the treatment was completed after 1 year. The patient had experienced no relapse [17].

Schuttelaar et al. reported another young patient with severe acne unresponsive to other treatments. They started him on infliximab 5 mg/kg intravenously at 8-week interval. A total of eight infusions were administered. After three infusions, they did not observe neither new lesions nor activation of the old lesions. After 4 months, they successfully treated negligible relapse of the acne with intralesional corticosteroids. No relapse was occurred at 1-year follow-up [18].

Electron beam processing has the ability to break the chains of DNA in living organisms and results in local destruction of cells. [19, 20]. The electron beam therapy delivers radiation primarily to the superficial skin lesions and spares the deeper tissues from radiation. Electron beam radiation has been used in the treatment of mycosis fungoides, basal cell carcinoma, squamous cell carcinoma, and AIDS-related molluscum contagiosum lesions and Kaposi's sarcoma [19–23]. The acute side effects of electron beam radiation are fatigue, itching, tanning, and burns. Long-term side effects include dry skin, decreased sweating, skin color changes, loss of scalp hair, and the development of dilated blood vessels [24].

Myers et al. reported a 53-year-old patient with acne conglobata and hidradenitis suppurativa who is unresponsive to oral doxycycline, oral ampicillin, triamcinolone intralesional injections, topical benzoyl peroxide 5% wash, clindamycin phosphate, 1% topical solution, betamethasone valerate 0.1% cream, and cyclosporine 5 mg/kg per day. After these therapies, the patient was started a total of eight treatments of modern external beam radiation over 2 weeks localized to the bilateral mandibular cheeks. Electron energies were 9 MeV. Daily fraction sizes were 2.5 Gy for a total of 20 Gy to each side of the face. Three weeks after radiation, the patient reported subjective improvement in cyst size, cyst drainage, pain, and self-esteem. He had no significant xerosis or pigmentary abnormalities status after radiation. The patient had experienced no relapse at 5-month follow-up [25].

Photodynamic therapy (PDT) is a kind of phototherapy that induces selective cytotoxic destruction by the activation of a nontoxic light-sensitive compound with light. Up-to-date PDT has been used for several dermatologic diseases, such as psoriasis, cutaneous T-cell lymphoma, and warts [26]. PDT with topical 5-ALA damages sebaceous glands, inhibits sebum production, kills *Propionibacterium acnes*, and obstructs the follicular openings [27]. The advantages of PDT include rapid efficacy, short recovery time, less destruction, and pain. Despite of these advantages, the local side effects of PDT are erythema, skin peeling, pain, burning, stinging, exfoliation, and post-inflammatory hyperpigmentation [27, 28]. It is obligatory to photoprotect after treatment for phototoxicity [29].

Yang et al. investigated the clinical effects of photodynamic therapy with topical 5-aminolevulinic acid for facial acne conglobata. They included 75 patients with facial acne conglobata. They divided the patients into photodynamic therapy (PDT) group with topical 5% aminolevulinic acid and red light for three times in a month and control group (n = 40) with the Chinese herbal medicine mask plus red light once a week. The patients were also administered topical metronidazole, oral doxycycline, viaminate, and zinc gluconate. Efficacy was assessed according to symptom score, cure rate, and response rate, 2 weeks after the final therapy course, and time points for assessment were selected as day 0, day 10, and day 20; day 34 for the treatment group; and day 7, day 14, day 21, and day 35 for the control group. They observed that PDT was more effective for pustules and papules than control group. The PDT group was associated with a higher cure rate, a lower symptom score, and response rate than the control group. They didn't observe systemic side effects. The erythematous swelling, increased number of cysts, pigmentation, and severe pain were the local side effects which they observed in the treatment group with PDT. They demonstrated that the treatment of acne conglobata with PDT is associated with a high cure rate, short treatment period, few side effects, and reduced scar formation [30].

Hasegawa et al. achieved to treat a case of acne conglobata by CO(2) laser ablation to remove the top of the sinuses and their tracts. After laser ablation, topical tretinoin therapy was also started simultaneously to prevent the appearance of new acne lesions. They proposed the CO(2) laser ablation with topical tretinoin as a powerful treatment option for acne conglobata [31]. They also reported another acne conglobata case, which they successfully treated by fractional laser after CO laser abrasion of cysts combined with topical tretinoin [32].

Liu et al. compared the effectiveness of encircling acupuncture combined with venesection and cupping and oral isotretinoin. A total of 26 acupuncture patients had their acupuncture courses once daily; venesection and cupping were applied twice a week. Patients of isotretinoin group were treated with oral isotretinoin 20 mg/d. The duration of study was 4 weeks. After 4 weeks, in acupuncture group and Western medicine group, 3 (11.5%) and 4 (15.4%) cases experienced remarkable relief in their signs, 14 (53.8%) and 11 (42.3%) had marked improvement, 6 (23.1%) and 7 (26.9%) had improvement, and 3 (11.5%) and 4 (15.4%) failed, with the effective rates being 88.5% and 84.6%, respectively. Overall, they didn't observe any significant difference between acupuncture and oral isotretinoin ($P > 0.05$). In terms of lowering serum IL-6 content, acupuncture was found superior than oral isotretinoin ($P < 0.05$) [33].

Author details

Fatma Pelin Cengiz[1]* and Funda Kemeriz[2]

*Address all correspondence to: fpelinozgen@hotmail.com

1 Department of Dermatoveneorology, Bezmialem Vakif University, Istanbul, Turkey

2 Department of Dermatoveneorology, Aksaray State Hospital, Aksaray, Turkey

References

[1] Whipp MJ, Harrington CI, Dundas S. Fatal squamous cell carcinoma associated with acne conglobata in a father and daughter. Br J Dermatol 1987;117:389–392.

[2] Zuo RC, Schwartz DM, Lee CC, Anadkat MJ, Cowen EW, Naik HB. Palmoplantar pustules and osteoarticular pain in a 42-year-old woman. J Am Acad Dermatol 2015;72:550–553.

[3] Braun-Falco M, Kovnerystyy O, Lohse P, Ruzicka T. Pyoderma gangrenosum, acne, and suppurative hidradenitis (PASH)-a new autoinflammatory syndrome distinct from PAPA syndrome. J Am Acad Dermatol 2012;66:409–415.

[4] Schackert K, Scholz S, Steinbauer-Rosenthal I, Albert ED, Wank R, Plewig G. Letter: HL-A antigens in acne conglobata: a negative study. Arch Dermatol 1974;110:468.

[5] Rapini, Ronald P, Bolognia, Jean L, Jorizzo, Joseph L. (2007). Dermatology: 2-Volume Set. St. Louis: Mosby. p. 449. ISBN 1-4160-2999-0.

[6] Jeong S, Lee CW. Acne conglobata: treatment with isotretinoin, colchicine, and cyclosporin as compared with surgical intervention. Clin Exp Dermatol 1996;21:462–463.

[7] Gollnick HP, Graupe K, Zaumseil RP. Comparison of combined azelaic acid cream plus oral minocycline with oral isotretinoin in severe acne. Eur J Dermatol 2001;11:538–544.

[8] Graham GM, Farrar MD, Cruse-Sawyer JE. Proinflammatory cytokine production by human keratinocytes stimulated with Propionibacterium acnes and P. acnes GroEL. Br J Dermatol 2004;150:421–428.

[9] Caillon F, O'Connell M, Eady EA. Interleukin-10 secretion from CD14+ peripheral blood mononuclear cells is downregulated in patients with acne vulgaris. Br J Dermatol 2010;162:296–303.

[10] Kimball AB, Kerdel F, Adams D. Adalimumab for the treatment of moderate to severe Hidradenitis suppurativa: a parallel randomized trial. Ann Intern Med 2012;157:846–855.

[11] Navarini AA, Trueb RM. 3 cases of dissecting cellulitis of the scalp treated with adalimumab: control of inflammation within residual structural disease. Arch Dermatol 2010;146:517–520.

[12] Fernandez-Crehuet P, Ruiz-Villaverde R. Acneiform eruption as a probable paradoxical reaction to adalimumab. Int J Dermatol 2015;54(8):e306–e308.

[13] Cleynen I, Verimeire S. Paradoxical inflammation induced by anti-TNF agents in patients with IBD. Nat Rev Gastroenterol Hepatol 2012;9:496–503.

[14] Shirakawa M, Uramoto K, Harada FA. Treatment of acne conglobata with infliximab. J Am Acad Dermatol 2006;55:344–346.

[15] Yiu ZZ, Madan V, Griffiths CE. Acne conglobata and adalimumab: use of tumour necrosis factor-α antagonists in treatment-resistant acne conglobata, and review of the literature. Clin Exp Dermatol 2015;40:383–386.

[16] Sand FL, Thomsen SF. Adalimumab for the treatment of refractory acne conglobata. JAMA Dermatol 2013;149:1306–1307.

[17] Vega J, Sánchez-Velicia L, Pozo T. Efficacy of etanercept in the treatment of acne conglobata. Actas Dermosifiliogr 2010;101:553–554.

[18] Schuttelaar M, Leeman F. Sustained remission of nodular inflammatory acne after treatment with infliximab. Clin Exp Dermatol 2011; 36: 668–679.

[19] Veness M, Richards S. Role of modern radiotherapy in treating skin cancer. Australas J Dermatol 2003;44:159–166.

[20] Sausville EA, Longo DL. Principles of cancer treatment. In: Fauci AS, Braunwald E, Kasper DL, Hauser SL, Longo DL, Jameson JL, et al., editors. Harrison's Principles of Internal Medicine. 17th ed. Available at: http://www.accessmedicine.com/content.aspx?aID=2888811. Accessed September 22, 2008.

[21] Griep C, Davelaar J, Scholten AN, Chin A, Leer JW. Electron beam therapy is not inferior to superficial x-ray therapy in the treatment of skin carcinoma. Int J Radiat Oncol Biol Phys 1995;32:1347–1350.

[22] Locke J, Karimpour S, Young G, Lockett MA, Perez CA. Radiotherapy for epithelial skin cancer. Int J Radiat Oncol Biol Phys 2001;51:748–755.

[23] Scolaro MJ, Gordon P. Electron-beam therapy for AIDS-related molluscum contagiosum lesions: preliminary experience. Radiology 1999;210:479–482.

[24] Lindahl LM, Kamstrup MR, Petersen PM, Wirén J et al.. Total skin electron beam therapy for cutaneous T-cell lymphoma: a nationwide cohort study from Denmark. Acta Oncol 2011;50 (8):1199–1205.

[25] Myers JN, Mason AR, Gillespie LK, Salkey KS. Treatment of acne conglobata with modern external beam radiation. J Am Acad Dermatol 2010;62:861–863.

[26] Lee Y, Baron ED. Photodynamic therapy: current evidence and applications in dermatology. Semin Cutan Med Surg 2011;30:199–209.

[27] Huh SY, Na JI, Huh CH, Park KC. The effect of photodynamic therapy using indole-3-acetic acid and green light on acne vulgaris. Ann Dermatol 2012; 24: 56–60.

[28] Hongcharu W, Taylor CR, Chang Y et al.. A-photodynamic therapy for the treatment of acne vulgaris. J Invest Dermatol 2000; 115: 183–192.

[29] Moseley H, Ibbotson S, Woods J et al.. Clinical and research applications of photodynamic therapy in dermatology: experience of the Scottish PDT Centre. Lasers Surg Med 2006;38:403–416.

[30] Yang GL, Zhao M, Wang JM, He CF, Luo Y, Liu HY, Gao J, Long CQ, Bai JR. Short-term clinical effects of photodynamic therapy with topical 5-aminolevulinic acid for facial

acne conglobata: an open, prospective, parallel-arm trial. Photodermatol Photoimmunol Photomed 2013;29 :233–238.

[31] Hasegawa T, Matsukura T, Suga Y, Muramatsu S, Mizuno Y, Tsuchihashi H, Haruna K, Ogawa H, Ikeda S. Case of acne conglobata successfully treated by CO(2) laser combined with topical tretinoin therapy. J Dermatol 2007;34:583–585.

[32] Hasegawa T, Matsukura T, Hirasawa Y, Otsuki A, Tsuchihashi H, Niwa Y, Okuma K, Ogawa H, Ikeda S. Acne conglobata successfully treated by fractional laser after CO laser abrasion of cysts combined with topical tretinoin. J Dermatol 2009;36:118–119.

[33] Liu CZ, Lei B, Zheng JF. Randomized control study on the treatment of 26 cases of acne conglobata with encircling acupuncture combined with venesection and cupping. Zhen Ci Yan Jiu 2008;33:406–408.

Chapter 13

Acne Rosacea

Burhan Engin, Muazzez Çiğdem Oba,
Zekayi Kutlubay, Server Serdaroğlu and
Yalçın Tüzün

Additional information is available at the end of the chapter

http://dx.doi.org/10.5772/65636

Abstract

Rosacea is a common chronic inflammatory cutaneous disorder with variable presentation and severity. Disease usually occurs between the ages of 30 and 50 years. Women are more commonly affected than men. Rosacea is divided into four subtypes: erythematotelangiectatic, papulopustular, phymatous, and ocular, and one variant: lupoid or granulomatous rosacea. Erythematotelangiectatic rosacea is manifested as flushing and persistent centrofacial erythema, and papulopustular rosacea as papules and pustules in a centrofacial distribution. With disease progression, phymas consisting of sebaceous gland hypertrophy can develop. Ocular rosacea can result in blepharitis and conjunctivitis. Diagnosis is made clinically. Management of rosacea consists of protective measures such as sun protection and gentle skin care and topical and systemic treatments to suppress inflammation and erythema.

Keywords: rosacea, acne, perioral dermatitis, rhinophyma, ocular rosacea

1. Introduction

Rosacea is a common chronic inflammatory cutaneous disorder with variable presentation and severity. Facial flushing, telangiectasia, papules, and pustules are the main features of cutaneous rosacea.

2. Epidemiology

Rosacea can be seen in any age, but the onset usually occurs between the ages of 30 and 50 years. Women are more commonly affected than men; however, the development of phymatous skin changes is more commonly observed in men. Although the disease is more common in fair-skinned people of Celtic origin, patients of any ethnic group can be affected [1]. Up to 1/3 of the patients report a family history [2]. Rhinophyma, bulbous nose due to increased connective tissue and hyperplastic sebaceous glands, is almost exclusively seen in men over 40 years of age [3]. The prevalence is highly variable as the methods used and the populations studied vary greatly from one study to another [4]. A Swedish study reported a prevalence of 10% with a female-to-male ratio of 3:1 [5]. Eye involvement may be observed in more than 50% of patients [1].

3. Pathogenesis

Pathogenesis of rosacea is not well understood. Abnormalities in innate immunity, role of cutaneous microorganisms, and UV damage and vascular dysfunction may play a role in pathogenesis of rosacea.

Recent studies have shown the dysregulation of innate immune response in rosacea. Due to an exacerbated innate immune response, patients develop inflammatory reactions to stimuli that do not affect normal individuals. Patients with rosacea have high levels of cathelicidin, an antimicrobial peptide with vasoactive and proinflammatory properties and local protease kallikrein 5 (KLK5), which controls the production of cathelicidin peptides in epidermis. Injection of mouse skin with cathelicidin peptides from patients with rosacea led to skin changes similar to those observed in rosacea confirming the hypothesis [6]. Toll-like receptors (TLRs) work by triggering inflammation in response to recognized microbial patterns and elevated TLR2 activity, leading to an increase in KLK5 level which may also contribute to enhanced inflammatory responses responsible for rosacea signs [7].

Some microorganisms have been proposed to stimulate inflammatory reaction in cutaneous rosacea. *Demodex folliculorum* is an obligatory parasite found in pilosebaceous unit. Although almost all adults are infested with *Demodex*, patients with rosacea have increased density of *Demodex* mites supporting a significant association between *Demodex* infestation and the development of rosacea [8]. Correlation of gastrointestinal *Helicobacter pylori* infection and rosacea is controversial. The prevalence of *H. pylori* infection is shown to be increased or not different in patients with rosacea compared to control subjects. Treatment of *H. pylori* infection with antibiotics has been shown to improve rosacea, but this may be the benefit of anti-inflammatory effects of the antibiotics used for treatment [9].

UV and sun exposure are among the exacerbating factors for rosacea. UV-B has been shown to induce cutaneous angiogenesis in mice. In skin, UV-B increases vascular endothelial growth factor (VEGF) and fibroblast growth factor 2 (FGF2) secretion from human keratinocytes promoting angiogenesis. UV irradiation also produces reactive oxygen species, causing a damage in dermal matrix and thus leading to inflammation [6].

Vascular hyperreactivity may also play a role in disease pathogenesis. Dermal expression of VEGF, CD31, and lymphatic endothelium marker D2-40 has been shown to be elevated in rosacea, leading to stimulation of vascular and lymphatic endothelial cells [10].

http://dx.doi.org/10.5772/65636

4. Classification and clinical features

Rosacea is manifested as erythematous flushing, papules, and pustules in a centrofacial distribution. Intermittent or chronic facial edema may also occur. With disease progression, some patients may develop yellow-orange plaques called phymas consisting of sebaceous gland hypertrophy [11].

There are four stages: pre-rosacea and stages I through III. Patients with frequent flushing are considered in pre-rosacea group. In stage I, there is erythema that lasts from hours to days and telangiectasias. In stage II, persistent erythema is accompanied by multiple inflammatory papules and pustules. In stage III, large inflammatory nodules and connective tissue hyperplasia occur [4] (**Table 1**).

Pre-rosacea	**Frequent flushing**
Stage 1	Transient facial erythema that becomes more persistent telangiectasias
Stage 2	Persistent facial erythema
	Papules, pustules
	Ocular changes
Stage 3	Large inflammatory nodules
	Tissue hyperplasia, fibroplasias

Table 1. Stage symptoms and signs [11].

The National Rosacea Society (NRS) has classified rosacea into four subtypes: erythematotelangiectatic, papulopustular, phymatous, and ocular, and one variant: lupoid or granulomatous rosacea.

4.1. Erythematotelangiectatic type

The erythematotelangiectatic type is the most common subtype of rosacea (**Figure 1**). It is characterized by flushing and persistent central facial erythema with sparing of periocular skin. The flushing of rosacea lasts longer than 10 min differentiating it from physiological flushing episodes. Telangiectasias are common but not essential for the diagnosis of this subtype. Stinging or burning sensations may be present [4].

4.2. Papulopustular type

Papulopustular rosacea is characterized by persistent central facial erythema: small, dome-shaped erythematous papules and surmounting pustules on the central face [4] (**Figure 2**). However, papules and pustules may also occur periorificially. The inflammation seen in papulopustular rosacea is similar to acne vulgaris, but comedones typical for acne vulgaris are absent in rosacea [12].

In a study, 15 patients with pustular rosacea and 15 age- and sex-matched control subjects were compared. A significantly increased growth of *S. epidermidis* was found in rosacea pustules and eyelid margins of rosacea patients suggesting a role of *S. epidermidis* in pathogenesis of pustular and ocular rosacea [13].

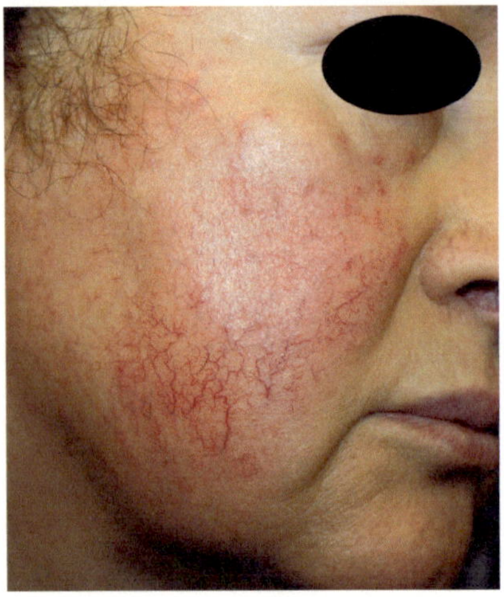

Figure 1. Erythematotelangiectatic type of rosacea. Prominent telangiectatic vessels and erythema on the cheek with characteristic sparing of periocular skin.

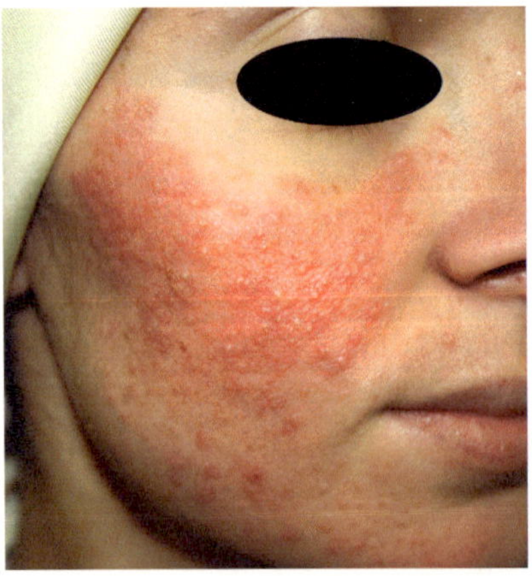

Figure 2. Papulopustular type of rosacea. Extensive papules and pustules on a background of persistent erythema.

4.3. Ocular rosacea

Ocular rosacea occurs in more than 50% of patients with rosacea. Eye involvement may follow, as seen in half of the patients, may precede as in 20%, or occur simultaneously with skin changes [12].

http://dx.doi.org/10.5772/65636

Patients with ocular rosacea may complain of foreign body sensation, dryness, itching, photophobia, and tearing. If the cornea is involved by the disease, the visual acuity may be decreased [14]. Blepharitis and conjunctivitis are the most common findings. Blepharitis is characterized by the eyelid margin erythema, scale, and staphylococcal infections. Hypopyon, scleritis, keratitis, and iritis can also occur. Rosacea keratitis is a severe condition and has a poor prognosis. It can lead to corneal opacity, scarring, and loss of vision. The severity of ocular rosacea symptoms is often not related to the severity of cutaneous manifestations [4].

4.4. Phymatous rosacea

Phymatous rosacea shows tissue hypertrophy manifesting as thickened skin with irregular contours and prominent pores. Involvement most commonly occurs on the nose (rhinophyma), but the chin (gnathophyma), forehead (metophyma), and ears (otophyma) may also be affected [4]. Rhinophyma occurs mostly in men with a male/female ratio of 20:1. Although rhinophyma is often accepted as a presentation of last stage of rosacea, it may occur in patients with few or no other features of rosacea. One diagnosis is a clinical one, and biopsy is only indicated to rule out alternative diagnoses or in suspicion of a malignancy such as basal cell carcinoma or squamous cell carcinoma [15].

4.5. Granulomatous rosacea

Granulomatous rosacea was classified by the expert committee as a disease variant characterized by discrete yellow, brown, red papules, or nodules on periorificial facial skin [12] (**Figure 3**). Patients do not often have persistent erythema or flushing of the face and may not have their disease distributed to convexities of the face [16].

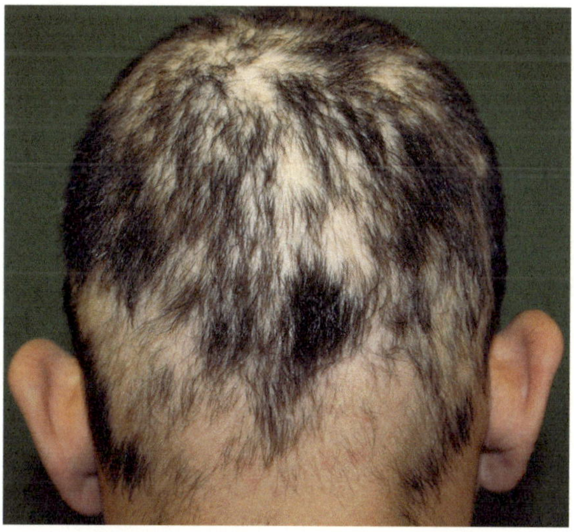

Figure 3. Granulomatous rosacea. Discrete yellow papules clustered periorficially.

5. Histopathology

In mild forms of rosacea, histologic findings are often limited to vascular ectasia and mild edema. A lymphohistiocytic infiltrate with perivascular and perifollicular distribution is observed in papulopustular form [17]. Solar elastosis is invariably found in histopathologic examination of biopsy specimens. In granulomatous variant, non-caseating epithelioid granulomas are seen within the dermis [18].

6. Diagnosis and differential diagnosis

Diagnosis of rosacea is made clinically; there is no laboratory test to confirm the diagnosis. A biopsy is only indicated to rule out alternative diagnoses [1] (**Table 2**).

Acne vulgaris
Seborrheic dermatitis
Keratosis pilaris
Dermatomyositis
Systemic lupus erythematosus
Photodermatitis
Sarcoidosis
Demodicosis
Haber syndrome
Basal cell carcinoma

Table 2. Differential diagnosis of facial rosacea [17, 19].

Acne vulgaris is the disease most commonly confused with rosacea, especially in middle-aged adults. Key distinguishing feature between acne vulgaris and rosacea is the absence of comedones in rosacea [4]. Patients with acne vulgaris are often younger patients, having oily skin with comedones, larger pustules, and less erythema with scarring [1].

Perioral dermatitis presents with micropustules and vesicles with scaling around the mouth. Seborrheic dermatitis often coexists with rosacea [17]. Scaling and erythema of the scalp, eyebrows, external auditory canals, and retroauricular folds serve as clues to the presence of seborrheic dermatitis [4].

The malar erythema of systemic lupus erythematosus can be difficult to distinguish from rosacea. Clinically, papules pustules and ocular symptoms are mostly absent in lupus [17]. Severe Demodex infection (demodicosis) may present with rosacea-like features, but flushing and telangiectasia are absent [4]. And also, photodermatitis is triggered by sun exposure and has similar skin manifestations to rosacea [4].

7. Associated diseases

Rosacea patients may have increased risk of developing certain diseases as evidenced by case-controlled studies. Further studies are necessary to confirm these associations.

Patients with rosacea are more likely to have dyslipidemia and hypertension. They are also at increased risk of coronary artery disease after adjustment for cardiovascular disease risk factors [20]. There is a possible association between rosacea and an increased risk of thyroid cancer and basal cell carcinoma [21].

Rosacea was associated with a significantly increased risk of glioma in a Danish nationwide cohort [22]. In the same Danish cohort, patients with rosacea had an increased risk of autoimmune diseases, including type 1 diabetes mellitus, celiac disease, multiple sclerosis, and rheumatoid arthritis [23].

8. Treatment

8.1. Protective measures

Protective measures are of utmost importance in management of rosacea patients of all subtypes. These include avoidance of triggers of flushing, gentle skin care, and sun protection.

Most sufferers report worsening of the disease by factors such as hot or cold temperature, wind, hot drinks, exercise, spicy food, alcohol, emotions, and menopause [24]. A variety of medications may exacerbate flushing such as vasodilative drugs, nicotinic acid and amyl nitrite, calcium channel blockers, and opiates [1].

Cleansers containing acetone or alcohol should be avoided. Usage of abrasive or exfoliant preparations and vigorous rubbing of the skin should also be discontinued [1].

Daily application of combined ultraviolet-A and ultraviolet B protective sunscreen with a sun protection factor of 15 or greater should be advised to every patient. Sun-blocking creams containing titanium dioxide and zinc oxide are usually well tolerated [1].

8.2. Erythematotelangiectatic rosacea

Erythematotelangiectatic rosacea is the most treatment-resistant subtype of rosacea. Flushing and burning are the most difficult features to treat. Non-cardioselective β-blockers such as propranolol 40 mg twice daily or nadolol 40 mg daily can be tried, but provide rather limited benefit [25].

Topical or oral medications described below for papulopustular rosacea are often used, but evidence supporting their role in erythematotelangiectatic rosacea is lacking [1].

Treatment of erythema and telangiectasia with vascular lasers or intense pulse light can help in improving flushing and burning [4].

8.3. Papulopustular rosacea

Systemic and topical antibiotics are effective in treatment of papulopustular rosacea. Patients with moderate-to-severe papulopustular rosacea at initial presentation may require systemic therapy to achieve clearance of inflammatory skin lesions followed by topical treatment to avoid relapses. Topical medications alone can be used to control milder disease.

Main topical agents utilized for the treatment of rosacea include metronidazole, sulfacetamide-sulfur, azelaic acid, and topical antibiotics (clindamycin, erythromycin) [26]. Three varieties of 0.75% metronidazole and 1% metronidazole and several brands of 10% sodium sulfacetamide with 5% sulfur and 15% azelaic acid gel are medications that have been approved by the Food and Drug Administration (FDA) for rosacea. All are indicated for the papules, pustules, and erythema [4].

Topical metronidazole used once or twice daily is effective in treatment of inflammatory papules and pustules and improving erythema of papulopustular rosacea. Azelaic acid is a well-tolerated preparation that also reduces papules and pustules. It is available in 15% gel and 20% cream forms, applied twice a day; 10% sodium sulfacetamide with 5% sulfur is used to treat acne, rosacea, and seborrheic dermatitis. It has beneficial effects in reducing both inflammatory lesion counts and erythema scores in papulopustular rosacea [27]. Topical erythromycin used for acne vulgaris can help in reducing symptoms but may prove irritant on skin affected by rosacea [24]. Clindamycin gel, also developed for treatment of acne, may be better tolerated. A combined formulation containing 5% benzoyl peroxide and 1% clindamycin has proved effective and well tolerated in a placebo-controlled trial [4].

Topical retinoids have been used to treat rosacea, but the true efficacy has not been established. Adapalen, a relatively well-tolerated retinoid, has been shown to be an alternative treatment agent in management of papulopustular rosacea [28].

Effective systemic antibiotics include tetracyclines (e.g., tetracycline or oxytetracycline 250 mg twice daily) and erythromycin 250 mg twice daily. Second-generation tetracyclines, such as minocycline and doxycycline, are also effective and offer the advantages of once daily administration and less gastrointestinal side effects [24]. Doxycycline shows anti-inflammatory effects at doses as low as 40 mg daily [29]. Azithromycin was proven to be as effective as doxycycline in a number of studies [4]. In one series, azithromycin proved beneficial after 4 weeks at 250 mg/day, for 3 days each week (Monday, Wednesday, and Friday) [30].

Oral metronidazole is an effective alternative treatment for rosacea. Metronidazole (200 mg) taken twice daily for 12 weeks has been proved to be as effective in improving the inflammatory lesions of rosacea as 250 mg oxytetracycline taken twice daily [4]. Abstinence from alcohol during metronidazole therapy is necessary to avoid disulfiram-like reactions. Although relatively safe, metronidazole has been associated with potential side effects such as neuropathy and seizures [24].

Oral isotretinoin is a treatment option for severe rosacea. The onset of action of systemic retinoids is slow when compared with the oral antibiotics. It is effective both in erythematotelangiectatic and papulopustular rosacea. Oral istotretinoin can also be used for granulomatous rosacea and rhinophyma. It has been shown that treatment-resistant patients taking isotretinoin experienced fewer papules and pustules, a reduction in erythema, and decreased nasal volume [31]. Daily doses of isotretinoin range from 0.2 to 1 mg/kg. It is usually given for 6 months. With low dose therapy, the common mucosal side effects of the drug are minimal and tolerable. However, due to its teratogenic effects, it is contraindicated in women of childbearing potential [4].

8.4. Ocular rosacea

Treatment of ocular rosacea depends on disease severity. Lid hygiene and warm compresses are the baseline treatment for all patients. For mild ocular rosacea, fucidic acid preparations and metronidazole gel are frequently used [4]. Systemic antibiotics such as oral tetracyclin or doxycyclin may be used in patients with a more severe involvement [32]. The keratitis associated with rosacea can be severe, and patients with potentially serious ocular symptoms should be referred to an ophthalmologist.

8.5. Rhinophyma

In patients with early rhinophyma, medical treatment with systemic isotretinoin may prove beneficial. In advanced cases, surgery is performed. Surgery can be done either as a complete excision or an incomplete excision made by cryosurgery, dermabrasion, electrosurgery, sharp blade excision, shaving with a razor, or laser surgery [32].

Author details

Burhan Engin*, Muazzez Çiğdem Oba, Zekayi Kutlubay, Server Serdaroğlu and Yalçın Tüzün

*Address all correspondence to: burhanengin2000@yahoo.com

Cerrahpaşa Medical Faculty, Dermatology Department, Istanbul University, Istanbul, Turkey

References

[1] Powell FC: Clinical practice. Rosacea. N Engl J Med. 2005;352:793–803. doi:10.1056/NEJMcp042829

[2] Del Rosso JQ: Update on rosacea pathogenesis and correlation with medical therapeutic agents. Cutis. 2006;78:97–100

[3] Buechner SA: Rosacea: an update. Dermatology. 2005;210:100–108. doi:10.1159/000082564

[4] Tüzün Y, Wolf R, Kutlubay Z, Karakus O, Engin B: Rosacea and rhynophyma. Clin Dermatol. 2014;32:35–46 doi:10.1016/j.clindermatol.2013.05.024

[5] Berg M, Liden S: An epidemiological study of rosacea. Acta Derm Venereol. 1989;69:419–423.

[6] Yamasaki K, Gallo RL: The molecular pathology of rosacea: J Dermatol Sci. 2009;55:77–81. doi:10.1016/j.jdermsci.2009.04.007

[7] Yamasaki K, Kanada K, Macleod DT, et al: TLR2 expression is increased in rosacea and stimulates enhanced serine protease production by keratinocytes. J Invest Dermatol. 2011;131:688–697. doi:10.1038/jid.2010.351

[8] Zhao YE, Wu LP, Peng Y, Cheng H: Retrospective analysis of the association between demodex infestation and rosacea. Arch Dermatol. 2010;146:896–902. doi:10.1001/archdermatol.2010.196

[9] Tan J, Berg M: Rosacea: current state of epidemiology. J Am Acad Dermatol. 2013;69:27–35. doi:10.1016/j.jaad.2013.04.043

[10] Gomaa AH, Yaar M, Eyada MM, Bhawan J: Lymphangiogenesis and angiogenesis in non-phymatous rosacea. J Cutan Pathol. 2007;34:748–753. doi:10.1111/j.1600-0560.2006.00695.x

[11] Culp B, Scheinfeld N: Rosacea: a review. P T. 2009;34:38–45.

[12] Wilkin J, Dahl M, Detmar M, et al: Standard classification of rosacea: Report of the National Rosacea Society Expert Committee on the Classification and Staging of Rosacea. J Am Acad Dermatol. 2002;46:584–587.

[13] Whitfeld M, Gunasingam N, Leow LJ, Shirato K, Preda V: Staphylococcus epidermidis: a possible role in the pustules of rosacea. J Am Acad Dermatol. 2011;64:49–52. doi:10.1016/j.jaad.2009.12.036

[14] Vieira AC, Höfling-Lima AL, Mannis MJ: Ocular rosacea—a review. Arq Bras Oftalmol. 2012;75:363–369.

[15] Lazeri D, Colizzi L, Licata G, et al: Malignancies within rhinophyma: report of three new cases and review of the literature. Aesthetic Plast Surg. 2012;36:396–405. doi:10.1007/s00266-011-9802-0

[16] Crawford GH, Pelle MT, James WD: Rosacea: I. Etiology, pathogenesis, and subtype classification. J Am Acad Dermatol. 2004;51:327–341. doi:10.1016/j.jaad.2004.03.030

[17] Webster GF: Rosacea. Med Clin North Am. 2009;93:1183–1194. doi:10.1016/j.mcna.2009.08.007

[18] Aroni K, Tsagroni E, Lazaris AC, Patsouris E, Agapitos E: Rosacea: a clinicopathological approach. Dermatology. 2004;209:177–182. doi:10.1159/000079886

[19] Fuller D, Martin S: Rosacea. J Midwifery Womens Health. 2012;57:403–409. doi:10.1111/j.1542-2011.2011.00156.x

[20] Hua TC, Chung PI, Chen YJ, et al: Cardiovascular comorbidities in patients with rosacea: a nationwide case-control study from Taiwan. J Am Acad Dermatol. 2015;73:249–254. doi:10.1016/j.jaad.2015.04.028

[21] Li WQ, Zhang M, Danby FW, Han J, Qureshi AA: Personal history of rosacea and risk of incident cancer among women in the US. Br J Cancer. 2015;113:520–523. doi:10.1038/bjc.2015.217

[22] Egeberg A, Hansen PR, Gislason GH, Thyssen JP: Association of Rosacea With Risk for Glioma in a Danish Nationwide Cohort Study. JAMA Dermatol. 2016;152:541–545. doi:10.1001/jamadermatol.2015.5549

[23] Egeberg A, Hansen PR, Gislason GH, Thyssen JP: Clustering of autoimmune diseases in patients with rosacea. J Am Acad Dermatol. 2016;74:667–672. doi:10.1016/j.jaad.2015.11.004

[24] Pelle MT, Crawford GH, James WD: Rosacea: II therapy. J Am Acad Dermatol. 2004;51:499–512. doi:10.1016/j.jaad.2004.03.033

[25] Wilkin JK: Effect of nadolol on flushing reactions in rosacea. J Am Acad Dermatol. 1989;20:202–205.

[26] Del Rosso JQ: Medical treatment of rosacea with emphasis on topical therapies. Expert Opin Pharmacother. 2004;5:5–13. doi:10.1517/14656566.5.1.5

[27] Gooderham M: Rosacea and its topical management. Skin Therapy Lett. 2009;14:1–3.

[28] Altinyazar HC, Koca R, Tekin NS, Eştürk E: Adapalene vs. metronidazole gel for the treatment of rosacea. Int J Dermatol. 2005;44:252–255. doi:10.1111/j.1365-4632.2004.02130.x

[29] Del Rosso JQ, Webster GF, Jackson M, et al: Two randomized phase III clinical trials evaluating anti-inflammatory dose doxycycline (40-mg doxycycline, USP capsules) administered once daily for treatment of rosacea. J Am Acad Dermatol. 2007;56:791–802. doi:10.1016/j.jaad.2006.11.021

[30] Fernandez-Obregon A: Oral use of azithromycin for the treatment of acne rosacea. Arch Dermatol. 2004;140:489–490. doi:10.1001/archderm.140.4.489

[31] Baldwin HE: Systemic therapy for rosacea. Skin Therapy Lett. 2007;12:1–5.

[32] Gupta AK, Chaudhry MM: Rosacea and its management: an overview. J Eur Acad Dermatol Venereol. 2005;19:273–285. doi:10.1111/j.1468-3083.2005.01216.x

Chapter 14

Ocular Rosacea

Aysun Sanal Dogan

Additional information is available at the end of the chapter

http://dx.doi.org/10.5772/66470

Abstract

Acne rosacea (AR) is a chronic cutaneous inflammatory disease of the midface. Ocular involvement occurs in 30–70% of patients. Although the incidence of this disease is seen highest between the ages of 30 and 50 years, it can also develop during childhood. The diagnosis depends on clinical findings such as meibomian gland dysfunction (MGD), conjunctival hyperemia, and corneal vascularization, and untreated cases can progress and lead to vision loss. Pathogenetic factors can be the altered the immune system, colonization of microorganisms, inflammation, abnormalities of sebaceous, and meibomian glands, environmental factors, and vascular dysregulation. Differential diagnosis from other ophthalmologic and dermatologic diseases is important. Management requires an interdisciplinary approach with a step-wise treatment algorithm. Patients should be informed about the chronic course of the disease and avoid the exacerbating factors. Caring about the lid hygiene and use of non-preserved artificial eye tears, topical ointments including antibiotics, anti-inflammatory agents are used when necessary. However, the mainstay of the therapy is the use of oral antibiotics for a long period. Surgical interventions may be needed in cases with a vision-threatening condition. During the long-term treatment period and disease course, the complications of medications should also be considered cautiously and patient should be followed up routinely.

Keywords: ocular rosacea, dry eye, meibomian gland, meibomian gland dysfunction, treatment

1. Introduction

Acne rosacea (AR) is the chronic inflammatory disease of skin typically involving the cheeks, nose, chin, and central forehead. The dermatological findings are transient or persistent erythema, papules, pustules, and telangiectasia. During the chronic course, these findings show exacerbations and remissions that may end up with progression. This dermatologic condition has been classified by National Rosacea Society into four subtypes based on the clinical features: (1) erythematotelangiectatic rosacea, (2) papulopustular rosacea, (3) phymatous rosacea, and (4) ocular rosacea [1]. Flushing, chronic inflammation, and fibrosis are present in dermatologic course. The presence of one of the findings: flushing, non-transient erythema, plaque, dry appearance, edema, papules-pustules, and telangiectasia on the face with burning sensation, ocular manifestations, and phymatous changes is indicative of rosacea, and these symptoms are graded as mild, moderate, and severe [2]. Ocular manifestations are defined as one of the secondary criteria [1].

Under the circumstances of existing acne rosacea, the diagnosis of ocular rosacea (OR) is made by the presence of inflammation of the ocular surface, accompanying redness, burning, and itching symptoms of the eye. The diagnosis is confirmed by the presence of corneal infiltration with meibomian gland inflammation, and accompanying skin findings of rosacea [3].

2. Epidemiology

AR is usually seen between ages of 30 and 50 years [4, 5]. The prevalence is reported from 4 to 22% that is more frequent in fair-skinned people [5–8]. The OR starts to be detected approximately 10 years after the diagnosis of AR, with an increasing incidence between ages of 40 and 50 years [5]. The ocular involvement occurs in 58–72% and interestingly the ocular signs may precede in 20% of rosacea patients [9, 10]. Because of mild cutaneous manifestations, the ocular findings may be underestimated in children. Therefore, the diagnosis is delayed with more ocular complications. In a case series, it was shown that only two of six children with ocular rosacea demonstrated cutaneous rosacea findings [11].

Although AR affects women more than men, ocular involvement is to be seen in both sexes equally [5, 12]. There is a family history in 15–30% of cases [13, 14]. Hence, with a suspicion of family history, the children should be followed up closely and should be kept in mind that the condition tends to progress in adulthood [15].

3. Pathogenesis

Although AR has no proven cause, scientific studies showed that there is dysregulation of vascular, immunologic, and nervous systems [16, 17]. Ocular surface is the mainly affected area with OR. Ocular surface compromises cellular components of the palpebral and bulbar conjunctiva such as corneoscleral limbus, cornea, eyelid margins, eyelashes, and tear film [18].

3.1. Altered immune system

Altered immune system may be one of the factors. It was postulated that a type IV hypersensitivity reaction may be responsible for the conjunctival inflammation in OR in which the reactant is unknown [19, 20].

3.2. Colonization of microorganism

Demodex folliculorum is a saprophytic mite that is found in normal flora of the skin. There are studies demonstrating that the Demodex density increased in rosacea patients [21, 22].

Bacillus olenorium serum immunoreactivity was detected in ocular rosacea patients. Its proteins cause high immune reactions [22, 23].

Staphylococcus epidermidis and *Propionibacterium acnes* that are found commonly in lid flora are accused microorganisms for their production of high levels of bacterial lipases [24].

In a study, *Chlamydia pneumoniae* antigen was detected in 40% of skin biopsies patient with rosacea [25].

Moreover, *Helicobacter pylori* IgG antibodies were found in 81% of the acne rosacea patients with dyspepsia, but there is a debate whether this is a coincidence or not [26]. The proteins produced by these pathogens might be responsible for the some aspects of rosacea.

The increased amount of free fatty acids produced by meibomian glands causes tear film instability and irritates the ocular tissues [27]. This increase may be due to biochemical abnormality of the meibomian gland secretions or lipolytic exoenzymes of bacteria which degrade lipids into free fatty acids [28].

3.3. Inflammation

OR was found to be associated with the increased tear fluid levels of several inflammatory mediators such as interleukin-1 (IL-1) and gelatinase B activity [29]. Matrix metalloproteinases (MMP), interferon-alpha (IFN-α), and inflammatory cytokines seem to be an important component of pathophysiology [30].

The meibomian glands of rosacea patients cause keratinization of epithelial cells, end up with thickening of secretions, plugging of the orifices, and trapping of the secretions [31].

3.4. Environmental factors

Many rosacea patients are aware of some factors that exacerbate their symptoms. Although these triggering factors differ for each patient: alcohol, sunlight, wind, temperature extremes, hot, and spicy foods, vigorous exercise, hot baths, medications that dilate blood vessels, menopause, and emotional factors (stress, anger, and embarrassment) can also play role in the pathogenesis [32–34].

3.5. Genetics

Rosacea is associated with familial predisposition [35]. In a study conducted in twin pairs, rosacea contribution has been reported equally by genetic and environmental factors [36]. The genetic predisposition showed single nucleotide polymorphisms in HLA-DRA and BTNL2 genes that support the concept of a genetic component for rosacea [37].

3.6. Vascular dysregulation and neurologic system

There is vascular dilatation and telangiectatic vessels and increased blood flow, causing erythema, flushing, and neovascularization [5, 34, 38], which is probably under control of the sympathetic system [39].

4. Diagnosis

The diagnosis of both dermatological rosacea and ocular rosacea is clinical. There is no single-specific test—even skin biopsy—to confirm the diagnosis.

Ocular involvement is varied and non-specific. Most of the patients refer to ophthalmologist with dry eye symptoms (**Table 1**). No correlation exists between the severity of the ocular manifestations and that of the skin lesions. However, in patients with increased flushing, ocular rosacea prevalence is higher [40].

Although rosacea is uncommon in pediatric cases, it deserves attention due to undiagnosed ocular rosacea that is common with severe ocular complication [41]. History of triggering factors should be investigated and dermatologist consultation is required.

4.1. Clinical feature

Both eyes are usually affected simultaneously, but unilateral or sequential involvements can also occur.

The primary and the starter of the ocular involvement is the meibomian gland dysfunction (MGD) [42]. Ghanem et al. reported that the most common ocular signs in patients with rosacea from the ophthalmologic clinic were meibomian gland dysfunction (MGD) in 85.2%, lid margin telangiectasias in 53.4%, blepharitis in 44.3%, and interpalpebral hyperemia in 40.9%. Accordingly, patients from the dermatology clinic were reported to exhibit MGD in 27.3%, chalazion/hordeolum, lid margin telangiectasia in 18.2%, anterior blepharitis in 13.6%, and pinguecula in 13.6% [9] Vision loss is a rare but devastating complication [43]. OR has been graded as mild, moderate, and severe (**Table 2**) [2].

Ocular symptoms
– dryness sensations (burning and stinging, feeling of a having foreign body sensation in the eye)
– irritation
– itching
– redness
– sensitivity to light (photophobia)
– tearing
– red and swollen eyelids
– blurry or decreased vision

Table 1. Ocular symptoms of the ocular rosacea patient.

Grade	Involved areas	Signs and symptoms	Recommended treatment
Mild	Eyelid margin, meibomian gland	Mild itching and dry eye sensation Fine scaling and erythema of eyelid margins Mild conjunctival hyperemia	Topical treatment only
Moderate	Ocular surface	Moderate burning, tearing, foreign body sensation Eyelid margin irregularities, erythema and telangiectasia Prominent conjunctival hyperemia, ciliary injection Hordeolum and chalazion formation	Topical, systemic treatment
Severe	Corneal involvement and decreased vision	Pain, sensitivity to light, blurred vision Severe conjunctival inflammation, madarosis and trichiasis Corneal involvement	Topical, systemic, surgical treatment

Table 2. Grading of ocular rosacea [2].

4.2. Symptoms

Feeling of dryness, irritation symptoms with burning and stinging and feeling of having foreign body sensation in the eye are common. Blurry vision, redness, sensitivity to light (photophobia), tearing, itching, red, and swollen eyelids are the other encountered symptoms.

4.3. Signs

It is not rare that the symptoms of the patient are not proportional with the ocular findings. Reduced fluorescein tear breakup time, punctate staining on the cornea, and bulbar conjunctiva (**Figure 1**). Superficial punctate keratopathy (due to tear film instability), dry eye disease, blepharitis, styes, MGD, eyelid inflammation-collaretes, telangiectasis, conjunctival hyperemia, conjunctival scarring, punctate epithelial keratitis, corneal infiltrate/vascularization, corneal thinning, corneal astigmatism, corneal ulceration, phlyctenules, phlyctenular keratitis, limbal pannus, episcleritis, scleritis, corneal melting, and perforation, iritis, periorbital edema, recurrent chalazia, pannus, neovascularization, trichiasis (**Figures 1–5**) [43–46].

4.3.1. Eyelid

The lipid layer produced by meibomian glands stabilizes the tear film and prevents evaporation. Abnormality of this function is the primary cause of the blepharitis and evaporative-type dry eye. Dry eye can be detected by decreased tear breakup times. There is inflammation, dilatation, and occlusion of the meibomian glands [31]. With pressure to eyelid margins, there is hardness to express the secretion, and usually occluded by toothpaste-like material namely meibomana. Hordeolum and chalazion are the signs of focal inflamed obstructive MGD. In chronic course, there will be telangiectatic vessels around the orifices of the meibomian glands. At the end, the ducts are fully keratinized and disappears leading the meibomian gland dropout.

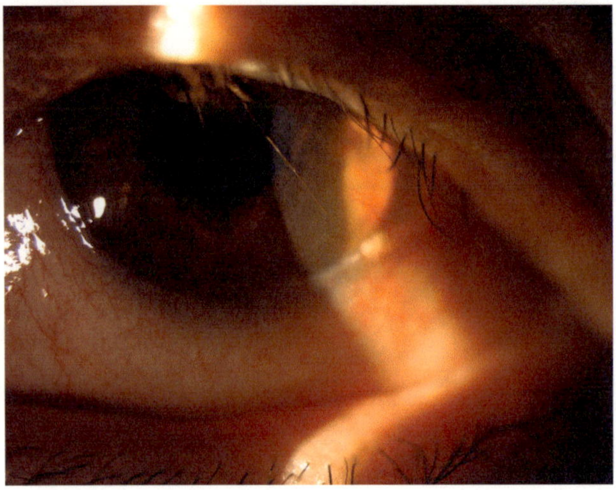

Figure 1. Ocular rosacea patient with irregular ocular margin, conjunctival hyperemia and trichiasis.

4.3.2. conjunctiva

Conjunctival hyperemia is the common finding. Hyperemia is mostly obvious in interpalpebral area. In 9% of OR, there is also conjunctival scarring [47].

4.3.3. cornea

Disease starts with inferior punctate epitheliopathy. Superficial vascularization of the peripheral cornea (especially triangular in shape and extending from inferior cornea) develops in

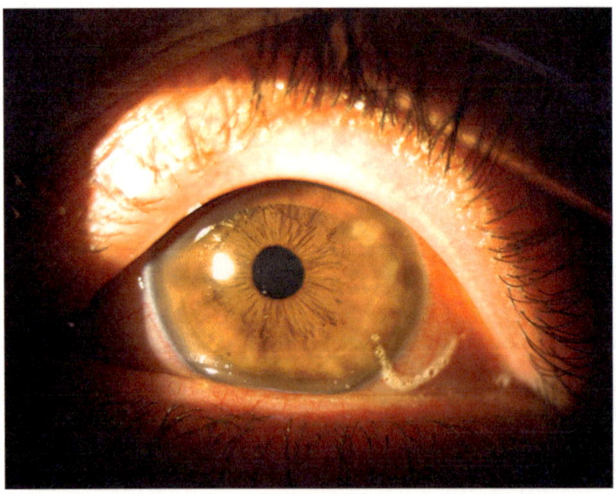

Figure 2. Ocular rosacea with sterile corneal infiltrate, lid telangiectasia, meibomian gland occlusion and foamy secretion.

http://dx.doi.org/10.5772/66470

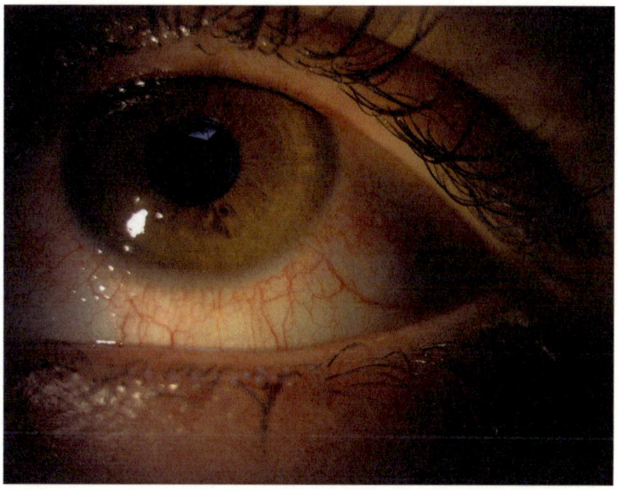

Figure 3. Bulbar interpalpebral conjunctival hyperemia with fine corneal vascularization.

untreated cases. In case of recurrent epithelium defects, one should be suspicious of OR also. Inflammatory episodes will end up with devastating problems, such as corneal scarring, thinning even perforation and sight threatening keratitis [48–51].

4.4. Ocular tests and imaging

Tests of evaporative dry eye are altered in OR. Tear osmolarity values, Ocular surface disease index (OSDI) questionnaire and corneal staining scores were significantly higher, and

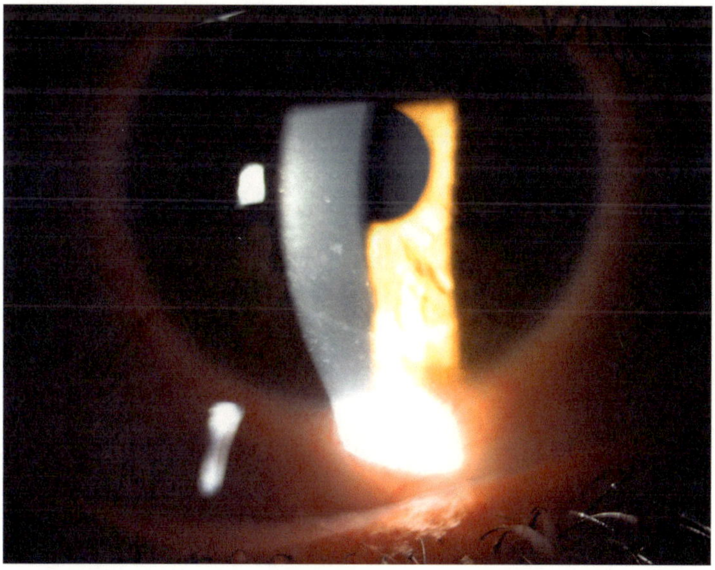

Figure 4. Ocular rosacea with severe dry eye symptoms and inferior punctate epitheliopathy.

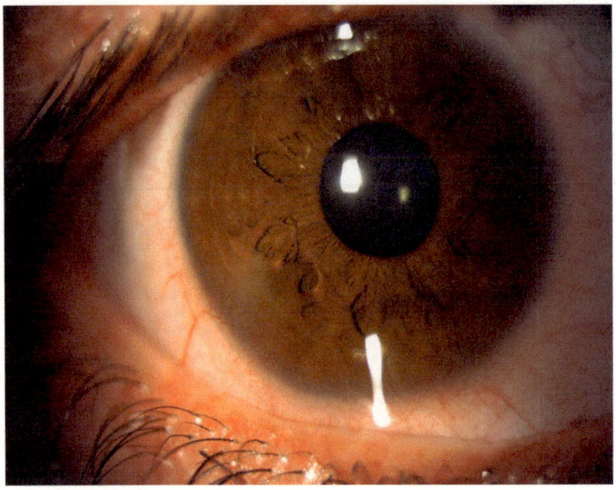

Figure 5. Corneal haze inferotemporally signifying healed corneal involvement of ocular rosacea.

Schirmer-I test and fluorescein tear breakup time were significantly lower, which all confirms tear hyperosmolarity and tear film dysfunction [52].

Dry eye in rosacea patients can also be diagnosed by tear meniscus measurement with optical coherence tomography (OCT) with considerable sensitivity and specificity [53]. Central corneal thickness, corneal hysteresis and corneal resistance factors were all significantly decreased in OR patients when compared to healthy controls [54]. Patients with OR show significant meibomian gland dropout which can be demonstrated by meibography (**Figure 6**)

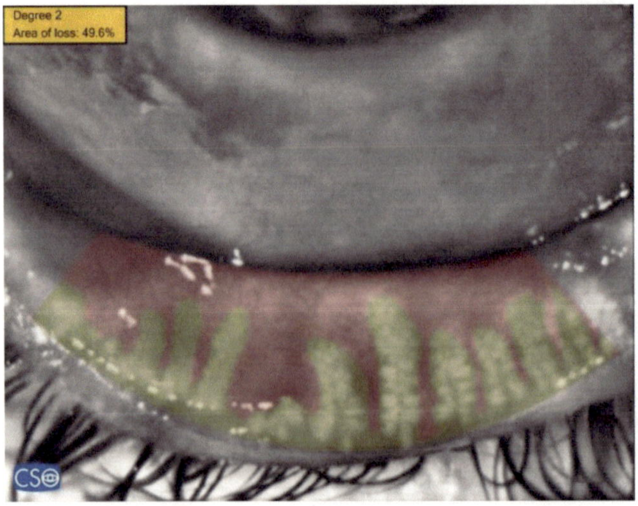

Figure 6. Ocular rosacea. Meibography, meibomian dropout.

[31, 42]. *In vivo* confocal microscopy findings revealed inflammatory changes of ocular surface and even Demodex infestations on eyelids [55, 56].

5. Differential diagnosis

5.1. From dermatological diseases

In patients with suspicion of OR, if facial dermatologic inflammatory changes exist, clinician would be aware of three main differential diagnosis [57]. These are as follows:

Acne vulgaris: The presence of comedones—which does not exist in rosacea—in young patients direct the clinician to diagnosis of acne vulgaris.

Seborrheic dermatitis: In seborrheic dermatitis, facial erythema is accompanied by yellowish scaling and prominent dandruff.

Perioral dermatitis: There is perioral involvement without flushing or telangiectasia.

5.2. From ophthalmological diseases

Ocular findings must be differentiated from the other causes of dry eye.

Corneal involvements must be differentiated from herpetic or bacterial keratitis and recurrent epithelial defects [48, 58, 59].

All forms of conjunctivitis are in differential diagnosis. Due to chronic course and leading to conjunctival scarring, chlamydial conjunctivitis deserves attention.

In severe OR, which ends up with inferior thinning and irregular astigmatism, it may resemble to keratoconus [51].

6. Management

For an effective therapeutic strategy, an interdisciplinary collaboration is needed between ophthalmologist and dermatologist. The stepwise approach is recommended.

- Inform patient about the chronic nature of their disease and requirement for regular follow-up.
- Avoid triggering and exacerbating factors. It might be advised to keep a daily diary to figure out triggering factors.
- Avoid wearing contact lenses and eye makeup when the symptoms are exaggerated.
- Lid hygiene: Hot compressing and MG expressions by mechanical massage to lids, lid hygiene cleaning solutions, eyelid scrubs massage to the tarsal plate [60]. This is the main approach and must be recommended to all OR patients

- Lubricants: Lubricants are used to decrease inflammatory mediators, and to provide symptomatic relief. Non-preserved artificial tears are recommended with a patient-individualized dosage [61]. The initial high dosages might be tapered gradually. OR is usually mild and responds well to lid hygiene and lubricants, but must be advised to do regularly to avoid exacerbations of symptoms.
- Topical antibiotics: Azithromycin 1.5% eye drops are effective for MGD treatment even with phlyctenular keratoconjunctivitis complicating OR [62, 63]. It has an anti-inflammatory effect as well as an antimicrobial effect. Topical antibiotic ointments (fucidic acid and metronidazole gel applied to lid margins), especially in the nighttime, are also effective to restore the flora.
- Mainstay of the treatment is the use of systemic antibiotics. Due to relapses, maintenance treatment may be 6 months. Low doses with longer duration of the antibiotic usage must be preferred to benefit from the anti-inflammatory effect without inducing resistance and other side effects.
  - Systemic tetracycline/doxycycline/minocycline shows the therapeutic effects by decreasing lid flora, inhibiting collagenase activity which prevents corneal thinning, inhibiting inflammatory mediators (i.e. MMP), decreasing concentration of free fatty acids [64–66].
  - Clarithromycin are also effective to *H. pylori* [67].
  - Metronidazole has anti-inflammatory, anti-microbic, anti-parasitic, and immunosuppressive effects [68].
  - Azithromycin 3 times per week for 4 weeks [69].
  - Erythromycin is appropriate for children <8 years old to avoid the untoward effects of tetracycline [70].
- Topical anti-inflammatory agents: Topical corticosteroids suppress the exacerbation episodes and are effective in prevention of the recurrent corneal erosions when used in combination with systemic doxycycline [71]. The application would be tapered and stopped after the symptomatic relief. Topical steroids should be used cautiously, minimal dose with minimal duration, under the supervision of the ophthalmologist. Instead of steroids, topical cyclosporine (with 0.05% concentration) might be the choice for a longer period of treatment [72].
- Dietary intervention with omega-3 fatty acids for 6 months is effective in decreasing the dry eye symptoms and signs in ocular rosacea [73].
- Surgical: Intraductal meibomian gland probing is shown to be a promising technique to improve dry eye symptoms related with OR [74]. Epilation of trichiatic lashes will eliminate the mechanical insult to ocular surface.

In cases of severe corneal involvement, surgical options are indicated [49]. Progressive epitheliopathy unresponsive to topical treatment with hazy epithelium extending centrally, indicating limbal stem cell insufficiency, is treated with limbal stem cell transplantation [75]. Thinning of the cornea and threatening perforation are treated with conjunctival flaps or amniotic membranes [43]. Little corneal perforations may benefit from cyanoacrylate glues. Minority people with untreated or resistant to treatment may need keratoplasty at the end of long-term OR [49].

Rosacea naturally waxes and wanes. However, because the damage from rosacea can be progressive, the long-lasting use of therapy has advantages. Due to the lack of prospective controlled studies, the optimum modality and duration for treatment and prevention of OR recurrence remain unclear. The duration of the treatment depends on the ophthalmologist's decision and the severity of the ocular involvement. There is a consensus to give treatment for several months, and tapering the doses within follow-ups.

7. Complications

Long-standing OR will end up with irregular eyelid margins and misdirected eyelashes (trichiasis). Untreated corneal involvement will lead to vision loss.

The long-term use of topical steroids may cause increased intraocular pressure, cataract formation, corneal thinning, and exacerbation of underlying herpes. Chronic use of systemic antibiotics makes necessary to control the hepatic functions.

Although it is recommended to use low dose with a long duration, clinician should be cautious about the potential side effects of oral tetracycline as gastrointestinal discomfort, vaginal yeast infections, photosensitivity, and decreased effectiveness of oral contraceptives. It is not appropriate for the children <8 years old, because of its accumulation in bone, color changes in teeth, and interfering enamel development [76].

Oral isotretinoin, which has both anti-inflammatory and immunomodulatory properties, has been used as a treatment for severe rosacea, particularly phymatous presentation by dermatologists [77]. In these cases, routine ophthalmologic follow-up should be recommended since the retinoids may cause blepharoconjunctivitis, worsening telangiectasias and may lead to severe keratitis [78].

8. Conclusion

Rosacea, mainly being a dermatological disease, may show ocular manifestations that sometimes may have severe consequences. The diagnosis mainly depends on the clinical findings and suspicion of the clinician. The evaluation and management should be performed by a collaborative approach by both dermatologist and ophthalmologist. The management should have a stepwise structure. The complications of both the disease and the treatment should be considered during the disease course.

Author details

Aysun Sanal Dogan

Address all correspondence to: asanaldogan@gmail.com

Ophthalmology Department, Diskapi Yildirim Beyazit Training and Research Hospital, Ankara, Turkey

References

[1] Wilkin J, Dahl M, Detmar M, Drake L, Feinstein A, et al. Standard classification of rosacea: report of the National Rosacea Society Expert Committee on the Classification and Staging of Rosacea. J Am Acad Dermatol. 2002;**46**:584–587. DOİ:10.1067/mjd.2002.120625.

[2] Wilkin J, Dahl M, Detmar M, Drake L, Liang MH, et al. Standard grading system for rosacea: report of the National Rosacea Society Expert Committee on the classification and staging of rosacea. J Am Acad Dermatol. 2004;**50**:907–912. DOİ:10.1016/j.jaad.2004.01.048.

[3] Vieira AC, Mannis MJ. Ocular rosacea: common and commonly missed. J Am Acad Dermatol. 2013;**69**:36–41. DOI: 10.1016/j.jaad.2013.04.042.

[4] Sobye P. Aetiology and pathogenesis of rosacea. Acta Derm Venereol. 1950;**30**:137–158.

[5] Berg M, Lidén S. An epidemiological study of rosacea. Acta Derm Venereol (Stockh). 1989;**69**:419–423.

[6] Halder RM, Brooks HL, Callendar VD. Acne in ethnic skin. Dermatol Clin. 2003;**21**:609–615. DOI: 10.1016/S0733-8635(03)00082-2.

[7] Tan J, Schöfer H, Araviiskaia E, Audibert F, Kerrouche N, et al; RISE study group. Prevalence of rosacea in the general population of Germany and Russia—the RISE study. J Eur Acad Dermatol Venereol. 2016;**30**:428–434. DOI: 10.1111/jdv.13556.

[8] Abram K, Silm H, Oona M. Prevalence of rosacea in an Estonian working population using a standard classification. Acta Derm Venereol. 2010;**90**:269–273. DOI: 10.2340/00015555-0856.

[9] Ghanem VC, Mehra N, Wong S, Mannis MJ. The prevalence of ocular signs in acne rosacea: comparing patients from ophthalmology and dermatology clinics. Cornea. 2003;**22**:230–233. DOI: 10.1097/00003226-200304000-00009.

[10] Bakar O, Demircay Z, Toker E, Cakir S. Ocular signs, symptoms and tear function tests of papulopustular rosacea patients receiving azithromycin. J Eur Acad Dermatol Venereol. 2009;**23**:544–549. DOI: 10.1111/j.1468-3083.2009.03132.x.

[11] Nazir SA, Murphy S, Siatkowski RM, et al. Ocular rosacea in childhood. Am J Ophthalmol. 2004;**137**:138–144. DOI: 10.1016/S0002-9394(03)00890-0.

[12] Spoendlin J, Voegel JJ, Jick SS, Meier CR. A study on the epidemiology of rosacea in the UK. Br J Dermatol. 2012;**167**:598–605. DOI: 10.1111/j.1365-2133.2012.11037.x.

[13] Donaldson KE, Karp CL, Dunbar MT. Evaluation and treatment of children with ocular rosacea. Cornea. 2007;**26**:42–46. DOI: 10.1097/ICO.0b013e31802e3a54.

[14] Rebora A. The red face: rosacea. Clin Dermatol. 1993;**11**:225–234.

[15] Kroshinsky D, Glick SA. Pediatric rosacea. Dermatol Ther 2006; **19**:196–201. DOI: 10.1016/0738-081X(93)90058-K.

[16] Webster GF. Rosacea. Med Clin North Am. 2009;**93**:1183–1194. DOI: 10.1016/j.mcna.2009.08.007.

[17] Steinhoff M, Schauber J, Leyden JJ. New insights into rosacea pathophysiology: a review of recent findings. J Am Acad Dermatol. 2013;**69**:15–26. DOI: 10.1016/j.jaad.2013.04.045.

[18] Yañez-Soto B, Mannis MJ, Schwab IR, Li JY, Leonard BC, et al. Interfacial phenomena and the ocular surface. Ocul Surf. 2014;**12**:178–201. DOI: 10.1016/j.jtos.2014.01.004.

[19] Hoang-Xuan T, Rodriquez A, Zaltas MM, Rice BA, Foster CS. Ocular rosacea. A histologic and immunopathologic study. Ophthalmology 1990;**97**:1468–1475. DOI: 10.1016/S0161-6420(90)32403-X.

[20] Faraj HG, Hoang-Xuan T. Chronic cicatrizing conjunctivitis. Curr Opin Ophthalmol. 2001;**12**:250–257. DOI: 10.1097/00055735-200108000-00003.

[21] Georgala S, Katoulis AC, Kylafis GD, Koumantaki-Mathioudaki E, Georgala C, Aroni K. Increased density of Demodex folliculorum and evidence of delayed hypersensitivity reaction in subjects with papulopustular rosacea. J Eur Acad Dermatol Venereol 2001;**15**:441–444. DOI: 10.1046/j.1468-3083.2001.00331.x.

[22] O'Reilly N, Gallagher C, Reddy Katikireddy K, Clynes M, O'Sullivan F, Kavanagh K. Demodex-associated Bacillus proteins induce an aberrant wound healing response in a corneal epithelial cell line: possible implications for corneal ulcer formation in ocular rosacea. Invest Ophthalmol Vis Sci. 2012;**53**:3250–3259. DOI: 10.1167/iovs.11-9295.

[23] O'Reilly N, Menezes N, Kavanagh K. Positive correlation between serum immunoreactivity to Demodex-associated Bacillus proteins and erythematotelangiectatic rosacea. Br J Dermatol. 2012;**167**:1032–1036. DOI: 10.1111/j.1365-2133.2012.11114.x.

[24] Dahl MV,,Ross AJ, Schlievert PM. Temperature regulates bacterial protein production: possible role in rosacea. J Am Acad Dermatol. 2004; **50**:266–272.

[25] Fernandez-Obregon A, Patton DL. The role of Chlamydia pneumoniae in the etiology of acne rosacea: response to the use of oral azithromycin. Cutis. 2007;**79**:163–167.

[26] Argenziano G, Donnarumma G, Iovene MR, Arnese P, Baldassarre MA, et al. Incidence of anti-Helicobacter pylori and anti-CagA antibodies in rosacea patients. Int J Dermatol. 2003;**42**:601–604.

[27] McCulley JP, Dougherty JM, Deneau DG. Classification of chronic blepharitis. Ophthalmology. 1982 Oct;**89**:1173–1180.

[28] Arita R, Mori N, Shirakawa R, Asai K, Imanaka T, et al. Meibum color and free fatty acid composition in patients with meibomian gland dysfunction. Invest Ophthalmol Vis Sci. 2015;**56**:4403–4412. DOI: 10.1167/iovs.14-16254.

[29] Afonso AA, Sobrin L, Monroy DC, Selzer M, Lokeshwar B, et al. Tear fluid gelatinase B activity correlates with IL-1alpha concentration and fluorescein clearance in ocular rosacea. Invest Ophthalmol Vis Sci. 1999;**40**:2506–2512.

[30] Barton K, Monroy DC, Nava A, Pflugfelder SC. Inflammatory cytokines in the tears of patients with ocular rosacea. Ophthalmology. 1997;**104**:1868–1874. DOI: 10.1016/S0161-6420(97)30014-1.

[31] Machalińska A, Zakrzewska A, Markowska A, Safranow K, Wiszniewska B, et al. Morphological and functional evaluation of meibomian gland dysfunction in rosacea patients. Curr Eye Res. 2015;**7**:1–6. DOI: 10.3109/02713683.2015.1088953.

[32] Goldgar C, Keahey DJ, Houchins J. Treatment options for acne rosacea. Am Fam Physician. 2009;**80**:461–468.

[33] Odom R, Dahl M, Dover J, Draelos Z, Drake L, et al. Standard management options for rosacea, Part 1: overview and broad spectrum of care. Cutis. 2009;**84**:43–47.

[34] Odom R, Dahl M, Dover J, Draelos Z, Drake L, et al. Standard management options for rosacea, Part 2: options according to subtype. Cutis. 2009;**84**:97–104.

[35] Abram K, Silm H, Maaroos HI, Oona M. Risk factors associated with rosacea. J Eur Acad Dermatol Venereol. 2010;**24**:565–571. DOI: 10.1111/j.1468-3083.2009.03472.x.

[36] Aldrich N, Gerstenblith M, Fu P, Tuttle MS, Varma P, et al. Genetic vs. environmental factors that correlate with rosacea: a cohort-based survey of twins. JAMA Dermatol. 2015;**151**:1213–1219. DOI: 10.1001/jamadermatol.2015.2230.

[37] Chang AL, Raber I, Xu J, Li R, Spitale R, et al. Assessment of the genetic basis of rosacea by genome-wide association study. J Invest Dermatol. 2015;**135**:1548–1555. DOI: 10.1038/jid.2015.53.

[38] Del Rosso JQ. Management of facial erythema of rosacea: what is the role of topical α-adrenergic receptor agonist therapy? J Am Acad Dermatol. 2013;**69**:44–56. DOI: 10.1016/j.jaad.2013.06.009.

[39] Metzler-Wilson K, Toma K, Sammons DL, Mann S, Jurovcik AJ, et al. Augmented supra-orbital skin sympathetic nerve activity responses to symptom trigger events in rosacea patients. J Neurophysiol. 2015;**114**:1530–1537. DOI: 10.1152/jn.00458.2015.

[40] Starr PA, Macdonald A. Oculocutaneous aspects of rosacea. Proc R Soc Med. 1969; **62**:9–11.

[41] Lacz NL, Schwartz RA. Rosacea in the pediatric population. Cutis. 2004;**74**:99–103.

[42] Palamar M, Degirmenci C, Ertam I, Yagci A. Evaluation of dry eye and meibomian gland dysfunction with meibography in patients with rosacea. Cornea. 2015;**34**:497–499. DOI: 10.1097/ICO.0000000000000393.

[43] López-Valverde G, Garcia-Martin E, Larrosa-Povés JM, Polo-Llorens V, Pablo-Júlvez LE. Therapeutical management for ocular rosacea. Case Rep Ophthalmol. 2016;**7**:237–242. DOI: 10.1159/000446104.

[44] Michel JL, Cabibel F. Frequency, severity and treatment of ocular rosacea during cutaneous rosacea. Ann Dermatol Venerol. 2003;**130**:20–24. DOI: AD-01-2003-130-1-0151-9638-101019-ART5.

[45] Chen DM, Crosby DL. Periorbital edema as an initial presentation of rosacea. J Am Acad Dermatol. 1997;**37**:346–348. DOI: 10.1016/S0190-9622(97)80389-1.

[46] Weisenthal RW, Afshari NA, Bouchard CS, Colby KA, Rootman DS, Tu EY, de Freitas D. Chapter 3: Clinical approach to ocular surface disorders. In: Cantor LB,Rapuano CJ, Cioffi GA, editors. Basic and Clinical Science Course, Section 8 (2014-2015). External Disease and Cornea. San Fransisco, CA; American Academy of Ophthalmology , 2014. P.37-81.

[47] Akpek E, Merchant A, Pinar V, Foster CS. Ocular rosacea: patient characteristics and follow-up. Ophthalmology. 1997;**104**:1863–1867. DOI: 10.1016/S0161-6420(97)30015-3.

[48] Jain V, Shome D, Natarajan S. Pseudodendritic keratitis in ocular rosacea causing a diagnostic dilemma. Indian J Ophthalmol. 2007;**55**:480–481. DOI: 10.4103/0301-4738.36493.

[49] Gracner B, Pahor D, Gracner T. Repair of an extensive corneoscleral perforation in a case of ocular rosacea with a keratoplasty. Klin Monbl Augenheilkd. 2006;**223**:841–843. DOI: 10.1055/s-2006-926720.

[50] Awais M, Anwar MI, Iftikhar R, Iqbal Z, Shehzad N, et al. Rosacea—the ophthalmic perspective. Cutan Ocul Toxicol. 2015;**34**:161–166. DOİ: 10.3109/15569527.2014.930749.

[51] Dursun D1, Piniella AM, Pflugfelder SC. Pseudokeratoconus caused by rosacea. Invest Ophthalmol Vis Sci. 1999;**40**:2506–2512. DOI: 10.1097/00003226-200108000-00024.

[52] Karaman Erdur S, Eliacik M, Kocabora MS, Balevi A, Demirci G, et al. Tear osmolarity and tear film parameters in patients with ocular rosacea. Eye Contact Lens. 2015;**27**:1–3. DOI: 10.1097/ICL.0000000000000211.

[53] Eroglu FC, Karalezli A, Dursun R. Is optical coherence tomography an effective device for evaluation of tear film meniscus in patients with acne rosacea? Eye (Lond). 2016;**30**:545–552. DOI: 10.1038/eye.2015.277.

[54] Yildirim Y, Olcucu O, Agca A, Karakucuk Y, Alagoz N, et al. Topographic and biomechanical evaluation of corneas in patients with ocular rosacea. Cornea. 2015;**34**:313–317. DOİ: 10.1097/ICO.0000000000000350.

[55] Leduc C, Dupas B, Ott-Benoist AC, Baudouin C. Advantages of the in vivo HRT2 corneal confocal microscope for investigation of the ocular surface epithelia. J Fr Ophthalmol. 2004;**27**:978–986. DOI: JFO-11-2004-27-9-C1-0003-4266-101019-ART02.

[56] Randon M, Liang H, El Hamdaoui M, Tahiri R, Batellier L, et al. In vivo confocal microscopy as a novel and reliable tool for the diagnosis of Demodex eyelid infestation. Br J Ophthalmol. 2015;**99**:336–341. DOİ: 10.1136/bjophthalmol-2014-305671.

[57] Culp B, Scheinfeld N. Rosacea: a review. P T. 2009;**34**:38–45.

[58] Ramamurthi S, Rahman MQ, Dutton GN, Ramaesh K. Pathogenesis, clinical features and management of recurrent corneal erosions. Eye (Lond). 2006;**20**:635–644. DOI: 10.1038/sj.eye.6702005.

[59] Derrar R, Daoudi R. Confusion between rosacea and bacterial keratitis. Pan Afr Med J. 2014;**18**:81. DOI: 10.11604/pamj.2014.18.81.4390.

[60] Geerling G, Tauber J, Baudouin C, Goto E, Matsumoto Y, et al. The international workshop on meibomian gland dysfunction: report of the subcommittee on management and treatment of meibomian gland dysfunction. Invest Ophthalmol Vis Sci. 2011;**52**:2050–2064. DOI: 10.1167/iovs.10-6997g.

[61] Auw-Haedrich C, Reinhard T. Chronic blepharitis. Pathogenesis, clinical features, and therapy. Ophthalmologe. 2007;**104**:817–826. DOI: 10.1007/s00347-007-1608-8.

[62] Doan S, Gabison E, Chiambaretta F, Touati M, Cochereau I. Efficacy of azithromycin 1.5% eye drops in childhood ocular rosacea with phlyctenular blepharokeratoconjunctivitis. J Ophthalmic Inflamm Infect. 2013;**3**:38. DOI: 10.1186/1869-5760-3-38.

[63] Murphy BS, Sundareshan V, Cory TJ, Hayes D Jr, Anstead MI, et al. Azithromycin alters macrophage phenotype. J Antimicrob Chemother. 2008;**61**:554–560. DOI: 10.1093/jac/dkn007.

[64] Del Rosso JQ, Thiboutot D, Gallo R, Webster G, Tanghetti E, et al. Consensus recommendations from the American Acne and Rosacea Society on the management of rosacea. Part 3: a status report on systemic therapies. Cutis. 2014;**93**:18–28.

[65] Sobolewska B, Doycheva D, Deuter C, Pfeffer I, Schaller M, et al. Treatment of ocular rosacea with once-daily low-dose doxycycline. Cornea. 2014;**33**:257–260.

[66] Jackson JM, Kircik LH, Lorenz DJ. Efficacy of extended-release 45 mg oral minocycline and extended-release 45 mg oral minocycline plus 15% azelaic acid in the treatment of acne rosacea. J Drugs Dermatol. 2013;**12**:292–298.

[67] Rebora A. The management of rosacea. Am J Clin Dermatol. 2002;**3**:489–496. DOI: 10.2165/00128071-200203070-00005

[68] Pye RJ, Burton JL. Treatment of rosacea by metronidazole. Lancet. 1976;**1**:1211–1212.

[69] Bakar O, Demirçay Z, Gürbüz O. Therapeutic potential of azithromycin in rosacea. Int J Dermatol. 2004;**43**:151–154. DOI: 10.1111/j.1365-4632.2004.01958.x.

[70] Miguel AI, Salgado MB, Lisboa MS, Henriques F, Paiva MC et al. Pediatric ocular rosacea: 2 cases. Eur J Ophthalmol. 2012;**22**:664–666. DOI: 10.5301/ejo.5000103.

[71] Dursun D, Kim MC, Solomon A, Pflugfelder SC. Treatment of recalcitrant recurrent corneal erosions with inhibitors of matrix metalloproteinase-9, doxycycline and corticosteroids. Am J Ophthalmol. 2001;**132**:8–13. DOI: 10.1016/S0002-9394(01)00913-8.

[72] Arman A, Demirseren DD, Takmaz T. Treatment of ocular rosacea: comparative study of topical cyclosporine and oral doxycycline. Int J Ophthalmol. 2015;**8**:544–549. DOI: 10.3980/j.issn.2222-3959.2015.03.19.

[73] Bhargava R, Chandra M, Bansal U, Singh D, Ranjan S, et al. Randomized controlled trial of omega 3 fatty acids in rosacea patients with dry eye symptoms. Curr Eye Res. 2016;**6**:1–7. DOI: 10.3109/02713683.2015.1122810.

[74] Wladis EJ. Intraductal meibomian gland probing in the management of ocular rosacea. Ophthal Plast Reconstr Surg. 2012;**28**:416–418. DOI: 10.1097/IOP.0b013e3182627ebc.

[75] Kim BY, Riaz KM, Bakhtiari P, Chan CC, Welder JD, et al. Medically reversible limbal stem cell disease: clinical features and management strategies. Ophthalmology. 2014;**121**:2053–2058. DOI: 10.1016/j.ophtha.2014.04.025.

[76] Gruber GG, Callen JP. Systemic complications of commonly used dermatologic drugs. Cutis. 1978;**21**:825–829.

[77] Park H, Del Rosso JQ. Use of oral isotretinoin in the management of rosacea. J Clin Aesthet Dermatol. 2011;**4**:54–61.

[78] Aragona P, Cannavò SP, Borgia F, Guarneri F. Utility of studying the ocular surface in patients with acne vulgaris treated with oral isotretinoin: a randomized controlled trial. Br J Dermatol. 2005;**152**:576–578. DOI: 10.1111/j.1365-2133.2005.06389.x.